INTELLIGENT MEDICINE

A GUIDE TO OPTIMIZING
HEALTH AND PREVENTING
ILLNESS FOR THE
BABY-BOOMER GENERATION

Ronald L. Hoffman, M.D.

A FIRESIDE BOOK
Published by Simon & Schuster

FIRESIDE
Rockefeller Center
1230 Avenue of the Americas
New York, NY 10020

Copyright © 1997 by Ronald Hoffman
All rights reserved,
including the right of reproduction
in whole or in part in any form.

FIRESIDE and colophon are registered trademarks
of Simon & Schuster Inc.

Designed by Irving Perkins Associates, Inc.

Manufactured in the United States of America

10 9 8 7 6 5 4 3

Library of Congress Cataloging-in-Publication Data is available.

ISBN 0-684-81082-4

Dedicated to the Class of '69

Contents

Part Three: Taking Charge of Your Health

Acknowledgments

"Intelligent medicine" is not something I can lay unique claim to. Rather, it springs from the collective consciousness of numerous health professionals, both conventional and alternative; from savvy American medical consumers, determined in their pursuit of excellence; and from the very spirit of the times, which attempts to reconcile valuable traditions with incredible breakthroughs as we usher in a new millennium. Thus, this book is merely a reflection of how, by virtue of being a baby boomer, a physician, a broadcaster, and a natural-foods retailer, my environment has shaped my thoughts on medicine and health.

Accordingly, I want to thank my parents, who, while unwittingly succumbing to the pitfalls of child rearing of their generation, described in this book, nevertheless provided me with a loving environment and imbued me with the thirst for knowledge that remains the engine for this enterprise.

I also want to thank my colleagues in the health profession whose intelligence, support, and fellowship I enjoy. Too numerous to individually acknowledge, their thoughts and writings are the daily staple from which I derive inspiration both for my clinical practice and for the information I share with listeners and readers. Specifically, I want to extend appreciation to the American College for Advancement in Medicine and the American Academy of Environmental Medicine as organizations that have nurtured my professional development.

I want to thank the patients and staff of the Hoffman Center, which has served as a living laboratory and a true crucible for the principles of intelligent medicine. The themes that I have been guided to in this book are a direct result of the challenging clinical dilemmas presented to me daily in the practice of medicine. The love and confidence patients and staff have shared with me have been an inspiration to keep striving toward better understanding of the fundamentals of wellness. I particularly want to extend gratitude to Anika Beech, my office manager, who has kept our crew steadfastly rowing past the rocks while letting me hear the Sirens sing.

I would like to acknowledge radio station WOR in New York and the WOR Radio Network for allowing me the great privilege of imparting health information to their many avid listeners. "Health Talk" is like a covenant that I renew daily by broadcasting the best and latest information I can. This challenging radio forum has inspired me to keep abreast of many of the medical issues that I share now with the readers of *Intelligent*

Medicine. A major impetus to me in the broadcast arena has been my agent and dear friend, Mrs. Betty Fredericks, whose late husband, Dr. Carleton Fredericks, was the irreplaceable prototype of all health broadcasters to follow.

I would also like to thank my mentor in the newest phase of my healthy endeavors — Sherpa, the manager of my retail health-food supermarket, Healthy Pleasures, in Manhattan. It is through daily interaction with Sherpa and the employees and customers of Healthy Pleasures that I have been initiated into an industry that has very much to do with influencing the health of America. The knowledge that I have gleaned through this new diversification of my professional career has been invaluable in the creation of *Intelligent Medicine.*

Now for the people more directly responsible for this book: Thanks to Elaine Pfefferblit, whose confidence in me launched my publishing career at Simon & Schuster. Loads of gratitude to my capable editor, Becky Cabaza, who patiently endured my writing extravagances and expertly guided me toward the finished product; acknowledgments to Suzanne Gluck, my agent, for capable stewardship of this project; and special appreciation to Robert Withers for dogged research and writing extraordinaire, without which this book would not have been possible. Acknowledgments, too, to Craig Silver for capable assistance in the preparation of this manuscript, and to Gladys Vasquez for her splendid cover design.

Finally, thanks of a special order go to my wife, Helen, who so fully appreciates and complements my chosen mission that I could scarcely imagine a better facilitator in the entire world.

Introduction

The past few years have been a rewarding time for me as a doctor. My own practice has grown, and I've seen exciting results from the practice of what I call "intelligent medicine" — the combination of conventional high-tech medical science with the best of alternative medical therapies, from nutrition to acupuncture. At the same time, I've been able to reach out to a broader group than the patients who come into our clinic. Through my nationally syndicated daily radio program, "Health Talk," I've been able to talk with many people throughout the greater New York City area, offering medical guidance and getting a real sense of the kinds of ailments that folks are coping with, and their experience with the health care system. Both in my practice and through my radio shows, I talk with patients with the same recurring kinds of needs and concerns — needs that are not being met by the standard health care system. That is why I am writing this book. It's for anyone who is concerned about the kind of health care they are receiving, or who wants to know how to optimize health and vitality through the middle years and beyond.

Over and over, I see or talk to patients with the same kind of problem: they are in their late thirties or early forties and are suddenly experiencing their first major health crisis — the first time that their body is letting them down — and it's often a terrifying experience. They are in pain, upset, and dissatisfied with the treatments offered by the conventional health care system — a medication that seems to have as many side effects as medicinal effects, or an invasive surgical procedure. They often feel they are getting inadequate information about the cause of their illness or how they can keep it from worsening. Often they do not receive the best course of treatment. I also see patients who are active, successful baby boomers who for some physical reason have lost the flexibility or get-up-and-go that sustains and enables their careers, their athletic pursuits, their lifestyles. More and more people are going to have these experiences, since every seven and one-half seconds from now until the year 2013, one more member of the baby-boomer generation will turn fifty. I sympathize with their pain and confusion because I myself had a similar experience a few years ago. This book is intended to offer help with these kinds of problems.

I use the term intelligent medicine to characterize the new vision of medical practice, which attempts to take the best elements of conventional, high-tech medicine and alternative practices and amalgamate them. Some people call this complementary medicine, some call it alternative medicine, some call it "holistic medicine." I prefer to call it intelligent medicine, because we are bringing real thought to bear on our prevention and treatment strategies, not just falling back on the conventional treatment, whether high-tech or alternative, in a knee-jerk reaction. For example, you might use state-of-the-art and antiulcer drugs or innovative antibiotic therapy to kill the causative bacteria for someone with an acute ulcer. After the fire is put out, you might then augment that treatment with a long-term dietary approach, or low-cost herbal therapy.

Another key aspect of intelligent medicine is that you are in charge of your own health and fitness. Of course, you will consult physicians and benefit from their expertise, but you will know enough about what is going on with your body to be able to make some intelligent choices about which programs and treatments you may want to embark upon, supported by your physician, and which you may not want to subscribe to. If you're coping with a disease, you should be able to get as much information as possible about your condition and thereby start to overcome the fear of the unknown that can be as debilitating as actual physical pain. A number of people came to consult with me after reading one of my previous books, *Seven Weeks to a Settled Stomach*, and said, "I wasn't able to make myself better, which is why I'm here, but at least I feel better understanding the problem, so I'm less emotionally upset by it." This is part of intelligent medicine. I tell my patients, "Look, here's what's going on in your body; I want you to have a clear picture of the processes." I try to clarify problems that are often more frightening if they're left unexplained, particularly for people whose symptoms allow them to fall between the cracks of the standard diagnoses.

This book will help you begin to use the intelligent medicine approach in maintaining and optimizing your own health. It will guide you through the maze of modern medicine, help you avoid the pitfalls of medical treatment, and manage your health risk factors. You can use it as a handbook to help you to cope with a variety of health problems, whether serious or minor, and to take full advantage of the best that high-tech medicine has to offer. At the same time, we will take a critical look at the excesses of modern medicine, and which high-tech treatments to avoid.

First, in Part One of the book, we'll look at the baby-boomer generation itself: its health legacy, its risks, and its opportunities for sustaining health and minimizing decline. This generation grew up at a time when medical science was making incredible discoveries and developing miraculous treatments: antibiotics, vaccines, pacemakers, surgical procedures. But somewhere along the way, the concept of wellness and quality of life was forgotten. At the same time, we are confronting new risks from environmental pollution, from our diet, even from medicine itself. But the new discoveries in nutrition, risk factors, genetic testing, and the like are giving us the tools to deal with them.

Then, in Part Two, we'll look at each of the body's "systems" — from the immune to the cardiovascular; from the respiratory to the muscular and skeletal. We'll review each system's components, how it works with others in the body, what can go wrong, how to avert trouble, how to troubleshoot if you've got an existing problem, and various possible therapies, including nutrition, alternative therapies, and high-tech possibilities.

Then, in Part Three, we'll look at the ways in which our environment and the foods, chemicals, medicines, and drugs we use or consume can affect our health and discuss how to manipulate our intake through diet and nutrition.

Finally, we'll present some strategies for dealing with illness and with the medical system: how to get the most effective care from doctors and clinics, and how to think about medications, surgery, hospitalization, and the medical alternatives. We'll follow up with a section of Resources to aid you in managing your health intelligently.

The good news is that our long-held notions about aging are rapidly being proved wrong. People are living longer now, but that's not the whole story. We are learning that debilitating decline is not inevitable. Medical scientists have worried that high-tech improvements in medical care would only result in a nation with more older people, most of them living with crippling, painful, debilitating ailments. However, it turns out that old people are living much more active, robust lives. The percentage of older Americans with chronic diseases like high blood pressure, emphysema, and arthritis has been steadly declining. Many people are staying mentally and physically agile well into their eighties and nineties. The baby-boom generation should continue to enjoy this trend. If we can get through midlife with few major problems, and through the years after sixty with relative health, then we stand a good chance of having healthy and happy lives as older people.

It's been an exciting process to write this book and to pull together in one place all of the current information that can help us maintain our health and vitality — from nutrition to high-tech medicine. And I join you in the hope that the future will see an increased interest in and support for the values of long-term wellness and intelligent medicine.

PART ONE

WHAT'S A BABY BOOMER?

CHAPTER ONE

Peter Pan Grows Up

Once upon a time, some of us lived as if there were no tomorrow. But we were surprised when the birthdays kept on coming, even though the Beatles made "when I'm sixty-four" seem to be light years away. Many in our generation believed that the world was ours, that we'd be the ones to make it a better place. But we discovered this was going to take more work than we'd thought. Most of us are still here, but no matter how we once felt about life and the future, we've all had to cope with changes.

Pete Townshend of The Who once declared, "Hope I die before I get old," but Townshend, now in his fifties, is still with us. He recently spent a year in physical therapy, cutting back on his guitar playing, to heal a shoulder damaged by RSI—Repetitive Stress Injury. He's supported a group called HEAR, for Hearing Education Awareness for Rockers, because he suffers from occupation-induced deafness. The organization educates people about the risks of deafness from high-decibel sounds, especially rock music.

Jane Fonda? Everyone knows her success story, her conversion from the diet pills and the diet fads of the sixties to the exercise and nutrition program that made her a best-selling author and a limber model for her own exercise videos. Whatever you may think of her past politics, no one can argue with her good looks and vitality.

Action movie stars like Sylvester Stallone and Arnold Schwarzenegger have become icons of health and physical fitness, swashbuckling their way through film after film, easily keeping up with the special effects with no perceptible diminishing of their top physical conditioning.

What do these celebrities and notables have in common? They're all baby boomers, born in that fateful period between 1945 and 1964 that changed the demographic face of America. And they have all had to cope with the changes that the body begins to register after the first thirty to forty years of life. Schwarzenegger, in fact, recently underwent heart surgery.

The first batch of baby boomers was born in May 1946—nine months after V-J Day—an unprecedented 233,452 American births. By the year's end, an all-time record of 3.6 million babies had been born in the United States, and the biggest baby boom in history was on. By the time the boom was over in 1964, the baby boomers, now one third of all Americans, had shaped every aspect of postwar America: they popularized "lite" foods, made jogging trendy, discovered the environment, and established the first Earth Day. They have lived through permissive child-rearing, fallout shelters, the Pill, drug experimentation, the sexual revolution, the weakening of the ozone layer, the cholesterol panic, the Beverly Hills diet, Eggbeaters, and irradiated foods, all of which may shape their unique health problems.

The baby boom is really a unique cultural phenomenon of twentieth-century America. It's like the Little Prince's elephant swallowed by the boa constrictor, squeezing its way along the line. For every milestone of this generation there's been a health event, from Dr. Spock's "new think" on child rearing to the first mass application of multiple immunization, the broad use of antibiotics for childhood diseases, the sexual revolution and the drug experimentation of the sixties, the gay revolution and drug burn-out of the seventies, and the jogging and exercise fads and new health consciousness of the eighties.

Further, these 76 million Americans, born into peacetime affluence, medical miracles, and great expectations, are gradually finding out, like all preceding generations, that their bodies are not only subject to wear and tear but are destructible. But we may not all realize that our physical health and vitality can change and improve, no matter what our age, just as we can change our mental outlook. Health and vitality are not the exclusive property of youth, but they are a gift that can be built on or squandered, renewed, or thrown away. Many of us have experienced the sudden shock of being diagnosed with a serious condition or disease after years of relatively uneventful good or fair-to-middling health. We then begin to take stock. "How could this happen to me?" we ask. "How did I get into this spot? What can I do to get out of it? What further shocks might the future hold, and what can I do to prevent them?"

These are some of the questions this book will help you answer. But first, let's take a closer look at the baby-boomer generation. This generation has enjoyed some unique advantages in terms of health and opportunity, but it is also experiencing some unique challenges to health and well-being. Most of these advantages and challenges affect nearly everyone's personal health picture.

Why We're Different

We grew up believing that a rich, exciting life was not only possible but somehow to be expected, and that with enough hard work or intelligent decision making we could create an enjoyable life. Looking to the future, we saw unlimited horizons. We wouldn't have to follow in our parents' footsteps, whether in careers, marriages, or gender roles. We would make our own choices. In fact, we were the generation that invented the word lifestyle.

This was all natural enough for a generation raised in the relative peace and affluence of the fifties and sixties. America, having just won the war that seemed likely to end all wars, came into its own as a world leader with awesome military and economic power, despite the threat of Communism. Postwar prosperity encouraged people to have a lot of kids, and Dr. Spock, apostle of the new relaxed and permissive child-rearing spirit, smiled benignly over our first squeals and tottering steps.

I was born to parents who had escaped from the horrors of the European Holocaust to the suburbs of Los Angeles, which seemed truly a City of Angels, a garden of Paradise. They felt that a new life was beginning and that their children would be raised in a new ideal society with every possible advantage. I think that many native-born Americans of our parents' generation, having lived through the Great Depression and World War II, felt the same sense of a nightmare ended and a new world beginning. In fact, suburbia was largely intended to be an ideal environment for raising children, a new idyllic, civilized way of living halfway between city grime and country backwardness.

The Age of Medical Miracles

At the same time there was a new and tremendous optimism in medicine — and some pretty amazing things were happening: new surgical techniques, an expanding range of antibiotics, and new vaccines that broke the backs of some of our most deadly and relentless enemies, from diphtheria to polio. The polio vaccine seemed like a miracle, a magic bullet, that came along just when it was needed — right in the middle of an epidemic. This was an era of tremendous expansion and consolidation, and real advances were made. It seemed that there was no disease that couldn't be conquered in time.

The great medical successes of this period marked our generation and its future for years to come. First, they created an atmosphere in which people began to believe that high-tech solutions — from designer drugs to ever more invasive surgery — could cure any disease and solve any problem, if we could only hit on the right technique or the right chemistry. That supported the unconscious bias toward curing disease rather than preventing it, toward fixing illness rather than promoting health. The idea was to conquer disease rather than establish health.

Second, these successes created a new attitude toward the medical establishment. There was a new confidence in medicine, and people were much more ready to entrust their children (the baby boomers) to the system. You can see this in the new approach to bearing children and feeding infants. Mothers-to-be began to expect to give birth in the hospital rather than at home. Perhaps as a result, there was a tremendous increase in the number of cesarean sections. Breast-feeding declined in favor of scientifically prepared formula-feeding, at the expense of the natural immunity conferred with mother's milk. Home birth and breast-feeding were seen as old-fashioned, outmoded practices. These were just two instances of a great cultural change.

If you came down with an illness, Mom wouldn't keep you home and feed you chicken soup. She'd take you to the doctor and he would fix you up. He'd take out your tonsils if you had a sore throat, give you an antibiotic if you had the flu, or pack a stuffy nose with cotton soaked with medicine and put you under a heat lamp. It might not be pleasant, but he'd fix you up. (I was the first kid in my class to have both glasses and leg braces. Like another noted baby boomer — Forrest Gump — I was incorrectly given a prescription for clumsy orthopedic braces, out of a sense that medical science could correct any of nature's little flaws.)

For better or worse, many of us came to believe that our doctors were next to infallible and always had the means to fix us up. This was really a major shift in perception — most of our grandparents had a healthy skepticism about the medical system. Now, when we reach a certain age and go to the doctor and find that something can't be fixed so easily, it's often a total shock. Worse, the procedures or drugs for the "fixing" can often lead to complications or worse problems.

Fortunately, these distortions of medical research and practice have finally started to turn around. Medical research now devotes a significant and increasing amount of attention to identifying risk factors in people's lifestyles and offering ways to prevent illness, not just fix it. People now realize that they need to pay attention to prevention and that when a doctor offers a drug or an operation "to fix you up," it's often wise to seek a second opinion.

The New Challenges to Health

It's a documented fact that older people are more concerned about health, and actually tend to lead healthier lifestyles, than the young. The baby boomers, who expected success and freedom in their lives, and a new and better world, are no exception. Medical science has offered many miraculous cures and procedures. Yet, we now confront new risks to health that our parents never knew.

THE PACE OF MODERN LIFE

We live in a culture that places unusual, even extraordinary, demands on us. Ten years ago, most stores were closed on Sundays. Now, all over America, Sunday is a shopping day. There is no longer a concept of the Sabbath as a day of rest. Labor Day has become the day to hit the stores for the sales. Professionals and business people work Saturdays and Sundays. Just getting to work can be a job in itself, involving a long auto or train commute. The airlines have their business class and frequent-flier programs for those whose day begins with a 6 A.M. flight to a distant city, and continues at 7 P.M. to another town.

Baby boomers have bought into the speeded-up pace of life with a vengeance. Born into affluent times, and with enormous expectations, they expect to wring the most out of life, whether through an eighty-hour work week or a vacation white-water rafting. The culture exalts youthfulness and the athletic ideal, so people go to gyms, swim laps, and run triathlons. It exalts material wealth and professional achievement, so people spend their evenings and Saturdays focused on work. It exalts family connection, so people try to keep up with their kids' schooling and activities. As a result, the rhythm of life, which should swing between relaxation and activity, can often seem like a perpetual race relieved by brief intervals of exhausted sleep.

Those daunting expectations — to work hard, play hard, look good, and enjoy every moment — put a kind of stress on the body and mind that can take its toll. It can lead to sleep disorders, decreased immune function, addictions, emotional burnout, or simple physical exhaustion. There are ways to maintain health and lead a fast-paced, active life, but this requires conscious attention and the right information.

ENVIRONMENTAL STRESS

It's no news that years of unchecked industrial growth and population increases have deeply altered our physical environment. Baby boomers do not live in the same world that their grandparents lived in. There are more chemicals in the environment, in food, in water supplies, and in the air. We put chemicals on our bodies in the form of hair dye, deodorants, perfume, makeup, and antiwrinkle cream. We dose ourselves with over-the-counter drugs. We build and decorate our homes and offices with synthetic materials that give off fumes and flakes. We live surrounded by increasing levels of electromagnetic radiation from appliances, TV sets, computers, and power stations. Some environmental dangers, like those from PCBs and asbestos, have been clearly documented. Others are being newly discovered or are the subject of speculation. Even when the risks are not always well established, they warrant our attention.

We do know that some chemicals and environmental stressors can cause specific ailments, like cancers, heart disease, and emphysema. Also it is possible that environmental factors contribute to the increase in autoimmune diseases. For example, researchers have noted a higher incidence of scleroderma in women who color their hair. Concerns have also been raised over the high lead content of hair preparations for both sexes, including the popular Grecian formula. However, the picture may be more complicated than a single-cause/single-effect model. There is some evidence that environmental pollutants may have a cumulative, interactive effect. Multiple factors make it all the harder to diagnose a cause and design a cure.

Chemical pollutants aren't the only problem. Higher noise levels are everywhere in our contemporary environment. Some are the result of urban, industrialized life and culture; some we voluntarily subject ourselves to. Muzak follows us from shopping malls to elevators and even seeks us out on the telephone when we're put on hold. Home entertainment centers and movie theaters offer us high-decibel "surround sound." We strap on our headphones before getting on a bus or setting off on a jog. These higher noise levels can cause a subtle and irreversible increase in deafness. It's been shown that the hearing of the average American youth is significantly less acute than that of the average youth of some rural Somalian tribes in Africa. And deafness is not the only danger of noise pollution. Recent studies have shown that higher noise levels can actually be immune suppressant.

Finally, combined environmental stresses may affect us in yet unknown ways. According to recent studies, something in the nature of urban life itself may be connected with the higher incidence of schizophrenia among lifelong city dwellers. The exact reasons are unknown, but there may be many — viral illnesses spread more easily in cities, there is increased risk to babies born to mothers who had the flu in their fifth month of pregnancy, there is a higher incidence of head injuries in the urban environment, and stresses like losing a job or a partner are more frequent.

Baby boomers are subjected to multiple forms of environmental stress — some entirely new, some at a much higher level than those our grandparents had to deal with a hundred years ago. We need to take these into account in making our plans for continued health.

WHAT DOES THE LABEL SAY?

Over the past hundred years, our diet has changed into something radically unlike what humans have ever survived on. For thousands of years, as we climbed up the evolutionary ladder, people survived on some combination of fresh fruits, vegetables, grains, fish, wild game, and free-range semi-domesticated animals. Now our fruits, vegetables, and grains are grown in soil pumped up with fertilizer and doused with herbicides and insecticides. Fish come from polluted waters. Domesticated animals are raised in factory-like environments, dosed with antibiotics and growth hormones. In fact, European medical scientists are so concerned about the presence of hormones and antibiotics in American meat products that this has become an issue in foreign trade. Further, we've added new things to our diet: sugars, processed fats and oils, chemical preservatives, artificial flavors and colorizers, sweeteners, and texturizers. In fact, Americans consume on the average several pounds of preservatives and chemical additives a year! We consume many foods, from margarine to "diet" marshmallows, that are nothing more than artificial creations of modern chemistry.

This shift in diet really began in our parents' generation and has accelerated in ours. We've seen some of the consequences — from diabetes to obesity to heart disease — and others are still being deduced, possibly including cancer.

It's not hard to figure out that the typical American diet can cause problems. Many doctors and researchers are now prescribing alternatives. What isn't always clear, however, is that even some of the alternatives may not be for the good. You may already be aware of the dangers of "yo-yo" weight reduction diets, wherein you starve for weeks, feeling weak and obsessed with food, then balloon up again the moment you relax the regimen. But you may not know that even the highly touted high-carbohydrate, low-meat diets can lead in some people to profound metabolic imbalances.

SHAKE IT UP, BABY

For thousands of years of evolution, the human animal was a walking animal. For most indigenous peoples, the way to get from point A to point B was to walk. Australian aborigines would pick up and walk for hundreds of miles, following their "songlines" that described the routes through unknown territories. In medieval Europe, pilgrims would walk across the continent to reach a holy destination. Even early in this century, in rural America, folks would think nothing of walking ten miles into town. Or they'd catch the horse and ride, exercising other muscles. Henry Ford changed all that. It's not surprising that exercise, or the lack of it, has become one of the major health issues of our day. We've seen the obvious effects of the sedentary life — muscle stiffness and joint pain — in members of our parents' generation. Gradually, we've learned that lack of exercise has other, more subtle effects, contributing to heart disease and even to reduced immune function.

While reducing healthful exercise for some, the industrial revolution brought new physical dangers for others. The body did not evolve to perform simple repeated motions over and over, but for years, hand laborers and assembly-line workers have suffered from various forms of repetitive stress injury, or RSI. The result can be muscle strain, arthritis, and nerve damage. No longer limited to factory workers, RSI affects office workers, executives, and professionals who spend long hours hunched over computer keyboards.

In what seems like a double whammy, many baby boomers find themselves suffering from too much exercise or the wrong kind. Our increased leisure and our new health consciousness have led many of us to throw ourselves into sports, workouts, and physical recreation with righteous intensity, seeking the high that exercise brings, and convinced we're doing the right thing. Too often, the result can be strained or torn muscles, injuries to joints and bones, physical debilitation, or RSI again. For too many, physical activity is still not a balanced, integral part of daily life.

CATCHING A BUG

While we've eradicated many crippling diseases or learned how to treat them, new threats are appearing. The world-wide pandemic of AIDS continues to spread from nation to nation and from population group to group. So far there is no cure in sight — only recently have advances in therapy with new protease inhibitor drugs suggested that the beginning of the end might be in sight. Tuberculosis, which had seemed such an outdated ailment that in recent years few scientists bothered to study it and research funds dried up, has suddenly revived and is spreading to new victims in scary, drug-resistant forms. Antibiotics, the miracle drugs of the fifties and sixties, are helpless against some of these scourges. What's worse, the use of antibiotics has become so widespread that drug-resistant bacteria have increased and our natural immune systems run the risk of being weakened. Antibiotics have even invaded our food supplies — chickens, pigs, and cattle are routinely given massive doses of drugs to ward off infections. European laws prohibit this practice. While the antibiotics in livestock may not make their way into our bodies directly, they do contribute to the growth of drug-resistant bacteria that pass from animals to humans.

The revival of old infectious agents, and the appearance of new ones, from HIV to the organisms that cause Creutzfeldt-Jakob disease, Legionnaires' disease, and Lyme disease, remind us that we can never be complacent about infections and that this generation has to cope with diseases our parents never knew or thought they'd conquered.

IT'S IN YOUR GENES

Research into the human genome promises exciting new opportunities for early diagnosis of risk factors and even for new therapies. Soon it may be possible, at birth, to assess a child's susceptibility to various risks such as heart disease. This offers the promise of early and lifelong management of potential health problems. There are no actual risks here, but there are new issues, some of them quite troubling.

For example, we are now able to identify gene markers for Huntington's disease, an irreversible and permanently debilitating disease that leads to severe neurological impairment and early death. The disease is passed on genetically, so that everyone whose parents or grandparents had the disease already knows they are at risk. Now, however, through gene testing, a person at risk can find out for sure whether or not he or she carries the gene that inevitably causes the disease. The question is: to test or not to test. Learning that you're free of the fatal gene could lift a shadow of fear from your life. But learning that you carry the gene is a sentence without appeal, since there are no treatments for detectable genetic diseases like Huntington's, Alzheimer's, and certain forms of breast cancer.

NO MORE LEECHES, BUT . . .

We can smile sadly at some of the ineffective therapies of past centuries, like the bloodletting that supposedly let "bad blood" escape but only weakened ailing patients. (Actually, microsurgeons who reattach hands and fingers have found a real use for leeches, in draining off blood from the tiniest blood vessels during an operation — the ones that are too small to stitch up.) But we should not be too complacent. Even now, we are still learning that many widely accepted therapies may be not only ineffective but actually dangerous, that some of our most effective treatments may cause insidious and unwanted side effects, and that some widely accepted treatments may actually cause illness or decline. This phenomenon even has its own Greek-based name: iatrogenic, or "physician-caused," illness.

Beside such specific risks, there are ways in which medicine has changed our whole climate of health. For example, this is the first generation to be raised on antibiotics. Our parents did not have access to these miracle drugs until well into adulthood. The antibiotic revolution really began with World War II, and not until after the war were antibiotics offered to the general populace. We have been exposed to antibiotics practically from birth, throughout childhood and on into adulthood. Many baby boomers are so accustomed to using antibiotics that they demand them from doctors at the first sign of illness. Many doctors acquiesce, even for illnesses that antibiotics cannot cure, like the flu. What is the effect of these long-term and repeated doses of antibiotics? In a sense, the baby boomers have been the guinea pigs in a long-term experiment. We do know that sustained use of antibiotics changes the intestinal flora: the bacteria that live in symbiotic balance in our bodies and affect the digestion and absorption of nutrients. There is evidence that repeated use of antibiotics affects the way our immune system works, replacing or inhibiting the natural immune response, and also encourages the development of drug-resistant bacteria.

Baby boomers have also been more heavily vaccinated than any other generation in history. In a way, that's been very good, because we've escaped some dangerous diseases and many lives have been saved. However, extensive vaccination may have indirect effects that we don't yet know about.

Simple Questions — Complex Answers

Some of these more recent syndromes and diseases, such as chronic fatigue syndrome and autoimmune disease, have been difficult to diagnose and identify, much less treat. It's been hard to trace some of these ailments to simple causes, like a virus, a gene, or an environmental poison. They probably have multiple contributing factors, which may include genetic predisposition, environmental chemicals, and even medical practices. It's very hard to say simply that it's the hair dye that causes scleroderma. But the hair dye might ratchet you up two more points on the risk scale, and that combined with smog, PCB residues, and mercury could be enough to push you over the edge. We are going to have to look at your whole health picture for answers to some of these problems. In fact, this is how we are now approaching some of the more "traditional" health risks. Heart disease, for example, appears to be a problem that's influenced by multiple factors: diet and nutrition, exercise, and environmental substances. One study, for example, has shown that small particulate matter in the air, like dust or pollen, is related to a high incidence of heart disease.

Some of these new and complex problems really point the way to an exciting new approach to medicine and to sustaining health. We are moving away from the reactive type of medicine, in which we wait for an illness to strike and then go to war against it — too often with aggressive procedures that may overwhelm the attacker but damage us in the process. There is a new vision of medicine in the making: a medicine that will look at our body and mind as an integrated whole, deeply connected to our environment and deeply influenced by our behavior. The more we understand the basic biologic processes on the cellular level, the more we can use "natural," low-risk therapies like nutrition and exercise, avoid illness and decline, and tune and optimize our health and vitality.

The New Age in Medicine

The baby-boomer generation in America now finds itself at a unique moment in history, confronting the inevitable process of aging but armed with a far greater knowledge of the body than ever before, and with the freedom to explore the potential for health and longevity. We now know more about the impact of diet on health and illness than ever before. Scientists are at this moment studying the effect of nutrients on organs and even on cells themselves. We understand better how to assess the risks for many kinds of diseases, including those that are genetically linked, and how to prevent them. We know that exercise not only strengthens the body but can prolong life and increase our resistance to disease. We can treat allergies and detoxify the body of harmful metals. We have profoundly sensitive tests to determine just where the immune system has gone haywire.

Now, more than ever, we have the tools and knowledge to build a future that maximizes our physical health and longevity and prevents unforeseen crises. We can begin to pursue excellence in health as active, empowered seekers.

CHAPTER TWO

Confessions of a Baby-Boomer Doctor

Many of my patients come to me when they are experiencing their first major health crisis—the first time their body is letting them down. They may be in their late thirties or early forties, and suddenly something takes them completely by surprise: a spinal problem, arthritis, an autoimmune disease, even a cancer. They are often devastated and can't understand how this could happen to them. They are sometimes hit even harder than some of my older patients with similar problems. Most of my patients who are sixty or seventy have already had surgery and some serious health problems, and they're also from a generation that has come to expect ups and downs in life—they've been through a world-wide depression and lived through a major world war.

But this generation, the baby boomers, has led a fairly sheltered existence, except for those who went to Vietnam, and a lot of them are quite devastated by their first health crisis. This is one of the reasons why chronic fatigue syndrome has made such an impression in the public mind. Someone who works hard; is upwardly mobile, successful, and active; has an active family life; and is pursuing meaningful goals suddenly finds that he or she can't do it anymore and just doesn't have the get-up-and-go that makes it all possible. Those who suffer from this syndrome feel as if life has just come to an end. Or someone develops, say, Graves' disease, which is a fairly common autoimmune disease that usually attacks young or middle-aged women, and she is shattered. She feels that this has come out of nowhere, that her body has just let her down. But these are often diseases that people can weather, and though they may go through some rough times, they can end up in two or three or five years and be quite well or with only slightly diminished capabilities.

But when it happens, they are in pain, in shock, upset, and often dissatisfied with the treatment they are getting from the health care system. People are offered powerful medications that may have unpleasant side effects, or they are offered invasive surgical procedures. Worse yet, they may be told that they're just getting old and will have to live with pain and reduced function. Too often, they are not offered enough real information about why an illness has developed, how they can keep it from worsening, or what they can do to get better.

I can easily sympathize with these concerns, because I have had my own minor brush with painful injury and with the anxieties of a sudden shock to the system. It came about a few years ago when I felt I was at the height of physical health and strength. Like many others, I had jumped onto the bandwagon of physical exercise that swept the country during the seventies and eighties. They say new converts are more fervent. Maybe because I had never been athletic as a teenager, or because as a doctor I knew the real benefits of exercise, I went at it with a vengeance. I swam, I ran, I worked out, I bicycled, I took up tennis and learned to play a lousy game, but I had a good time. And I still do all these things.

But this experience sent me into a tailspin. I had been training for triathlons and had been running that morning, doing wind sprints. As I approached my house I slipped on some wet grass near a sprinkler and fell really hard. The instant I hit the ground I felt a tremendous pain in my shoulder. I got up thinking, "Hey, this really feels bad, maybe the shoulder is dislocated" — and I discovered I couldn't even lift the arm, it was so painful. And I had to do a radio broadcast that afternoon. I did the broadcast, but at the end I said to my wife, "You know, maybe I should go to the hospital and get an X-ray, because it could be dislocated, and if you leave an arm dislocated for too long, it just doesn't heal right."

We went to the hospital for the X-ray, and as a doctor I was very officious and probably a little bit arrogant about it, and I started giving orders: "I'd just like this checked out, because it might be dislocated." By this time my arm was practically immobile. After the X-ray was developed, I hurriedly asked, "What's the result?" And they said, "Well, doctor, it's not dislocated. It's *fractured.*"

Now I've seen all kinds of horrendous X-rays, with bones sticking out of arms and things like that. But when I heard the word *fractured* and saw the X-ray of what looked like a snapped matchstick *and it was me,* a wave of weakness overtook me. Within a few seconds I found myself lying down on a gurney and getting smelling salts. Uncharacteristically, I had just fainted dead away. Of course, I had seen so many people with much worse injuries, but the realization that this drama was being played out within my own body was just too much to take in.

This was really my first confrontation with mortality and physical vulnerability. I'd been enjoying all the athletics — feeling my body get stronger, building up my endurance, pushing myself. And unconsciously, somehow, I probably felt that I couldn't be hurt, that I was somehow invulnerable. I had no apparent handicaps and no special susceptibilities to any illness or chronic condition. Suddenly I was told that a part of me was irrevocably broken, that I would take a scar to my grave, and that there might be a certain amount of irreversible damage.

It turned out to be a long recovery, and I went through all the classic psychological stages of denial and adjustment and anxiety. The funny thing was that I *knew* about all that stuff from textbooks, and I'd witnessed my patients experiencing all kinds of anxieties and fears. But this didn't make it any easier for me. I first went through a sense of tremendous regret and guilt, saying to myself, "*How* could I have done this? *How* could I have ruined my body like this? This is going to ruin my life." I knew that an injury like this could have long-term or permanent effects, that it could limit the range of motion of my arm, and that it could affect my professional work, to say nothing of all the athletic activities I'd become such a nut about. I thought, "It's never going to be the same; I'm never going to play tennis again; I'm never going to be able to swim, run, do all the things I like to do." And in my darker moments I wondered just how I was going to function as a doctor if this meant that I would have trouble with certain procedures. I remembered that sometimes I had wondered how patients could be so anxious about problems that weren't really life-threatening. Well, now I was going through the same trauma myself, and I desperately wanted someone to assure me that I was going to be all right.

The first doctor I consulted took a quick look at my shoulder and then looked over my X-rays very carefully without saying anything. Finally he looked up with what I thought was almost an air of disappointment, and said, "I don't think you're going to need surgery for this." He added, "That's not too bad a fracture — just come back in six weeks and we'll take another X-ray." I was very relieved, of course, but it seemed to me that after he found out that surgery wasn't called for, he lost interest. He told me, "Let's just keep it in a sling and don't move it, and use some pain medication." I asked him, "Is there anything I can do to facilitate the healing?" He said, "In a couple of weeks, just start making little circles with your arm, like this." I asked, "Is there anything else?" and he said, "No, that's it." All in all, we had had about four minutes of interaction. Finally I came out with what I was really worried about: "Do you think I'm going to be a hundred percent healed?" His response: "You won't be a hundred percent, but you'll proba-bly be pretty near to it. But we won't really know for a few months." Not only had he not offered me any sort of proactive role in the healing process, but he left me hanging, with my worst fears still unanswered. And I'd really been looking for something that would build up my confidence, some kind of benediction, like "If you really work on this you're going to be fine."

But I just couldn't leave it at that. I was still anxious, and I really wanted to do something to help the healing process. So I sought out an orthopedist I knew of, who also had the knowledge of a physical therapist about how to deal with injuries. She wasn't so focused on the surgery issue, but she *was* concerned with what *I* could do to facilitate healing. She immediately said to me, "You must begin a therapy program, and you have to get someone to assist you in moving your arm as far as possible, because you could lose your range of motion if you don't." This turned out to be much harder than it sounds, because I quickly found that even having someone else lift or raise my arm was torturously painful.

But she gave me the opportunity to get involved in my healing process as well as the hope and confidence that I would get results. And even though it was excruciating to do these exercises, I persisted. She told me what was safe to do and what wasn't, and she pushed me and encouraged me. In her office, when she stretched my arm back to where it should be, tears came to my eyes, but I stuck it out. I really wanted to be able to return unencumbered to my regular lousy game of tennis.

But several times during the recovery phase I truly despaired. I just couldn't believe that I was going to get better again. I had to keep reminding myself that nature and the healing process would take their course, and in fact I did recover nearly all of my function. I can still swim well enough, and still knock the tennis ball around, albeit with a trace of stiffness now and then.

I certainly would have preferred to forego the whole experience, but it taught me something about what some of my patients have had to go through and how they've felt as they have confronted their own accidents and crises. I can certainly assure them with a little more warmth and encouragement than before that the body does heal, that recovery is possible, and that we can be resilient in the face of these crises. Of course, surgery was not recommended in my case, but I was able to get better with the help of a medieval medical device (an arm sling), a little encouragement, and the simple (but painful!) therapy of exercise.

Why digress and tell you my own story? I just want to make clear that when I say baby boomers have been sheltered, and react in shock to major illness, I'm not at all unsympathetic. I've been there, and I know what it feels like. I know from personal as well as professional experience that you can come back from some very serious problems. Sometimes it takes high-tech solutions, but sometimes the simplest, low-tech therapies are the answer. And sometimes it just takes time, or an adjustment to lifestyle. We may well experience ups and downs in our health, as well as sudden crises. But if we take a balanced, long-term approach to staying well, and apply the principles of "intelligent medicine," we should be able to come back from the crises and smooth out the rockier roads.

In fact, it's no longer a matter of speculation that our belief systems and our attitudes toward health and illness have a great deal to do with how we weather crises, how well we bounce back from injuries, and ultimately with our own success in maintaining wellness and vitality over the years. Many recent studies have shown that mental attitude has a powerful effect on recovery from illness. State of mind has even been shown to have a measurable effect on immune response. These studies don't surprise me —

I've long been as interested in the psychology and philosophy of medicine as much as in the science and the procedures.

In fact, I had never intended to go into medicine when I was young. In high school I was a science whiz, but when I got to college I had a reaction against the objectivity of hard science. At that point, I became interested in anthropology because I wanted to study people. Of course, one of the major tenets of anthropology is cultural relativism: the differences between societies and the things we can learn from cultures that are very different from ours. One of the first lessons I learned from studying different cultures was that the beliefs and practices of any society, anywhere in the world, have an internal validity. No matter how strange they seem to us, another society's belief systems work for that society — they sustain the community and the individuals within it. This applies to beliefs about wellness, disease, and healing practices.

I studied healing systems that from our standpoint look absurd or unscientific but have tremendous validity for the people who participate in them, and because of that they work. Of course we've also discovered that many traditional healing methods, like herbal treatments, have a scientific basis in plant chemistry. While we don't want to eschew high-tech medicine, there are valuable lessons we can learn from traditional societies. Despite curious and "nonrational" belief systems, many societies have adapted to their environments in remarkable ways, and in some ways they have sustained qualities of life that we seem to have lost. In the use of herbs and in the respect for nature, there are values that may still be of benefit to us. After all, the aboriginal peoples of Australia have survived in that ecosystem for perhaps thirty to forty thousand years, while our Western European culture seems to be on the verge of permanently damaging the ecosystem of the entire world after just a few hundred years of colonial and industrial expansion. And what we've done to our environment and to our diet can literally make us sick.

Even the negative side of traditional belief systems has lessons for us. People who believe that a curse has been laid on them will get sick and die — unless a powerful shaman comes to the rescue. Aboriginal peoples who see a European doctor coming at them with a weird device like a stethoscope, or giving them some strange concoction like penicillin, can actually get worse, believing they've been attacked by magic or poisoned. By the same token, someone who is terrified of chemotherapy, who feels he or she is being poisoned, is much less likely to improve with this treatment. It becomes a self-fulfilling prophecy: they are poisoned. Consequently, when we work with people who have different belief systems, we have to engage their healing faculties. Healing is as much a process of engaging people's healing apparatus as it is of mechanically defeating disease.

I developed an interest in traditional healing systems as a result of my studies in anthropology, and a willingness to accept the importance of belief systems in the healing process. In fact, I don't think I could have gone directly into medicine without engaging in some of this soul-searching and philosophical questioning along the way. How has this affected my practice? I remain very open-minded. I look to high-tech medical science for the good that it has to offer. And I look to developing and alternative therapies to see what they have to offer. It was important for me to study Western science, to get that M.D. degree, to go through my postgraduate training. But I've never lost my general philosophic openness toward new and alternative methods that work. And my experience in the medical profession has strengthened my conviction that how we think about wellness, illness, and healing has a great deal to do with our success in maintaining health.

CHAPTER THREE

A New Look at the Body

The doctor of the future will give no medicine, but will interest his patient in the care of the human frame, in diet, and in the cause and prevention of human disease.

THOMAS A. EDISON

Something interesting happens when I take a family medical history from some of my patients. They will talk about their grandparents from Russia, or the Caribbean, or rural America—grandparents who often lived into their nineties. What's more, they stayed pretty active and healthy into old age. Were they wealthy? No, they were farm people, or working people; they did hard physical labor all their lives. What did they die of? No one really knows. It seems they died of old age—simple as that.

But my patients' parents, of the same genetic stock, are encountering all kinds of problems: they have cancer in their fifties or heart attacks in their sixties. They develop diabetes. The parents are usually better off financially than the grandparents. They haven't had to work as hard, and they retire when they're sixty or sixty-five. Yet, they have more serious health problems than the grandparents, who perhaps lived through deprivation or poverty and perhaps never had the opportunity to retire. My patients are reflecting on this and asking, "What is it about my parents' lifestyle that has put them in jeopardy?" This is a typical experience, and the only thing we can really point to is the American way of life: smoking; drinking; the high-fat, high-sugar diet; minimal physical activity; the habit of driving a car instead of walking; the whole suburban dream that has somehow gone awry.

It's clear we need to take a closer look at some of the typical American health risks if we're going to mount an effective campaign against decline and illness. Each chapter in Part Two of this book will examine the major risks that can affect the different systems of the body. But first let's look at some typical examples of how baby boomers can get into trouble and how they can get out.

How Things Can Go Wrong

I see a lot of patients like Ellen, who first appeared in my office complaining of fatigue, spaciness, mood swings, and occasional "shakiness." She told me that she was hungry all the time and couldn't seem to help putting on a few more pounds every year, even though she was trying to eat a healthy diet. Ellen had just turned forty and did seem to be carrying some extra weight, mostly around her waist, which is a tip-off for a metabolic imbalance we call Syndrome X. Her complaints were real, though she half-wondered whether she should be seeing a psychiatrist because of her mood swings, even though she had a happy, stable family life and enjoyed her work in publishing.

I asked Ellen what she thought a healthy diet was. She had granola with fruit for breakfast, a no-fat muffin and fruit juice in midmorning, and a light salad for lunch. By midafternoon she was starved and fatigued, but she drank tomato juice or ate crackers and forced herself to put off eating until dinner, when she'd usually have a big pasta dish with lots of whole-wheat Italian bread on the side. The fact was that although her fat intake was relatively low, she was eating exactly the sort of high-sugar, high-carbohydrate diet that would naturally induce food cravings and weight gain. She was flooding her bloodstream with high levels of sugar when she ate, which gave her immediate energy but then invoked her insulin reserves to lower the blood sugar levels. She would then have a crash — no energy, spaciness, shakiness.

I put Ellen on my Salad and Salmon Diet (see chapter 16), and she soon began feeling better and gradually lost weight. Fortunately, we were able to arrest a process of decline that could have had some very serious consequences, including heart disease and diabetes. But not everyone takes the necessary steps in time. Ellen was in the middle stage of a syndrome I call sugar disease. This manifests itself in different ways in different individuals, and at different stages of life. In younger years, it often appears as hypoglycemia, or low blood sugar, which is marked by a whole array of shifting symptoms: spaciness, fatigue, mood swings, sugar craving, headaches, tremors, depression, hot flashes, abdominal pain, panic attacks, and even more.

In the middle stages, sugar disease progresses to Syndrome X, which is marked by weight gain, especially around the midsection; elevated blood pressure; elevated cholesterol and triglycerides; fatty deposits on arterial walls; immune suppression; and insulin resistance. This latter complication typically leads to the third stage of sugar disease: full-fledged adult-onset diabetes. (For more details on this syndrome, see chapter 6.)

Ellen's sugar disease is one example of a medical concept called *diathesis*—a syndrome of decline that extends over years. It's a way of looking at disease over the course of a lifetime and is a much more sophisticated way of understanding disease than to simply say that so-and-so "contracted" diabetes in her fifties. The idea is that you don't have just a disease that suddenly strikes you but an unfolding pattern of vulnerabilities that may manifest itself at various times as various diseases.

For example, an allergic diathesis might be characterized in childhood by infantile colic, which subsides, but is followed by childhood eczema, develops later into adult asthma, and perhaps later in life appears as chronic obstructive pulmonary disease, causing cardiac strain and ultimately death. This is a way of looking at the disease potential of an individual and what his or her weak spots are. Genetic predispositions play a part in diathesis, but so do health habits and lifestyle. The great value of this concept is that we can be aware of these syndromes, offer early warning, and recommend changes in diet or lifestyle, or intervene with nutrient supplements to ward off the final-stage disease.

The concept of diathesis is given lip service in medical schools, but more often as theory than as a principle to apply in clinical practice. In the examining room, doctors are much more likely to say simply that you have a disease or don't have one, or sometimes that you don't have one—yet. You're just auditioning for the part! Actually, the concept of diathesis is very much in line with the theory of some non-Western traditional medicines. A doctor practicing traditional Chinese medicine may examine a patient and say, "Ah, very weak spleen," and this could be part of a life-long theme for the patient. It doesn't mean that the spleen got kicked by a horse one day and all of a sudden became a problem, but rather that the person has a constitutional problem, which can generate many different difficulties. We can apply the same principle using the high-tech diagnostic techniques of Western medicine. In a new patient I look for the potential for a diathesis to occur, to see what kinds of genetic or behavior patterns might indicate one type of decline or another, and which preventive approaches we should take.

Turning Things Around

As you read through this book, or look up specific chapters, bear in mind the concept of diathesis: that we're not looking simply to ward off specific diseases but to shift whole patterns of decline. One of the great things about this approach is that certain basic adjustments, such as dietary changes, can affect a whole range of outcomes, from improving cardiovascular health to preventing diabetes and maintaining good vision.

We're also learning that it's possible to backtrack from high-risk health patterns, recover from behavior-caused illness, and arrest or slow physiological decline. I have patients in their forties who are savvier than they were in their twenties or thirties and as a result feel healthier and more energized than ever before. Some of my patients have made significant adjustments in their lifestyles to conquer illness or slow decline. I also have patients who are not in decline but come to me because they want to "optimize" their health; take a proactive, preventive stance; and build their energy and stamina to an optimal level. Both goals require a willingness to compromise, to pay more attention to the body and its needs, and to take a more active or proactive interest in developing a healthy, prevention-conscious lifestyle. It also means taking a more active, engaged, and responsible role in dealing with the medical system and in choosing treatments, physicians, and sometimes alternative caregivers.

This book really comes out of a paradigm shift in medicine, both in technology and in philosophy. We increasingly have a sophisticated technology to identify risk factors for disease. More and more physicians, their patients, and even health insurance companies are subscribing to the philosophy that prevention is worth more than cure and that it's a viable goal to optimize our physical well-being and energy levels, our longevity, and our physical performance.

In the next part of this book, we'll take a closer look at each of the different systems of the body to understand how to reduce the risks of decline and optimize health from each of these different perspectives. I say "different perspectives" because the different systems of the body that are studied in medical school aren't really different "things" but different ways of looking at the whole mind/body complex. There are intricate and subtle relationships between the digestive system and the immune system, for example, that we are only now beginning to understand. I like to think of each system as a different window into the whole health of a person. I continue to find it a fascinating experience to look through these windows and to help people make beneficial adjustments to their health and well-being. I think you'll find the view just as fascinating.

PART TWO

THE SYSTEMS

CHAPTER FOUR

Self and Nonself: The Immune System

- A young woman comes into my office with an assortment of vague symptoms, including a rash on her face and joint pains. She's on the verge of tears because her doctor has diagnosed lupus, a deadly disease that can attack crucial bodily organs, seemingly at random, and can lead to death.

- A hard-working, highly stressed 36-year-old television producer suffers colds that last two to three weeks. They occur with increasing frequency every couple of months, regularly turn into sinus infections, and now require spiraling doses of antibiotics to treat them. On top of this, he contracted a bad case of the flu, and three weeks later he still doesn't feel back to normal. In desperation he asks, "Doc, I can't understand what's happening to me. It's as if my immune system is collapsing. Do you think I should take the AIDS test?"

- A stockbroker tells me at her annual checkup that she feels weak and exhausted whenever she's at work — she feels as if she's "losing her edge." But on weekends she starts to recover, and by Sunday afternoon she feels fine. This has been happening ever since her company moved to new quarters in a prestigious new office building, raising the company's profile in the industry. She doesn't know whether there's something physically wrong with her or whether she's having a nervous breakdown or some kind of midlife crisis.

- A new patient comes in who has had a successful kidney transplant but is taking so much medication to prevent rejection of the organ that he has developed Kaposi's sarcoma, a rare type of opportunistic cancer that typically occurs in AIDS patients. And he has to take additional medication to prevent other infections like the form of pneumonia caused by *Pneumocystis carinii*. He's relieved that the transplant is working, but now he's plagued with new illnesses.

- I'm treating a cop — a detective who's worked his way up in the ranks — who is overwhelmed by anxieties from his job and by asthmatic attacks that seem to get worse when he's under pressure. This is starting to affect his self-confidence and his performance on the job.

What do all these people have in common? They are all suffering from imbalances of the immune system. And these represent only a few of the disorders that are generally accepted as immune related. Even heart disease seems to be mediated through an immune-system response, and there is evidence that the natural decline of immune function with age may be related to the increased rate of cancer in those over sixty.

Still, we've achieved some of the greatest of our medical advances by enhancing or modulating the immune system. We've used vaccination to completely eradicate smallpox and to protect children from illnesses like polio and diphtheria that plagued us only forty or fifty years ago. We've mounted a worldwide assault on infectious diseases in the developing world, drastically reducing mortality from childhood diseases in many countries. Thanks to modern antibiotics, we've successfully avoided scourges like the flu epidemic of 1918 that killed hundreds of thousands of Americans.

At the same time, though, we've seen the proliferation of new and deadly diseases, from Legionnaire's disease to AIDS. As populations move across porous national borders, and as air travel links every part of the globe, obscure microbes from Amazonian jungles or the African veldt can move out into the world arena. Many of them live in symbiosis with their animal hosts but can leap to humans, where they may turn deadly. AIDS, the hanta virus, the Ebola virus, and Creutzfeldt-Jakob (mad cow) disease all seem to have taken this path. Moreover, we are inundated with pollutants, preservatives, and new and strange foods from around the world that may be putting our immune system in a state of constant alert. Industrial pollutants, smog, and second-hand smoke challenge the immune system's ability to absorb and neutralize toxins. In the industrialized world, immune system imbalances are on the rise, from annoying allergies to deadly autoimmune diseases. Cancer rates are rising, too. At the same time, some of our most amazing medical miracles, like the replacement of vital organs, are thwarted by the primitive and powerful action of our immune systems.

For some forty years, we've been using antibiotics to help knock out bugs that our immune systems can't easily handle. Yet, our very success with antibiotics has led to new challenges to our health. Old scourges like tuberculosis, which we thought we had conquered, are back in new, virulent forms that are resistant to every drug we've used to combat them. And this is not an isolated case. Our overuse of antibiotics is shaping the evolution of bacteria and viruses around the world, so that more and more diseases are becoming resistant to the basic antibiotics. Baby boomers, the first generation raised from childhood on antibiotics, are at particular risk. We are forced to develop new and sophisticated drugs just to keep up, and these are increasingly expensive and often have dangerous side effects. We are now looking at the possibility that the "age of antibiotics" may have been a temporary and short-lived respite from the scourge of infectious disease.

As a result, the notion of strengthening the immune system has almost superseded the belief in divine protection. People used to wear amulets to ward off evil spirits. Now they gulp down vitamins to strengthen the immune system — the shield against disease. While the immune system has been studied for a century, it has in the time of the baby boomer been propelled from an obscure niche of medicine to extraordinary prominence in both medicine and the popular imagination. Although few people really understand the workings of the immune system, recent advances have convinced baby boomers that it is now possible to enhance their natural defenses against infections, cancer, and other serious diseases as well as hasten their recovery from minor ailments. In many cases they are right.

The huge upsurge of interest in the immune system has inspired the creation of a "Body Wars" exhibit at Epcot Center. The exhibit is very well done and shows the components of the immune system, but it's based on the typical martial imagery that people use to describe immune function. People talk about invaders, spies, skirmishes, defending armies of lymphocytes, and so on. This imagery makes sense in some ways, but we shouldn't be limited by it. Some patients can use the martial imagery as part of guided imagery to help them fight disease, but the invader/army image has become a limiting stereotype.

Another stereotypical view is that we have to "build up our immunity" as if it were on a dimmer switch and we should just turn up the juice. What we really want to do is balance elements of the immune system. Autoimmune disease, for example, is immunity gone berserk. It's really an excessive immune response — the flip side of weakened resistance. But an individual can have both an autoimmune disease and a weakened immune response to outside invaders. So we can't just say your immunity is too high or too low. It makes more sense to think of the immune system as being properly balanced or out of balance and out of order.

The immune system mediates our response to infection and disease, but it also enables a healthy coexistence with the microbes and "foreign substances" of the world. The immune system does "defend" us — it's a barrier, a shield to protect us from threatening parasites and microbes. But the immune system also enables the body to integrate materials and organisms from outside so it can simultaneously and selectively fend off some invaders while accommodating itself to harmless or useful agents. In fact, we live in synergy or at least peaceful coexistence with many bacteria, microbes, and even insects. We should be able to tolerate common creatures in the environment like dust mites and roaches without their sending our immune systems into a tizzy. People have lived with these creatures for thousands of years. We've evolved with them, and yet for people with allergies they can be a real problem. Somehow their immune systems have failed to adapt to their presence.

The intestinal flora are a good example of immune adaptation. These are bacteria that live in the intestine, usually without harming us, sometimes even assisting with the digestion of food. We adapt to the bacteria of our geographical region and develop a kind of "nonaggression pact." So a person living in Mexico City may be able to eat fruit from an outdoor stand and be fine, while a tourist from the United States can come down with diarrhea and illness caused by the local bacteria. And the Mexican citizen could come down with intestinal illness after eating vegetables from a New Jersey farmers' market. The lymphatic tissue of the gut, which harbors cells of the immune system, becomes adjusted to the presence of local bacteria and tolerates them in a kind of symbiotic way, but it will mount a severe reaction against unfamiliar bacteria in a foreign environment. Antibiotics can distort this natural balance, wiping out the "friendly" bacteria, and leaving the gut open to colonization by strangers.

These examples suggest that our immune system balances or "harmonizes" our own physiology with outside influences. We shouldn't view microbes and infection simply as the enemy but as a necessary source of information to prime the immune system. We might do well to look at the immune system as a way of processing information, distinguishing between self and nonself, rather than simply as a kind of Star Wars defense against external threats.

In this view, sickness becomes not the enemy but a natural process in the ebb and flow of optimal immunity — something like a boot camp for white blood cells. Efforts to vanquish disease by developing vaccines and using antibiotics at the slightest pretext may leave the immune system incompletely programmed and may result in the development of unforeseen consequences such as the bizarre autoimmune diseases that we are currently seeing.

From Cowpox to T Cells: How the Immune System Protects Us

Though a clear understanding of the immune system has begun to emerge only in this century, people have been trying to harness its power for millenia. Molds containing the antibiotic tetracycline have been found in the preservatives used to embalm ancient Nubian mummies. In the Middle Ages, Chinese physicians tried to confer resistance by scratching the skin of their patients and applying smallpox scabs from other patients. (Unfortunately, their patients were as likely to contract the disease as to acquire resistance.) Two hundred years ago, in England, Dr. Edward Jenner discovered that he could safely confer resistance to smallpox by scratching the skin and applying cowpox scabs from an infected animal. The cowpox did not infect humans but did confer immunity to smallpox. This was the first effective vaccination. By the early nineteenth century, smallpox vaccination was commonplace in Europe, though no one knew how it worked or how to extend the principle to other diseases. Finally, in the late nineteenth century, Dr. Louis Pasteur developed the germ theory of infection and demonstrated that killed cells from an infected animal could confer immunity upon another animal.

We now know that vaccination works through the so-called humoral aspect of immune response, through a release of antibodies into the bloodstream. When a bacterium or other foreign agent enters the body, it activates B cells, which originate in the bone marrow, to produce substances called gamma globulin antibodies, or immunoglobulins. These are specialized chemical compounds, each designed to attack and destroy one specific type of foreign microbe. Once the infection has been conquered, enough of the activated B cells remain to enable the body to quickly produce more antibodies, in case of reinfection. Vaccination works by introducing a small amount of material, called antigen, which induces the antibody response. For safety, and so as not to induce the infection we are trying to guard against, the antigen can be made up of killed microbes, or protein fragments, or even related nonthreatening microbes like cowpox. Once the B cells have been activated and the antibodies produced, they stand guard to quickly wipe out any microbes that bear the specific antigen, so that they can't get a foothold in the body and cause infection.

In the twentieth century, doctors and researchers have developed a wide range of vaccinations to guard against some of the most dangerous and life-threatening diseases, from diphtheria to polio. This has been one of the great triumphs of modern medicine, but researchers are still looking for new vaccines against everything from Lyme disease to AIDS.

But there's another whole side to the immune system, the so-called cell-mediated immunity. Late in the nineteenth century, Elie Metchnikoff, an eccentric Russian zoologist and a contemporary of Pasteur, began to explore this kind of immunity. Studying specialized digestive cells in the starfish, he observed them reaching out with amoeba-like extrusions to capture and absorb foreign particles. In a mental leap of sheer genius, Metchnikoff speculated that similar cells—he later called them phagocytes—might serve as biological defenders against intruders. In his later research at the Pasteur Institute, Metchnikoff established that phagocytes are among the white blood cells, or leukocytes, known to cluster at the site of wounds and infections and that they play a significant part in resisting bacterial infections. Phagocytes are omnivorous—they'll consume all kinds of foreign material, from smoke particles to bacteria to cancerous cells. The discovery of cell-based immunity did not lead immediately to any new forms of therapy. However, it did prove a valuable diagnostic tool, since white blood cell counts can indicate whether an infection is present or how advanced it is.

The last twenty years or so have seen an explosion of knowledge about the immune system, much of it fueled by research into AIDS. We have identified different types of white blood cells: natural killer cells, the B cells that produce antibodies, and the specialized T cells that can target and kill specific microbes. (T cells are the ones infected by the HIV virus.) We've identified a group of chemical messengers called cytokines that different cells of the immune system use to communicate with each other and with other systems of the body. We've discovered subsets of T cells, "helper Ts" that react to a single specific foreign agent and start the immune reaction; "killer Ts" that directly attack infectious agents; and "suppressor Ts" that turn off the immune reaction when the infection has been conquered. We now know about factors such as sugar, or environmental toxins like mercury, that can inhibit the functioning of white blood cells, and other factors that can enhance them. And we've begun to learn about the intricate interplay between the immune system, the nervous system, and the endocrine system.

But for all this, we've become much too dependent on a single crutch — antibiotics — to do the work of the immune system. And this tool is becoming less and less effective. We can no longer simply look at the "invading" microbes, and come up with magic bullets to kill them. We have to look more closely at the body's own response to microbes and foreign organisms, and whether it offers them an inviting or difficult environment to grow in. This chapter will offer an approach to natural immune enhancement, based on our current knowledge. Let's take a look at how we can use this knowledge to maintain health and enhance our resistance to disease.

Immunity Under Siege

Despite the advances of modern medicine, we are living in an age that presents staggering risks to our immune system. In the global village, microbes can spread from continent to continent and from community to community more easily than ever before in history. Our polluted industrial environment is filled with toxic chemicals that challenge the immune system. Many of us lead high-stress lifestyles, with inadequate nutrition, sleep, and exercise — all of which can debilitate the immune system. Even our social environment comes into play: there is evidence that living in a warm, close-knit, stable community and with the extended family can enhance immunity and provide natural "vaccination" against common diseases through early exposure in infancy. But whether we live in suburbs or cities, too few of us enjoy this kind of stable, supportive community. The nuclear family shelters us from some early exposure to disease but can also leave gaps in our immunity. Our very pleasures can weaken us: the vast array of imported and foreign foods challenge our immune system's ability to adjust and become acclimated to them. And too many people challenge their immune systems directly with cigarette smoke, alcohol, and sugar. Our diets of processed, packaged foods lack essential nutrients that help the immune system do its work. Finally, we must all deal with the decline in immune function that is a natural consequence of aging. Baby boomers can't take for granted the robust immune response we may have enjoyed in youth.

As a result, diseases and syndromes of impaired immune function, almost unheard of before the 1940s, have been on the rise in industrialized nations, especially during the past thirty years. They are still exceedingly rare among indigenous peoples. R. K. Chandra, a nutritional researcher at the University of Nova Scotia, has used a beautiful illustration to describe what is happening to the immune system. He shows an open umbrella (the immune system), protecting us from the "rain" of environmental risks. And then he shows a tattered umbrella, full of holes caused by poor nutrition, lack of exercise, and self-inflicted damage to the immune system, with the threatening agents raining in. Whether we think of the immune system as an umbrella or a defensive army, it's crucial, for our health, to maintain and support it. Let's look at some of the specific risks we face and how to guard against them.

Aging: Best to Plan Ahead

Just like other organs and body parts, the immune system weakens with age. The decline begins at about age thirty. The thymus, which produces T cells, is the size of a walnut in children, shrinks by puberty to the size of a pea, and nearly disappears by the age of fifty. By old age, we have only about one-fourth of the T cell activity of youth. We become more susceptible to bacteria and viruses, and it gets harder to fight them off. We become more vulnerable to the proliferation of cancer cells. Fortunately, the bone marrow can effectively produce B cells, which in turn produce antibodies, well into old age. However, the aging B cells make fewer antibodies. While some immune functions weaken, others can become overactive, leading to an increase in autoimmune reactions. The endocrine system seems to play a part in this.[1]

On top of the natural decline, many elderly people are at increased risk because of limited, inadequate diets that do not contain enough of the immune-supporting nutrients. Since our need for these nutrients grows with age, even the standard Recommended Dietary Allowance may be inadequate.

Some of us have an extra edge against disease, however, since the vigor of the immune system is partially inherited. There are people who just don't seem to get sick. One Japanese study found rare genetic markers — perhaps coding for resilience — in a group of people over the age of 100 — and the absence of other markers that are linked with disease.[2] Most of us, however, need to augment our natural immunity.

Pollution and Domestic Chemicals

We are learning that chemicals, petroleum byproducts, and toxic heavy metals can suppress the immune response. Industrial byproducts and hazardous wastes are increasingly polluting our environment with these materials, but some may be present in ordinary household chemicals and products, such as cleaning fluid and paint thinner.

Heavy metals like cadmium, lead, and mercury are everywhere in the industrialized world, and all cause immune suppression in addition to their other toxic effects. Mercury is a special concern. Not only is it poisonous in itself, but studies have shown that mercury amalgam fillings in teeth may contribute to immune suppression and to the development of antibiotic resistance.

Other pollutants that affect the immune system include polycyclic aromatic hydrocarbons — the kinds of petroleum byproducts that were produced in massive quantities by the burning of the oil fields in Kuwait and that can also be released by ordinary household chemicals. In fact, tests of immune function are increasingly turning up responses to chemical pollution that mimic the patterns of other immune deficiency diseases, such as HIV infection and chronic fatigue syndrome. On top of this, too many Americans compound existing environmental risks by "self-pollution" through smoking, alcohol abuse, and drug abuse.

Malnutrition: Even for the Well-fed

From Biblical times through the Middle Ages to the present day, famine has been followed by plague and pestilence. Immune systems weakened by malnutrition have always provided fertile ground for infection. Today, malnutrition is common in underdeveloped countries, but it exists in fractions of every national population. In the industrialized West, it's common among the poor and among hospitalized patients. Studies of illness around the world have identified deficiencies of vitamins and trace elements as the cause of immune weakness and even death by infections. Immunologist R. K. Chandra has pointed out that the pattern of infections in malnourished people mimics the patterns of immune deficiency disorders such as AIDS.[3] Working backward, scientists have found that tests of immune response are very sensitive indicators of nutrient deficiencies. It seems that the cell-mediated immune response — along with the effectiveness of phagocytes, natural killer cells, and T cells — is most profoundly affected by malnutrition.

The word malnutrition makes us think of starving children in famine-ridden parts of the world. Yet, even well-fed American citizens can suffer from malnutrition. The past forty years have seen a steady decline in the basic nutritional content of the American diet. Processed foods have had important vitamins and minerals processed out of them. Vitamins may be added back into processed foods in such a haphazard way that they do more harm than good. An *excess* of some foods can also lead to immunosuppression. The most common example in affluent societies is an excess of fat in the diet, which can lead to increased respiratory infections and is associated with higher risks of multiple sclerosis and certain cancers.[4]

There is even some evidence that the progressive decline of immune function with age may be due in part to nutritional deficiencies. People older than sixty-five may eat less, and as lean body mass decreases with age, blood levels of many nutrients fall. Studies have shown that vitamin and mineral supplements can reverse or arrest the natural decline of immune function. Supplements have a clear effect in hastening healing and preventing bacterial infections after operations, and they can increase the effectiveness of flu vaccinations, which are intended to evoke an antibody response.[5] Good nutrition turns out to be one of the best ways of strengthening the immune response, and we will look at this in detail below.

Since the immune system will inevitably, if gradually, decline, we must plan to bolster it. We have to make an action plan for immune health. More and more people are watching their diets and jogging or working out to strengthen the cardiovascular system and guard against heart attacks. We have to take the same kind of proactive approach to supporting the immune system. Fortunately, we don't have to learn a whole new set of tricks, because the same good diet and exercise that supports the immune system will help give us a healthy heart. There are some immune-specific prevention measures, though, and we'll learn about them in this chapter.

Nutrition and Immunity: Building the Base

A good diet is the best place to begin bolstering immunity. It's critical to create a good biochemical environment to support the complex cellular and subcellular processes of the immune system and to avoid dietary stressors that can weaken the immune response. Diet and nutrition can affect the immune system in myriad, complex ways. Fortunately, we can boil down the most crucial factors into a list of nutrition dos and don'ts, and we can offer a list of dietary supplements that will provide additional support for immune function.

Curiously, surgeons are among the specialists who first became interested in nutrition to prevent disease. Infection is one of the major risks in surgery. In fact, wounds are among the simplest models of immune system activity. If you cut yourself, white blood cells migrate to the wound, both to fend off infection and to consume damaged cells. Surgeons have found that good diet and nutrient support before surgery can contribute greatly to easy recovery and avoidance of postsurgical infections.[6]

Nutrition Don'ts

SUGAR: ON THE TABLE, IN THE BLOOD

One of the most immune-suppressive foods is sugar, or any food that induces high levels of blood sugar. A quick rise in blood sugar to higher than normal levels can paralyze our immune response. We can see this in diabetics, who are unable to process blood sugar normally and as a result are much more prone to infection. You can actually see this effect under a microscope. If you look at normal, living white blood cells, they move about vigorously across the microscope slide. It's a fascinating demonstration to take a drop of blood from someone who's just eaten a sugary, high-carbohydrate meal and put it under the microscope. In the presence of sugar, the white blood cells look round and puffy and move sluggishly. I've shown this phenomenon to some of my patients who are embarking on a new dietary program — it really makes them sit up and take notice!

Scientifically speaking, we say that high blood sugar inhibits neutrophil chemotaxis. Neutrophils are the most common type of white blood cells, and they are normally drawn by chemical messengers (the process called chemotaxis) to the site of wounds or injuries to "gobble up" the dead tissue. High blood sugar slows down this process, so that the fragments of dead tissue linger, ripe for infection. Sugar also inhibits vitamin C absorption, so that a given blood level of vitamin C has less of a protective effect against infection.

We have to watch more than the sugar levels in desserts and soft drinks. Foods that we might think of as healthy, such as fruit juice or trail mix, can increase blood sugar levels beyond the optimum level. In fact, the food doesn't have to contain refined sugar to have this effect. Any food that rapidly raises blood sugar, such as alcohol or simple carbohydrates, will produce the same effect. Eating a big plate of white spaghetti will rapidly raise the blood sugar. This is why complex carbohydrates, such as whole grains and beans, are better for you — they release their sugar content much more slowly, so that blood sugar levels don't swing wildly up and down.

CALORIES

Beyond sugar and high blood sugar, it appears that excessive caloric intake of any kind seems to impair immunity. We see this in studies of rats showing that lean, slightly underfed rats are less prone to infectious disease, malignancies, and autoimmune disease — and they actually live longer. Why this occurs is unclear, but it appears that excess food may burden the body's detoxification pathways and thereby tie up energy required for immune response. Alternatively, the toxins that build up when wastes are not easily eliminated may suppress immunity. We do see a similar effect in patients suffering from anorexia nervosa. Even though they severely undereat, they sometimes show a robust immune response.[7] It's as if there were an evolutionary advantage to boosting immune response in times of famine. However, extended undereating, with insufficient nutrition, will ultimately weaken immune response.

FAT

The biggest source of excess calories in the American diet is fat, which may indirectly suppress immune response in other ways. Studies show that high blood cholesterol levels in animals are associated with increased susceptibility to infection. T cell response is weakened, and phagocytes seem to be less active in doing their job of consuming foreign particles and dead tissue. It's true that obese people suffer more than others from infections. In laboratory studies, animals show enhanced cellular immunity on a low-fat diet.

There is also evidence that a high level of dietary fat is related to reduced activity of natural killer (NK) cells.[8] These NK cells are the first line of defense against tumors and inhibit the spread of cancerous cells throughout the body. One study showed that lowering the amount of fat in the diet caused a significant increase in NK cell activity.[9] The implication is that high-fat diets may increase the risk of cancers, and there does appear to be some correlation with some types of cancer, including uterine cancer, prostate cancer, possibly breast cancer, and even certain skin cancers. It's theorized that the dietary fat may affect hormone secretion.

One type of fat does seem especially harmful: trans-saturated or hydrogenated artificial fats, normally found in margarine and vegetable shortening but rarely found in nature. Cell membranes are normally composed of fats, and these artificial "trans-fats" seem to damage immunity by filling up the cell membrane at the expense of natural fats and possibly by interfering with the ability of cells to communicate with one another. There is

evidence that the use of hydrogenated fats is related to an increased incidence of cancer, and we can certainly note a general increase in cancer that
just happens to coincide with the introduction of these artificial fats earlier
in the twentieth century.

Roy Wolford's book *The 120-Year-Old Diet* advocates reducing calories
and undereating to extend life. There does seem to be some logic to this. If
obesity and high-fat diets reduce the immune response, the contrary should
be true, and a low-calorie, low-fat, low-sugar diet should keep the immune
system functioning at top form.

Nutrition Do's: The Basic Immune-supporting Diet

This sets us up for the ideal immune-supporting diet: low-fat, low-
cholesterol, and low-sugar, with plenty of complex carbohydrates like whole
grains and beans. Sufficient protein is important, since protein deficiency
can suppress immune function. Some nutritional studies have been done
with cancer patients undergoing surgery who experience extreme immune
suppression caused by the surgery, the blood transfusions, the anesthesia,
and malnutrition caused by the cancer itself. It turns out that protein, RNA,
and omega-3 fatty acids, as found in fish oil, are helpful in boosting their
immune response.[10] Other studies with animal subjects have also shown
that fish oil helps recovery from immune challenges.[11] It seems Grandma
was on to something with her cod-liver-oil tonic!

The best immune-supporting diet is really our basic Salmon and Salad
Diet outlined in chapter 16, which is good for cardiovascular health and
general health as well as for the immune system. But we are learning that
vitamin and nutritional supplements can play an important role in maintaining immune health, and can slow or even arrest the natural decline with
age. In particular, studies have shown that supplementing diets with vitamins and minerals that exceed the Recommended Dietary Allowances
improves measures of immune response and increases resistance to infectious disease.[12] The body especially demands nutrients that assist with the
rapid protein synthesis of antibodies and the production of T and B cells. In
one study, R. K. Chandra gave nutritional supplements to elderly people and
found that they had half the number of colds, flus, and other infections,
compared with a group that didn't receive the supplements, and recovered in
half the time. Other studies have produced similar results.[13] Studies done at
Tufts suggest that it's not a single nutrient but a synergistic or cumulative
effect of several nutrients that makes the difference.[14] Let's take a look at
some of the principal nutrients that help support the immune system.

• *Vitamin A and the carotenoids* are crucial nutrients for immune health.
Vitamin A is required for lysozyme, an antibacterial enzyme found in tears,

sweat, and saliva. Vitamin A regulates and protects the surface of epithelial cells that line the body's digestive tract and other passages and surfaces, including the skin, cornea, mucous membranes, lungs, and bladder. In animal studies, vitamin A inhibits cancer growth by stimulating killer T cells to eradicate mutant, precancerous cells.

The carotenoids, including beta-carotene, are precursor nutrients, which are converted in the body to vitamin A as they are needed. By itself, beta-carotene enhances the cell-mediated side of the immune system, stimulating the production of T and B cells, macrophages, and natural killer cells. As an antioxidant, beta-carotene can also absorb the dangerous oxidized particles in the body called free radicals that can suppress the immune function by damaging the cell receptors that recognize foreign antigens.

Recent large-scale prevention trials performed with Finnish smokers and American physicians have disappointed proponents of the use of beta-carotene for cancer prevention. However, the tests used beta-carotene alone, which may explain the results. Critics of these studies point to the necessity of utilizing beta-carotene along with companion carotenoid nutrients, as well as other antioxidants, to achieve immune enhancement and protect against free radical damage. They also point to the rigorous task assigned to beta-carotene: that of preventing cancer in heavy smokers for the relatively short duration of the trials themselves—a few years, rather than the decades during which the subjects had been smoking. The truth is that all studies of beta-carotene *in foods* have shown it to have pronounced cancer-protective and immune-enhancing characteristics. This suggests that we need to unlock the potential of the carotenoids and other phytonutrients. New efforts are under way to reformulate supplements with broad-spectrum carotenoids and individual phytonutrients with daunting names like lycopene and zeazanthine.

DOSAGE: Mixed carotenoids, 5,000–20,000 I.U.; Vitamin A, 5,000 I.U. As little as 30–60 I.U. a day of vitamin A supplement has been shown to enhance immune response, though the RDA is 5,000. Some people don't easily convert beta-carotene to vitamin A, so it's important to have both in the diet or as supplements.

• *The B vitamins* are essential cofactors in cell metabolism, and they may regulate the activity and rapid proliferation of the white blood cells of the immune system. Folic acid, pantothenic acid, pyridoxine, riboflavin, and vitamin B_{12} all play an important role in sustaining immune function. Of all the B vitamins, pyridoxine, or vitamin B_6, has the most profound effect on the immune system. Low levels can globally suppress immunity, inhibiting both antibody production and cell-mediated immune response. Curiously, vitamin B_6 deficiency is one of the most common of all vitamin deficiencies, especially among the elderly, who typically have a reduced immune response. Studies have shown that supplements of just 15 milligrams a day can increase immune response. Most B-complex supplements contain 50 milligrams of vitamin B_6.

• *Vitamin C* is probably best-known of the nutrients that affect immunity. A whole literature of studies shows the effect of vitamin C in increasing immune activity and reducing the incidence of infection. This includes Nobel prize winner Linus Pauling's 1976 study on vitamin C and the common cold. It's true there's plenty of resistance to the late Pauling's enthusiasm for vitamin C in the medical and scientific community, but his studies speak for themselves. And his aren't the only ones. One double-blind study by I. M. Baird showed that even the relatively small dose of 80 milligrams a day of vitamin C had a statistically significant effect in reducing the rate of infection by colds.

Another interesting study was of the incidence of respiratory infections in long-distance runners, people who run marathons and ultra-marathons. These runners tend to have a much higher incidence of colds and upper respiratory diseases following a race because of the physical stress on the lungs. The study found that runners given vitamin C supplements had half the incidence of post-race infections compared with runners who received a placebo.

We also know that vitamin C reduces infection and the symptoms of other viral infections, including mumps, herpes, measles, and flu. Like beta-carotene, vitamin C is a powerful antioxidant and may promote immunity in this way. Studies also suggest that vitamin C may work by boosting levels of interferon, which fights viral infections, and by activating the phagocytes and T cells that attack bacteria. There's a high concentration of vitamin C in phagocytes. Though colds are viral, vitamin C helps fight the secondary bacterial infections that can extend the course of a cold and make symptoms worse.[15] There's evidence that vitamin C can also promote antibody production. Large doses of vitamin C, as espoused by Linus Pauling, may help reverse the natural decline of immunity with age.

• *Vitamin E* is another antioxidant that has a documented effect on supporting immune cell activity and increasing resistance to infections. White blood cells have a higher concentration of vitamin E than do red blood cells, and vitamin E has been shown to increase activity of phagocytes and T cells. Vitamin E also suppresses the hormone called prostaglandin E_2, which has been linked to age-related declines in immune response.[16]

Several studies have shown that even moderate supplementation of vitamin E can reduce the statistical rate of infections among healthy older people. In animal studies, high doses of vitamin E given to elderly animals have caused their immune response to equal that of younger individuals. So this is one more nutrient that may help in slowing the natural decline of immunity with aging. In fact, we could look at this from another point of view: the elderly simply have a greater need for certain nutrients, like vitamin E, just as children require a higher than normal intake of other nutrients.[17]

DOSAGE: 200–400 milligrams daily. **Warning:** megadoses in the range of 1200 mg daily or higher may inhibit immune function, especially in the young.

• *Zinc* is one of the most important nutrients for sustaining and boosting immune response. It's an ingredient in a hundred different enzymes, including one that works to assemble DNA strings during cell division. So it's essential for immune response, which is directly dependent on the rapid reproduction of T cells and other white blood cells. It promotes activity of the thymus gland, where many immune functions take place. Zinc can increase the activity of natural killer cells that attack tumorous and precancerous cells, and increases the production of antibodies in response to infections. It can speed up the healing of wounds, and there is even evidence that elemental zinc can directly kill viruses.[18]

There is a natural decline in zinc blood levels with aging, and several studies have shown that zinc supplements can correct and even reverse the immune suppression that occurs with aging. Older people often have a reduced response to vaccines because of the reduced antibody production associated with reduced levels of thymic hormone. There's evidence that zinc can restore thymic function as well, thereby restoring this aspect of immune function. It's interesting that zinc supplements produce a greater effect in the elderly than in the young.[19]

One of the most fascinating effects of zinc on immunity is its ability to shorten the duration and reduce the symptoms of the common cold. Studies have shown that elemental zinc, in lozenge form, directly attacks the rhinovirus that takes hold in the tissues of the throat and mouth.[20] If taken early enough, the zinc can halve the duration of a cold.

DOSAGE: For general supplementation, the USRDA of 15 milligrams a day should probably be doubled, but taking more than about 80 milligrams a day may actually suppress immune function.

DOSAGE FOR COLD SUPPRESSION: 180-milligram lozenges of zinc gluconate (containing 20–23 milligrams of elemental zinc), up to 12 tablets a day until symptoms cease, or up to seven days.

• *Selenium* is a trace metal in the environment, but a necessary dietary element. Its deficiency can cause liver disease, muscular disease, and even degenerative disease of the heart. Selenium is also an important nutrient for maintaining the health of the immune system, and it is an essential component of one type of antibody that fights bacterial infection.[21]

Selenium in concert with vitamin E has an antiinflammatory effect, and some studies suggest a role in preventing cancer growth. Indeed a recent study showed that doses of 200 micrograms of selenium daily halved the rates of prostate, breast, and colon cancer in human subjects. Selenium is also a component of an important antioxidant enzyme, glutathione peroxidase, which typically decreases in blood level with age. In a University of Helsinki study, an organic selenium supplement plus vitamin E was given to a group of retirement home residents, who then became less depressed, fatigued, and hostile; were more active; took more initiative; and had better appetites than residents in the control group, who did not receive the supplement. So here's another nutrient with the potential to arrest or reverse the natural decline in immunity with aging.

DOSAGE: This is a trace element, so the optimum amount is hard to quantify. The suggested dosage is 50–400 *micrograms* daily. Doses in excess of 800 micrograms per day can be toxic.

• *Other metals*, as nutrients, can also affect immune function. Deficiencies in copper, iron, and magnesium can cause immune suppression. An excess of copper or iron can *increase* susceptibility to infection. In response to infection, the body automatically removes iron from the blood serum and redistributes it to cellular storage sites in order to restrain bacterial growth. Magnesium is necessary for the robust production of antibodies, and deficiencies are widespread. If you think you may have immune impairment, you might ask a nutritionally oriented doctor to check your blood levels of these minerals. Not everyone needs or can tolerate extra doses of these nutrients, so they need to be prescribed by a qualified nutritionist.

• *Nucleotides and nucleic acids* are the materials that make up RNA and DNA, the genetic programmers of cell division. A sufficient dietary source, usually from protein, is necessary to support the growth and rapid division of immune system cells. A diet without nucleotides causes decreased immune cell function and decreased resistance to infection.[22]

• *Fish oil*, which is rich in the omega-3 oils, has been shown to have a powerful immune-modulating effect. It's particularly helpful with autoimmune problems. The omega-3 oils in fish oil work by affecting the prostaglandin mechanism. The prostaglandins are a group of hormones, some of which enhance immune function, while others put the brakes on. Fish oil tends to put the brakes on immune reactions and can therefore help with the overactive immune response that causes autoimmune problems and allergies. It can also be used to help reduce the amount of debilitating immune-suppressive drugs that are required for people with organ transplants.

POSSIBLE DOSAGE: 2–3 1,000-milligram capsules twice daily, as approved by a qualified nutritionist.

Exercise and Immunity: The Hidden Benefits

The effect of regular physical exercise — 30–40 minutes, three or four times a week — is just as powerful as the effect of good nutrition in supporting the immune response and slowing its decline with age.

It's true that moderate physical exercise temporarily suppresses some immune functions, including T cell activity and antibody production. But the effect does not linger, and over time a pattern of moderate exercise actually increases antibody response and resistance to tumor formation while increasing the white blood cell count, including levels of specialized immune cells like the natural killer cells and messenger hormones like interferon. The body adapts to moderate physical stress, if it's repeated over time, by increasing immune function. In one study, women who engaged in moderate physical exercise were found to actually have lower rates of cancer than those who did not exercise, possibly because of increased immune system vigilance against tumor cells and precancerous cells. The

NUTRIENTS THAT CAN AFFECT THE IMMUNE SYSTEM

NUTRIENTS AND BEST FOOD SOURCES	EFFECTS
Omega-6 fats (corn, safflower, soybean oils)	Excess disrupts immune system; high levels may suppress rejection of transplanted organs but promote tumor growth
Omega-3 fats (fish oil, canola oil, flaxseed oil, purslane)	May inhibit spread of cancer cells; can increase the activity of white blood cells; dampens down autoimmune reactions
Nucleotides, including DNA and RNA (all plant and animal foods)	Can decrease risk of fungal and bacterial infections
Arginine (nuts)	Enhances immunity in malnutrition, cancer, etc.; speeds surgical recovery; may accelerate herpes growth
Zinc (meat, eggs, poultry, seafood)	Deficiency suppresses maturation of immunological cells; excess suppresses immune response
Iron (liver, red meats, leafy vegetables)	Early life deficiency can cripple immunity; high levels can foster infectious organisms
Selenium (seafood, whole-grain cereals, meat, egg yolk, chicken, milk, garlic)	Needed for the formation of antibodies and enzymes that participate in immunity; excess can impair immune response
Vitamin A (dark green and deep yellow vegetables and fruits) (good to obtain through beta-carotene, body makes its own, nontoxic amounts)	Deficiency increases risk of infection; excess is toxic
Vitamin B_6 (whole grains and greens)	Deficiency impairs cellular and hormone-regulated immunity
Folic acid (organ meats and greens)	Needed for cell division; deficiency impairs immunity; pregnant women, elderly, and inner-city children often deficient

top quarter of women who exercised had about one-sixteenth the incidence of cancer found in women in the sedentary bottom quarter.

It's also interesting that many of the longest-surviving AIDS patients are people who pursue a vigorous exercise program. Some of the benefits may be indirect: regular exercise can reduce the anxiety and depression associated with HIV infection, and it's known that depression directly suppresses immune response. The improved mood that comes with exercise can have a beneficial effect on interlocking hormonal, neurological, and immune functions. However it works, the benefits are real and have been demonstrated in several studies.[23]

The key to exercise benefits is moderation and regularity. Professional or

HEALTHY LIFESTYLES BOOST IMMUNE RESPONSE

A recent Japanese study has shown that healthy habits have a direct effect on the blood levels of natural killer cells — the immune cells that are our first line of defense against tumors and metastasis, or the spread of cancer cells through the bloodstream to different parts of the body. It's already been observed that high dietary fat, stressful life events, and a sedentary lifestyle all lower NK cell activity. In the Japanese study, a questionnaire was used to rate sixty-two healthy male office workers on each of these health practice factors:

1. Cigarette smoking (not smoking)
2. Consuming alcohol (not every day)
3. Eating breakfast (every morning)
4. Hours of sleep (7–8)
5. Hours of work (less than 10)
6. Physical exercise (at least once a week)
7. Nutritional balance
8. Mental stress (keeping stress levels moderate)

A good health practice group and a poor health practice group was identified for each factor. The results? The good health factors all correlated with increased NK cell activity, with the factors related to smoking and exercise producing the most significant increase. The men with all good overall habits showed significantly higher NK cell activity compared with those in the poor habit group. The implication is that good health habits have a cumulative effect — the more you follow them, the better the results.[24]

amateur athletes who engage in strenuous exercise or train intensely over long periods of time do have some special risks. They are actually more susceptible to infection and colds, probably because of the immune-suppressive effect of the exercise. We can measure lower numbers of T cells and lower levels of antibodies after a strenuous training session, while other white blood cells remain at high levels. Strenuous exercise increases oxygen flow through muscles, which generates a higher level of oxidizing free radicals that can damage tissue and prevent immune cells from recognizing their targets. Inhaling large amounts of polluted, ozone-tainted air can also increase free radicals and oxidant levels in the blood, and strain the immune system. People who regularly exercise strenuously need higher levels of antioxidant nutrients, especially vitamins C and E.

Also at some risk are people who go on exercise binges, engaging in strenuous exercise for short periods and then stopping cold. This kind of short-term stress weakens the immune response without giving the body a chance to establish a balance. People who are accustomed to regular exercise and then stop may also experience some degree of immune suppression. Studies show that animals who aren't allowed to exercise freely can develop constricted blood vessels and symptoms resembling rheumatoid arthritis. A regular, moderate exercise program, with sufficient rest, and sufficient antioxidant nutrients, will provide the most effective long-term support to the immune system. A 30–40 minute exercise session three or four times a week — swimming, jogging, or a workout at the gym — will do the trick.[25]

The Mind–Body Connection

Doctors have long known, and popular wisdom has held, that mental attitude has a lot to do with recovery from illness and maintaining health. A patient who has the will to live has a big advantage in recovering from serious illness. Norman Cousins has told the world about how he recovered from cancer by taking a daily dose of funny movies. We're now finding out just how intimately mood and mental attitude are related to health and how closely intertwined are the immune system, the nervous system, and the endocrine (hormonal) system on a deep biochemical level.

We've learned that certain hormonal neurotransmitters, which help convey electrical impulses in the brain and nervous system, are also crucial messengers between different cells of the immune system, and that immune reactions can directly stimulate hormonal and nervous system responses on a preconscious level. Immunologists have become fascinated with parallel functions of both the brain and the immune system: both can learn from outside stimuli, and both can make the important distinction between that which is "self" and that which is "nonself," the brain on the macro level, and the immune system on the cellular and molecular level. And both can act instinctively, based on what they've "learned," to protect us. For a while now, some immunologists have been working in the field of *psychoneuroimmunology*. And some are beginning to look at the nervous system, the endocrine system, and the immune system as one complex, interactive field, the study of which is *psychoneuroimmunology*.

Fortunately, we don't have to practice pronouncing these jawbreakers to benefit from this branch of medicine. Let's take a look at some of the key discoveries and how we can use them to support immune health.

Stressed Out? Or Stressed Just Right?

Stress has gotten a bad name over the past few years. In some ways we have become a nation of people with a stress phobia. Overstressed, stressed out, burned out — it's part of our daily vocabulary. I see patients who are really upset that they have stress in their lives. With some, the only thing they seem to be stressed about is stress itself. We tend to forget that Hans Selye, who first explored the deleterious effects of excessive stress, also noted the positive effects of a manageable amount of stress. Stressing the muscles causes them to strengthen; stressing the mind causes us to learn and adapt. We need a certain amount of physical stress to keep the body in optimum condition. And this goes for the immune system, too.

This said, drastically reducing stress can have very clear benefits for some people. I have had several patients who decided to quit the job, get out of the fast lane, and work full time on bolstering their immune systems. I'm very supportive of this. As a young student I used to observe a venerable Chinese herbal physician who was given to oracular, impressive pronouncements like "Ah, organs very weak, you must lie down, one month, no get up, no move, only go to bathroom and to table to eat." When people followed his advice, some would have fair to middling results, some would have trouble with spouses or jobs, and some would have very good results, because only this kind of drastic prescription would get them to slow down enough to get better. In fact, Chinese medicine is much more supportive of rest and rehabilitation. Chinese hospital stays are much more prolonged than in the West; they are more like an old-fashioned spa cure, with light activity that includes t'ai chi and housekeeping chores. Our medical system and our culture itself don't encourage this kind of approach to treating illness. But this doesn't mean that we can't deal with stress in creative ways, even if we can't take off a month from work to rest and let the immune system do its work. And Western medicine is making some very interesting discoveries about how stress affects the immune system.

Studies have shown that extreme, traumatic stress clearly depresses immune function. In one study, reduced T cell counts were found in men who were suffering from profound grief because their wives were dying of cancer. Other studies have shown depressed immunity and increased rates of tumor growth in rats who were subjected to repeated shocks that they could not escape from. Stress that is profound and chronic is that which most weakens the immune system. Yet, studies of illness levels in people who have experienced stressful events — like death in the family, job loss, taking out a mortgage, or moving to another city — have come up with mixed results. Stressful events do correlate to weakened immunity and susceptibility to infection. But of people who experience the same kind of stress, some tend to get sick and some don't. It is probable that different people handle their stress differently, and this may affect their immune health.

Other studies have shown that certain kinds of stress can actually enhance immunity. Rats who are subjected to shocks that they can escape from have a heightened immune response. Medical students who are studying for exams usually don't get sick until *after* the exams, when the stressful period is over. This fits in with the notion that mild or manageable stress can actually be good for us.

Conditioning the Immune Response

A fascinating discovery in the area of mind-body medicine is that the immune response can be a conditioned response, just as Pavlov conditioned his dogs to salivate at the sound of a bell. In a key experiment at the University of Rochester, psychologist Robert Ader gave rats saccharine water before they received an immune-suppressive injection, and he discovered that eventually the rats would have an immune-suppressive reaction to drinking the saccharine water alone, without the injection. The implications of this fact are enormous — it means that neural and psychological events can directly affect the cells of the immune system, and it implies that we may be able to use psychology or conditioning to enhance our immune response to diseases.

In fact, experiments have shown this to be true. Clinical studies at UCLA and elsewhere have shown that cancer patients who participate in support groups, where they talk over their feelings and the problems they're facing, experience a strengthening of some aspects of immune response, and overall have a better rate of recovery. At the University of Pittsburgh, psychologist Sandra Levy and her colleagues found that women with breast cancer whose personal relationships with husbands and physicians were supportive had improved immune cell activity. And psychologist James Pennebaker, found that students who merely kept journals in which they wrote about their feelings and any disturbing or traumatic events had measurably better immune functions.

Other researchers have looked at meditation, relaxation, guided imagery,

IMMUNE HEALTH CHECK LIST

———— ❧ ————

———— Do I get some sort of regular exercise, 30–40 minutes, at least three times a week?

———— Do I eat a healthy low-fat, low-sugar diet?

———— Do I eat organic foods when possible?

———— Does my diet contain sufficient amounts of carotenoids, vitamins C and E, zinc, and selenium?

———— Do I drink more than one or two alcoholic beverages a day, if a man, or more than two or three a week, if a woman?

———— Do I smoke?

———— Do I have some effective means of dealing with normal or extraordinary stress in my life?

———— Do I get sufficient sleep? An average of seven or eight hours a night?

———— Am I subjected to any persistent environmental hazards or pollutants at work or at home?

———— Is my drinking water free of pollutants and excessive chlorine?

———— Do I live near any industrial sites?

———— Do I have a lot of mercury amalgam dental fillings?

———— Do I get the flu every winter or more than two or three colds a year?

———— Do I get repeated colds or flu attacks? Do they linger for weeks and weeks or require antibiotics to deal with secondary infections?

———— When I get the flu, do I run a real fever and have strong symptoms that run their course, or do I run only a low-grade fever with lingering symptoms?

———— Have I had any chronic or persistent infections that don't ever clear up for good?

———— Do I get frequent bladder or yeast infections?

———— Do any wounds I get heal quickly, or do they tend to heal slowly and get infected?

———— Do I often feel ill after eating certain foods?

humor, and even hypnosis as ways of modulating immune response. Studies have confirmed the positive effects of these activities on immune response. To mention just one, residents of a geriatric nursing home who were taught relaxation techniques and guided imagery showed increased activity of immune cells and had better control over recurrent herpes infections.

Acupuncture: A New Tool for Immune Support

One of the most fascinating areas of current research is the study of how acupuncture, the traditional medical treatment of China, can help modulate the immune system. Studies have shown that acupuncture treatment can assist in the treatment of diseases like chronic hepatitis infection, not just in reducing symptoms but in actually hastening the end of the infection and normalizing the body's immune response. How is this possible just from a needle stuck into the flesh? Well, it appears that acupuncture may work by stimulating specific portions of the autonomic nervous system, which in turn causes responses in the immune system. One study has even found that acupuncture stimulation can cause a significant rise in blood levels of interferon, one of the immune system's messenger hormones. The effect lasts for several days and is much safer than other methods of boosting interferon.[26] Interestingly, the acupuncture point used in this study has traditionally been used to treat symptoms and infections of the head and upper respiratory tract, including the common cold, headache, dentalgia, pharyngitis, rhinitis, and tonsillitis.

   The point is that we now have a range of "new" tools, from meditation to guided imagery to support groups, that have a clear medical benefit for treating immune suppression, whether caused by stress, state of mind, or other reasons. Anyone who is concerned about maintaining immune health should seriously consider these.

Trouble-Shooting: Testing and Diagnosis

The explosion in knowledge about the immune system has led to a search for tests that will indicate very specific problems with the complex range of cells and hormones that make it up. Let's take a look at our current tool kit for testing immune health.

T CELLS AND T CELL RATIOS

The HIV epidemic has made T cells part of everyday language, since they are the primary target of the AIDS virus. It's the very low T cell count that indicates when HIV infection has matured into AIDS. But T cell counts can give us important information about other problems with the immune system. T cells are grown and prepared in the thymus gland and travel throughout the bloodstream. There are actually several subsets of T cells: helper Ts, which identify foreign cells and set the immune response into motion; natural killer Ts, which attack foreign invaders; and suppressor Ts, which "turn off" the immune reaction after it's been successful. The suppressor T cells are essential to keep the immune system from starting to attack the body's own tissues.

When we're testing for T cell levels, we're especially concerned with the helper/suppressor ratios. In AIDS, for example, helper cells that promote the immune response are decreased, and at the same time suppressor cells that turn off the immune response are increased. This combination is a double whammy that weakens the immune response overall. In certain types of allergic or autoimmune conditions, helpers are increased and suppressors are reduced, indicating that the immune system is overactive.

THE ANERGY PANEL

This is a simple test that measures the cell-mediated branch of the immune system, which works through the activity of all the different kinds of white blood cells. A set of prongs is prepared with killed versions of common antigens, or bits of foreign protein, from infectious agents like TB, diphtheria, tetanus, and *Candida*. Most people show a bump or swelling at each prick-point, typically delayed over 48 hours. If the reaction doesn't occur, that indicates a condition of anergy, or reduced immune response.

We can also test independently for natural killer cells, which are important in cancer suppression.

IMMUNOGLOBULIN (ANTIBODY) TESTING

These are tests that measure the humoral branch of the immune system, which defends the body through the release of chemicals called antibodies. Low levels of gamma globulin, an important antibody, are particularly common in people who are susceptible to bacterial infections. Kids who are susceptible to ear infections often have reduced levels of gamma globulin.

Several new tests are available for IgA, or immunoglobulin A, which is normally present at the surface of tissues such as the vagina, the bladder, the nasal passages, and the inside of the GI tract. Low IgA levels can indicate heightened susceptibility to infection of these tissues. The simplest IgA test measures the presence of the antibody in saliva. Not many doctors do this test, which I think is unfortunate, since it's a very simple indicator of immune health. But many doctors do not think of testing for immune problems as part of their diagnostic routine.

There is also a simple blood test for IgE, or immunoglobulin E, which at high levels is linked with allergic reactions.

Catching a Bug: Infection and the Immune System

Most of us think about how well our immune system is working only when we catch a cold, come down with the flu, or catch a bug that's going around. But in fact, our immune system is constantly active, keeping all tissues and cells of the body under surveillance, patrolling the bloodstream, destroying precancerous cells, skirmishing with foreign bacteria and viruses, and absorbing smoke particles and environmental pollutants. But most of this action takes place without our being aware of it. Only when a virus gets a substantial foothold do we feel the side effects of an immune reaction: fatigue, achy muscles, headache, upset stomach, high fever. The symptoms make us want to stay home, curl up in bed, and do nothing—an adaptive reaction that helps the body devote maximum energy to fighting the bug. Within a few days or a week, our immune system has shaken off the threat, and we start to feel normal again, though we're usually a little weak for a while.

In this section, we'll look at a few of the special issues relating to infection and the immune response, and some of the common misconceptions about the process.

The End of the Antibiotic Age?

The first antibiotic, penicillin, was discovered in the 1920s as an accidental mold on a laboratory dish. More of these bacteria-killing molds were discovered, and by the 1950s, researchers had begun to synthesize artificial ones. Pharmaceutical companies were turning them out by the ton, not only for treating disease in people but for preventing infections in cattle and poultry. These were truly miracle drugs, and the baby boomer generation was raised on them. Yet, right from the start, some researchers were warning against their overuse, and as early as the 1950s the phenomenon of drug resistance began to appear as bacteria mutated into new genetic forms that penicillin and other antibiotics couldn't touch. The fact is that the increased use of antibiotics automatically increases the spread of resistant strains of microbes, and the past forty years has seen a race between constantly mutating microbes and researchers trying to come up with new antibiotics to combat them. Antibiotic overuse has become a world problem, and an increasingly mobile population now carries its microbes and resistances across the globe. Bacteria are wondrously adept at passing on antibiotic resistances to their progeny. In fact, the process doesn't depend entirely on natural selection, as we might expect. Bacteria can pass genetic material that confers resistance directly from one bacterium to another, and even between different species. The process is so insidious that antibiotics given to farm animals can induce resistance not only in the animals who received them but in other livestock on the farm and in farm workers themselves. And bacteria that become resistant to one antibiotic are likely to confer resistance to several others as well.

It is not too alarmist to say that we may actually be looking at the end of the antibiotic age as we have known it. Already we are discovering new strains of old diseases for which we simply do not have any effective antibiotic treatment, or have one that is prohibitively expensive or as dangerous as the disease itself. You've probably heard of the new strains of tuberculosis in American cities that are resistant to multiple antibiotics and can be treated only by combinations of three or four extremely expensive synthetic drugs. Well, this is only one example of a growing trend. Overseas, and in developing countries on our continent and around the world, new strains of multiple-drug-resistant infections are cropping up — deadly diseases that have no real cure and can be "treated" only by quarantine.

Though a few voices are crying in the wilderness about this problem, and the medical community is becoming more aware of it, too little is being done. Antibiotics are massively overprescribed and overused here in the United States, and even more so in many countries where they are available without prescription. They are often consumed in quantities too low to eradicate an illness but just high enough to elicit resistance.

What can be done? First of all, we should scrupulously avoid any unnecessary antibiotic use. Too many Americans are in the habit of automatically calling up their doctors and demanding antibiotics when they get a cold or the flu, and too many doctors feel pressured to prescribe them, knowing that a patient can easily get them somewhere else. But antibiotics are completely useless against viruses — the kind that cause colds and flu. (Sometimes colds or flu can develop secondary bacterial infections, such as pneumonia, which do call for legitimate antibiotic treatment.) So if your doctor recommends going to bed and getting some rest as a treatment, don't argue that you need antibiotics. Even if you think you "can't" be sick for business reasons, the antibiotics will never, ever, cure the flu. But they will assuredly increase the risk of resistant bacteria in the future. They are also likely to kill off beneficial bacteria in the gut and increase the likelihood of opportunistic infections like *Candida* (yeast), which move in when the normal intestinal flora have been destroyed.

The misuse of properly prescribed antibiotics can also induce resistant strains of bacteria. Normally, it's necessary to take antibiotics for seven to ten days, even after symptoms of the illness have disappeared, to make sure that all of the disease-causing bacteria have been eradicated. If you stop taking an antibiotic too early, the drug has most likely wiped out only part of the bacterial population — the part that's most susceptible to the antibiotic. The bacteria that remain are those which are most successful at resisting the antibiotic, and they can survive and multiply, passing on their resistant characteristics. Even if the infection doesn't take hold again immediately, it will be less treatable with antibiotics in the future.

Besides avoiding unnecessary antibiotic treatment for ourselves, I think we have to be concerned as citizens about the massive dosing with antibiotics of livestock, agricultural crops, and even fish in fish farms. Dosing crops or livestock can prevent infections and permit raising fish or animals in much more crowded quarters, thus increasing the "efficiency" of the operation and the final market yield. This lowers food prices, but even if traces of antibiotics don't linger in the food itself, they can create resistant bacteria in the agricultural environment that can then be passed to humans.

There's no question that we should take more precautions to prevent the spread of resistant strains of bacteria. But it may actually be too late, on the worldwide scale. In years to come, we may be forced to return to measures like quarantine and prevention that were in use nearly a century ago. More optimistically, we certainly should be turning our attention to ways of supporting our natural immune system and avoiding things that weaken it.

NUTRIENTS THAT FIGHT INFECTION

Besides the immune-boosting nutrients we've already mentioned, there are some natural foods and nutrients that can help fight infections directly.

Garlic shows a broad-spectrum activity against seventeen different strains of fungal infections and may be even more effective against pathogenic yeast infections like *Candida* than Nystatin, the commonly prescribed drug. *Dosage:* Three or four chopped, crushed, or chewed cloves a day, or two or three nonodiferous garlic capsules.

Grapefruit seed extract, a product incorporated into many natural infection-fighting formulas, has specific activity against *Candida* as well as a wide variety of organisms, including *Staphylococcus, Streptococcus,* and *Pseudomonas. Dosage:* One or two capsules two or three times daily, not with food.

Fighting the Flu

Sometime in the fall we start to hear the first predictions of the flu season and the name of the latest viral mutation. By December or January we have the grim flu watch on the news, telling us which state is hardest hit so far, and how it's spreading across the country. All this is accompanied by vivid advertisements for cold and flu remedies, which are now a multibillion dollar enterprise, though many of them are ineffective. Well, we all assume that it has something to do with the cold weather. But it's curious to me that this epidemic coincides with the beginning of America's nonstop feast and holiday season, which starts with Thanksgiving and continues on through New Year's Day, by which time an enormous number of people have been stricken by the flu bug. It's just possible that all of the excess holiday food and drink has taken its toll on the immune system. The sugar, the fat, the alcohol, along with the sleep deprivation from "shopping till you drop"—these are all known to suppress immune function. It's not that the people have caught the bug, but that the bug has caught up with them.

We've already talked about how antibiotics are useless against the flu itself, though they are called for in the less common instances of secondary bacterial infections. But using antibiotics to try to treat the flu is not the only common erroneous practice. There is growing evidence that using aspirin or acetaminophen to reduce a fever during a flu attack may be counterproductive. Fever is one of the body's natural defenses, and driving up body temperature can inhibit reproduction of some viruses and help burn away toxins. Reducing a fever with acetaminophen may actually extend the length of illness. I generally avoid taking fever-reducing drugs when I do get the flu. I let the fever build up to a nice, intense level, perhaps around 102°F. I definitely feel wretched but find that the flu episode is usually pretty short-lived.

Actually, many elderly patients cannot mount a fever successfully. They may be very sick, but with a temperature of perhaps only 99.5°F, whereas younger, robust individuals may run a very high fever and show a very vigorous response to a virus, which they will then expel more quickly. Generally, people who can't mount a fever have longer courses of illness, and people who do mount a fever get rid of an infection relatively quickly. Some caveats: Over 103°F, a fever can become dangerous in an adult and should be reduced. In the elderly or in those with a weak heart, a high fever can put too much demand on the circulatory system and should be kept at a lower level. Children have a much greater tolerance for fever than adults do.

Should You Get the Flu Shot?

Then there's the question of the flu shot. Every autumn we start to hear announcements about when it will be ready and who should take it. Flu vaccines are a relatively new phenomenon, and there are certainly some people who should take them. Diabetics, people who have emphysema or chronic lung disease, and people who are susceptible to pneumonia or other secondary infections should definitely get a shot. Since flu viruses mutate wildly, a new vaccine has to be made up every year to protect against the new dominant strain. Some people do have some side effects from the shot, such as malaise or mild flu symptoms for a day or two. If you do get the vaccine, get it early in the season so it has time to boost your immunity before there's any risk of exposure to the flu.

Some people want the vaccine just to avoid the inconvenience of getting the flu, but I think they are misguided. Having the flu or some other viral infection may actually serve as part of the natural regulation of the immune system. Having a healthy immune system doesn't mean that you never get sick with a virus. When you get a viral infection your body mounts a healthy, normal, immune response, and you get a fever, which adjusts the metabolism and literally burns up toxins. You could think of it as a kind of "boot camp" or training session for the immune system, which will increase your natural resistance.

Health care workers are often encouraged to take the flu vaccine on the theory that they are exposed to a lot of sick people and run a higher risk. I see plenty of sick people, but I've never gotten the shot, and I get the flu about once every three years. For a normally healthy person, I think this is a perfectly normal pattern and probably better for you in the long run.

It's worth remembering that optimal immunity does not mean never getting sick. It means getting sick and responding in a supple fashion, without long, lingering consequences. I think of the immune response as being like an oriental martial art. In judo or tae kwon do or aikido, the object is not to form an impregnable wall against the invader but to respond in a flexible, fluid way to the attack and use the attacker's own force to subdue him. That's really a good way to think about immunity — in terms of suppleness of response, rather than an rigid barrier against diseases.

Simply going ahead and taking to bed when sick is one of our best natural responses. When animals get sick, they have the sense to go off by themselves and curl up in a ball and wait it out. But too often, we humans try to take drugs or symptom-suppressing medications to keep us on the go. We try to short-circuit the natural response to illness in ways that may actually extend the course of disease or weaken our resistance.

I think it's interesting that sitting and reflecting are so discouraged in Western culture that we don't want to do it even when we're sick. In a way, illness can be a kind of forced meditation. It's often the only time when we feel that it's OK to stop and do nothing without feeling guilty. And this is certainly what our body wants us to do — it's the message of viral fatigue.

Chronic Fatigue Syndrome — Beyond the Hype

Ten years ago, if you went to your doctor and said that you were tired all the time and couldn't work, you'd probably get sent to a psychiatrist and get a prescription for an antidepressant. Then some doctors and researchers identified a multisymptom, multisystemic syndrome they called chronic fatigue syndrome, or CFS. Attention really built when a whole group of people working at a hospital in England came down with symptoms. People would suddenly get hit with this, and they'd feel terrible, with low-grade fever, sore throat, sleep disturbances, headaches, muscle aches, and depression. They'd have no energy; they'd be dead in the water. The problem was that no one could find a single causative agent that could be identified in every case of CFS. Many who suffered from this showed evidence of infection with the Epstein-Barr virus, and some with human herpesvirus 6, but not all. And no one could explain a mechanism for the weird mix of symptoms.

Therefore, many people in the medical field simply denied that CFS existed. They said it was depression or some other psychiatric problem. They derided it as "yuppie flu," probably because it was the well-educated, successful victims who had the persistence and self-confidence to insist on getting a clear diagnosis. But now the pendulum is swinging the other way. The Centers for Disease Control and Prevention have established symptomatic criteria for a diagnosis, though there's still no distinctive single marker, like a virus. This puts CFS in the same category where AIDS was before the HIV virus was identified. But there seems little question that CFS is a unique syndrome, distinct from depression. It causes distinct patterns of blood flow disruption in the brain that are different from the patterns associated with clinical depression, and distinct hormonal changes involving the hypothalamus, pituitary, and adrenals.

Doctors have now discovered CFS, but unfortunately it gives them a very convenient category for patients with complex symptoms and for whom they offer no very effective mode of treatment. Nowadays, a doctor may see a patient with complex symptoms and simply give a test for Epstein-Barr virus. This is a complex test with four or five aspects, which will show up with at least partial positive readings for 95 percent of the population. Then, in a compassionate tone they can say, "Your test is back; it is positive for the Epstein-Barr virus. Your complaints are legitimate, you've got a chronic virus that we don't know very much about, and we're looking very hard for a cure. In the meantime, keep resting, take a multivitamin, and good luck."

But I think that often when doctors give that diagnosis they're not doing their homework. They're not looking for issues like food allergies, nutritional deficiencies, overgrowth of intestinal pathogens, chemical toxicity (a common cause of chronic fatigue), and other causes. I've seen Lyme disease misdiagnosed as CFS; some chronic infections with the parasite *Giardia* can also masquerade as CFS. Doctors are not giving the patient enough options for improvement. It's also very common for extreme fatigue to have multiple causes — some environmental, some hormonal, some viral, some nutritional. It's a complex subject, and I've written a whole book on it: *Tired All the Time*. A good diagnosis really has to take multiple factors into account and to be followed by a multipronged approach to treatment.

How does this relate to the immune system? Well, CFS does seem to derange many aspects of immune function — or whatever is causing it does. T cell counts are often abnormal, and there's an increased production of cytokines such as interleukin and interferon (both of which incidentally, have induced the symptoms of CFS when given artificially to patients). So it seems that CFS is at least in part an immune disregulation. The stage may be set by some weakening of the immune system through chemical exposure or poor diet, and then the unknown Agent X (which could be viral, bacterial, parasitic, chemical, psychological, or a combination of factors) comes on the scene and pushes the immune system over the edge into disregulation.

Researchers are now involved in the hunt for a virus, but so far the quarry has been elusive. Viruses seem to proliferate in these patients, but that may be an effect rather than the cause. Epstein-Barr virus may be a marker rather than a trigger, a chronic viral infection perhaps activated because the immune system is less vigilant, but not necessarily the instigator. I can say, having treated many patients with chronic fatigue syndrome, that it's essential to look for multiple causes and offer multiple treatment options, including nutritional treatment that supports immune regulation.

AIDS: Coming to Terms

It is a terrible irony that during our age of unprecedented medical knowledge and technological achievement, one of the worst scourges of human history was raging out of control. That would have been very hard to predict before 1980, when this disease first became known as AIDS. This is one disease that a lot of people encounter in midlife — it's felling a lot of baby boomers. It's one of the principal reasons why many in this generation are prematurely having to face the prospect of mortality, and it's touching people who thought that because of their "safe" lifestyle they were somehow immune. In my practice I've seen several "innocent" middle-class people who unknowingly contracted HIV infection from their spouses, from a fleeting period of sexual experimentation in their lives, or from a casual sampling of IV drugs during college in the seventies. (Of course, this is not to say that people who have contracted this terrible infection by any other pathway, unless they deliberately flouted known prevention measures, are any less innocent victims.)

Though AIDS research has led to a real explosion of knowledge about how the virus attacks the immune system, a remarkable number of questions still remain unanswered. We do know that HIV causes AIDS, but we don't know why some individuals are more resistant to infection in the first place and why other individuals, once infected, show a slower progression to disease.

We also don't know why AIDS seems to stimulate certain parts of the immune system at the same time massive sections of it are being destroyed. We would expect AIDS patients to show fewer allergic reactions as the immune system weakens. Yet, for some reason, AIDS patients become more allergic as they get sicker. This does reinforce our picture of immunity as a complex and multifaceted system of checks and balances, not something like a light switch that we turn on and off.

Another mystery about HIV is how to measure the progress of the disease in a patient. What do we monitor? Do we pay attention to clinical symptoms and infections, or simply count T cells? I have patients with extremely low T cell counts who seem healthy and are doing quite well, and other patients with moderately good T cell counts who are sick and suffering. The question remains, will all patients with HIV infection succumb to the disease? To date, some individuals have been HIV positive for ten years or more and have relatively stable T cell counts, and new drug therapies utilizing protease inhibitors seem to be turning the corner on the epidemic.

Is there a fear of testing? No doubt about it. People have all kinds of avoidance reactions to getting tested for HIV. From my perspective, the time when you should get tested is just as soon as you start thinking about the possibility. If for any reason you have some question or doubt about possible exposure to the virus, get a test. It's easy — don't wait around thinking about it and building up anxiety.

In fact, I have referred patients to psychologists for help in resolving their anxieties about whether to get the test or not. The basic question is, "Do you want to know or do you not want to know, and why are you walking around with this uncertainty?" My advice is to get the test, because it puts an end to all the anxiety and questioning. Besides, anyone who really is HIV positive needs to get to work on adjusting his or her lifestyle, getting medical support, and working things out with loved ones. Some people who are at risk say, "Why should I take the test; it isn't 100 percent accurate anyway." But this is just denial. Of course, there's the occasional very rare false positive, but a system of confirmation is available.

For someone who is HIV positive, it's crucial to seek out a doctor who is experienced with the disease and to participate in some kind of support network. From our experience in dealing with HIV-infected patients, we're learning a lot about the nature and limits of current therapies for the disease. We're learning that with AIDS, as with other chronic and refractory diseases, natural methods have a role to play. High-tech medicine can't provide all the answers. An increasing number of studies are indicating that nutrition, exercise, psychological affirmation, guided imagery, and the like can help with quality of life and avoidance of opportunistic infections. Hopeful new developments suggest that soon AIDS may become a disease that can be stopped in its tracks with the right combination of antiviral agents.

Unneeded Immunity: The Allergic Reaction

It's spring, the flowers are blooming, and you or someone you know is sneezing away — eyes red, nose running — as the pollen wafts through the air. And in August, when the grasses are waving in the open country, it's no better. Millions of Americans suffer from hay fever, a type of immune response that's called an allergic reaction. Hay fever is merely annoying, but other types of allergic reactions, as to poison ivy, can cause extreme pain and discomfort. Some people react to bee stings or shellfish with an intense allergic reaction that can lead to suffocation and death. Others suffer from mysterious chronic symptoms that may be caused by allergies to foods or even to certain kinds of microbes in the gut. We'll deal with food allergies in chapter 9 and respiratory allergies in chapter 13, but any discussion of immunity ought to touch on this strange and seemingly useless phenomenon.

Today, an estimated 20 percent or more of the United States population is allergic to something. Allergies like hay fever and asthma are most common, but many children and some adults are allergic to various foods. The medical costs are not insignificant: asthma alone was responsible for $3.6 billion in direct medical expenses in 1990, the last year for which these figures were available. This represented nearly 1 percent of all health care costs. Even more chilling, 43 percent of asthma cases involved a visit to an emergency room, a hospital stay, or death.

Simply defined, an allergy is an abnormal immune reaction to otherwise harmless living or nonliving matter in the environment. We call the substance that causes an allergic reaction an allergen or an antigen. In the body, whether inhaled, eaten, or absorbed through the skin, the allergen triggers an immune response. The body begins to produce antibodies against the allergen, just as it would against an invading microbe. It's the immune response itself that causes the problem.

The typical antibody that's released in an allergic reaction is a special type called immunoglobulin E, or IgE, which signals other cells of the immune system to release a compound called histamine. Histamine is a normal component of cells, but in the allergic reaction it circulates in high amounts through the bloodstream, where it constricts small muscles around air passages, increases the flow of mucus, and causes blood vessels to leak fluid into tissues. Hay fever brings about a runny nose and fluid in the windpipe, and the resulting coughs and sneezes are an attempt to expel the allergens from the breathing passages. With asthma, constricting muscles in the windpipe can choke off the flow of air. Some allergens, like drugs, chemicals, skin products, and poison ivy, cause a secondary T cell reaction, releasing toxins into the tissues and inducing inflammation.

In extreme cases, an allergic reaction can cause an explosive release of chemicals by the immune system, leading to a sudden drop in blood pressure, shock, reduction of oxygen to the brain and heart, and suffocation as swelling vocal cords cut off air to the lungs.

The IgE antibody found in elevated levels in people with allergies is also produced in response to parasites like intestinal worms. It's theorized that IgE developed as humans evolved in the presence of parasites, since the release of histamines that it causes makes worms themselves go into spasm and become unable to attach to the gut wall. And it's interesting that allergic reactions seem to be on the rise in the industrialized world, where parasites have become less common. We may be plagued by an immune defense that is losing its natural enemy in the environment.

Allergies: Fact and Fancy

We don't often think of allergies as an immune disorder, probably because of the wild variety of symptoms that can be evoked and the range of systems that can be attacked. Researchers disagree widely about how many people really suffer from allergies; the typical caricature of the holistic doctor is someone who finds an allergy lurking behind every symptom. I certainly wouldn't go that far, and I don't test every patient of mine for allergies. Still, normal diagnostic analysis will often suggest a possible allergic component to certain types of symptoms, such as itchy eyes, nasal congestion, frequent colds or bronchitis, itchy skin, hives, or severe gastrointestinal problems. And when people are chronically ill but no one's been able to identify an infectious agent or other clear cause, I do think of a possible allergic component. Other kinds of problems, such as arthritis, can definitely be influenced by allergies, though most people are unaware of this.

I consider possible allergic reactions when I see some kinds of mental symptoms, fatigue, digestive problems, chronic stomach pain or upset, and especially symptoms that wax and wane with changes in diet or location. If you're fine when you go on vacation to the beach but sick at home; or fine at the office during the week but worse at home, this can indicate the presence of allergens in one of these places.

I don't automatically do allergy testing with a new patient, but if I see a symptom that suggests this, I will. It's easy to test for IgE antibody levels, and a high level linked with possibly allergic symptoms is a good marker. If the symptom is refractory, I will try an elimination diet; or perhaps go directly to allergy testing, in which we prick the skin with a panel of common allergens; or do a challenge test with a suspected allergen. I've had many satisfied patients who were very pleased to find out that their seemingly intractable problem could be solved by avoiding an allergen.

I sometimes think that there's a subconscious resistance, rooted in our whole approach to disease and treatment, to the idea that food allergies can cause medical problems. We're conditioned to think that if you're sick, you should *take* something — maybe something expensive or "powerful." It goes against the grain to think that you might get better by *avoiding* something, especially something as everyday and "wholesome" as wheat or milk. Yet, these are two of the most common food allergies. We'll look at food allergies in greater detail in chapter 9.

Treating Allergies

One interesting approach to treating allergies is to directly modulate the immune system, to try to restore it to balance. There are expensive, high-tech, immune-enhancing therapies and simpler nutritional approaches. One therapy proposed for asthma is the use of intravenous gamma globulins, or IgG. This was very naively headlined on one TV program as "a new cure for asthma that has changed the life of many." What the show didn't mention was the cost of the therapy, which could be close to $30,000 per year. With five million kids suffering from allergies and asthma in this country, this type of therapy is clearly not going to solve everyone's problems, but it is an option for severe, life-threatening asthma. You might wonder, "Why give immunoglobulins? I thought the whole problem with allergies was too much of an immune response." Well, that's true. But gamma globulin in a very large intravenous dose (much larger than that used to prevent hepatitis), gives the immune system a potent jolt, and causes a kind of "makeover" of immune response and a lower response to allergens.

We can do the same thing much less expensively by giving immune-boosting vitamins and nutrients to patients with allergies. Vitamin A, vitamin C, vitamin E, zinc, and selenium can help bring the immune system back into balance. In my office I sometimes use an asthma drip, an intravenous "cocktail" of nutrients that are particularly helpful. It contains vitamin C, which acts as a natural antihistamine; pantothenic acid, a B vitamin that supports adrenal function; and magnesium, which is helpful in patients with chemical sensitivities; as well as zinc, selenium, and glutathione — a powerful antioxidant. Magnesium is especially helpful with asthma sufferers. Many people with chemical sensitivities turn out to have magnesium deficiencies. Magnesium also has a relaxing effect on respiratory tissues: the smooth muscles of the bronchial tubes don't go into spasms as much. Documented studies in emergency room medicine suggest that giving magnesium intravenously is as effective as other types of emergency treatments and can sometimes eliminate the need to admit patients to the hospital because their symptoms are reduced.

Another approach to treating allergies is immunotherapy. The idea is to induce a tolerance to an allergy-causing substance by injecting or having the patient ingest small amounts of the allergen, and gradually increasing the dosage. The results vary from person to person, but I've personally observed neutralization of violent allergic reactions to bee stings and food allergies, and I've seen it work with chemical sensitivities as well. Immunotherapy should be performed only by a trained allergist, who can carefully control doses and monitor the immune response.

Autoimmune Disease: Too Much Immunity

The first job of the immune system is to distinguish between "self" and "nonself," and all further immune responses follow from that primal distinction. Immune cells are constantly on the prowl, looking for markers of foreign matter — the antigen — that marks the bacteria, viruses, parasites, and other substances that make their way into the body. There is a built-in tolerance for the body's own cells and tissue; they're passed over untouched. But what if something should go wrong with the primary distinction of self and nonself? This is the failure that leads to autoimmune disease. The perception process goes awry, and the immune cells pick out some bit of the body's own protein, or other living matter, and identify it as foreign — a dangerous intruder. Then the whole arsenal of immune response gets called into play, and the immune system begins to target and destroy some of the body's own cells. The results can be merely painful and annoying, or devastating. In rheumatoid arthritis, the immune system causes painful swelling and stiffness in joints. In multiple sclerosis, the target is the myelin protein that sheaths the nerves, and the result is loss of sensation and paralysis. In lupus, which affects mostly women, the immune system goes to war against multiple organs and organ systems, sometimes in sequence, causing skin rash, hair loss, kidney damage, arthritis, fluid around the heart, and inflamed lungs.

Autoimmune illness should be a special concern of baby boomers for several reasons. First, many autoimmune diseases typically appear in midlife, perhaps linked with the natural decline of immunity with age. Even more significant, autoimmune conditions seem to have become especially rampant in recent generations, especially in the industrialized West. Yet, they were rare or unreported before the 1940s and are still rare in indigenous cultures. Even when corrected for improved diagnostic techniques, the rates of increase for autoimmune syndromes seem to be reflecting new patterns of disease peculiar to life in postindustrial society.[27]

According to current estimates, at least 5 percent of adults in Europe and North America — two-thirds of them women — suffer from an autoimmune disease, many from multiple syndromes. We are also learning that autoimmune disease can complicate many other conditions whose primary cause may have nothing to do with impaired immune function. Chronic hepatitis, for example, involves an autoimmune mechanism, though it's initially caused by a viral infection. There are even indications that rampant autoimmune activity may play a role in arteriosclerosis, which is the number one killer in the United States.

Why the big increase in autoimmune illness? Well, we certainly have to look at environmental factors: the increase in overall pollution levels, the sheer number of new chemical pollutants and products in the environment, the increase in food processing and food additives, the varieties of drugs and medicines. These all present new challenges to our immune system. These are compounded by the growing nutritional deficiencies of our contemporary diet, especially in the antioxidants that trap metabolic waste fragments in the bloodstream, and by a whole constellation of impaired digestive and eliminative functions that open the pathways for foreign antigens to enter the bloodstream.[28]

We might also need to look more closely at the possibility that we trigger autoimmune disease by what we put in the body. Millions of people are walking around today with foreign material in their bodies, implanted in medical procedures. Silicon breast implants were once thought to be inert, but women who have them are sometimes at a higher risk for autoimmune disease. People have plastic and titanium hip replacements, plastic surgery, and dental work that puts foreign matter deep in the tissue, in contact with the bloodstream. Mercury alloy fillings, when tested in animals, have clearly depressed their immunity. And there's some speculation that root canal work that allows chronic tooth infections to persist unnoticed may trigger immune disruption.

Genetic factors and infections apparently play a part in setting off autoimmune disturbances. But recent discoveries have also begun to trace the immense influence of mental and emotional stress on autoimmune syndromes. It's long been observed that stress can worsen autoimmune disease, and fear of a relapse can actually trigger one. We've now learned that stress affects the hypothalamus-pituitary gland axis in the brain, which leads to secretion of hormones that promote inflammation, which in turn causes the release of cytokines, which stimulate immune cells. We've also identified nerves that connect directly to lymph glands (where immune cells are activated) and to immune cells in organs.[29]

We're finding that the complications of impaired immune function cut across every branch of medicine and every system of the body. The list of illnesses that have an autoimmune component is constantly increasing and ranges from hyperthyroidism to ulcerative colitis and even to some forms of baldness. All share the common characteristics of an immune response that attacks the body's own tissue.

What can be done about this growing problem? One answer lies in supporting the immune system at the same deep biochemical level. Let me give an example of one case where this was effective. A young woman came in to my office in a panic because she had just been diagnosed as having lupus. Lupus is a serious autoimmune disease, which often progresses to kidney failure and early death. It's usually treated with powerful corticosteroids. Meg had gone to a doctor after experiencing a variety of symptoms, including a skin rash on her face and some vague joint pains. These are suggestive of lupus, so the doctor had done a simple test for lupus, which came out positive. Meg was terrified, imagining a whole cascade of events that would lead to an early death. So she called me and asked, "Can you do anything about this?"

But I didn't perceive that she had an active form of the disease. The test for lupus does not itself define the disease: There's a whole gradient of illness from slight, nonspecific autoimmune syndrome to full-blown lupus. So I said, "First of all, let's not assume that you have lupus. You have a positive anti–nuclear antibody [ANA] test [a test that defines an autoimmune susceptibility], which does not indicate you have any particular disease. But I suspect you have some kind of mild, early-onset autoimmune problem, not lupus."

I then tested her for food allergy and discovered that she had a variety of them, which were causing a heightened immune response. She eliminated the problem foods, and I advised her on a healthier diet and gave her a protocol of immune-supportive vitamins. I also prescribed fish oil and borage oil, which have a dampening effect on autoimmune disease. For example, they reduce inflammation in rheumatoid arthritis and appear to reduce symptoms of lupus as well. So with her improved diet, the supportive nutrients, and reduced food allergies, we watched as her successive ANA tests got lower and lower, her lupuslike symptoms receded, her skin rash improved, and her joint pain improved. Instead of finding herself on the path of an irreversible progression of disease, Meg found that she could take control over the process if she did the right things. This was a dire prognosis that we prevented from coming to pass.

This is not an isolated case. I see many people in my practice who elude specific diagnosis but may have some of the early features of autoimmune illness, which hasn't yet emerged into a distinct disease. These are people with the joint stiffness and skin rashes that might be characteristic of lupus, or the blanching fingertips that suggest Raynaud's syndrome. But they don't have full-fledged manifestations or full-blown symptoms, and not all the lab tests correlate. I find that this is the stage where a particular kind of physician can often intervene and restore immune balance. Holistic doctors are often the best choice for patients dealing with symptoms that seem to elude diagnosis, or an illness that goes unaltered by conventional therapies.

The Future of Immune Therapy

This is an exciting time for immunologists — so many breakthroughs and discoveries are happening yearly. The whole vision of the field is changing and expanding. We can expect some of these new discoveries to lead to new breakthroughs in high-tech medicine and to new support for the "low-tech" nutritional approach to immune therapy. One area where we should look for real breakthroughs is the treatment and prevention of cancer.

Cancer and the Immune System

One important function of the immune system is to keep the tissues of the body under constant surveillance and to destroy precancerous cells. Cells are constantly dividing and replicating throughout the body, and out of thousands and thousands of cell divisions some few cells are bound to replicate imperfectly. They are mutants, in a sense, and some of them are capable of multiplying uncontrollably and becoming tumors or cancerous cells. Many people harbor these precancerous cells in their body at the time of death, even if they don't die of cancer. Autopsies show that 90 percent of men have cancer cells in their prostate at the time of their death.

The immune system provides a whole array of specialized cells and compounds that can recognize and destroy these accidents of nature. These include natural killer cells, macrophages, and the compounds called gamma interferon and tumor necrosis factor. For most of our lives, our immune defenses scour our blood and tissue for precancerous cells and eradicate them effectively. However, the immune system does decline with age and becomes a little less vigilant, less effective in destroying them. As you might expect, the number of cancers rises with old age. But what's tragic is the high incidence of midlife cancer. Scarcely a baby boomer has not been touched by the tragic story of a classmate who's not there at the class reunion. There are women who die of breast cancer at the age of thirty-six, men who die of colon cancer in their early fifties. This isn't part of the natural course of things.

Under certain conditions, and we've noted them, the immune system can lose its natural vigilance against precancerous cells. Nutritional deficiency, stress, and environmental toxicity can all cause the natural killer cells and other white blood cells to fall asleep on their watch and let some precancerous cells survive for a little too long, until they get out of hand. Weakened immunity also permits viruses to flourish more easily, and there is some evidence that many cancers may be caused by viruses. This is be particularly true of leukemia, a cancerous proliferation of the very white blood cells that are supposed to be protecting the body. We're learning that immune-strengthening measures may be crucial in protecting us against many cancers, especially in midlife.

There are also interesting developments in high-tech methods for boosting the immune attack on cancer. One reason tumors can evade the immune system is that they so closely resemble normal human tissue at the cell surface that they don't provide antigens that will trigger the immune response and serve as targets for killer T cells. But promising experiments isolated small amounts of tumor antigen, grown outside the body, that will evoke an immune response. The idea is to then "vaccinate" the body against tumors by reintroducing enough of the antigen to evoke a strong immune response against the tumor or cancer.[30] Other researchers have experimented with removing natural killer cells or T cells from the body and "educating" them or "souping them up" so that they will react more strongly against cancers, and then reintroducing them to the body. At least one clinical trial has showed promising results against melanoma with this method.[31]

The good news is that the older you are when you develop cancer, past a certain age, the less likely it is to be a rapid, virulent cancer. Breast cancer in postmenopausal women is a less serious disease than in menopausal women, and cancer in very aged patients is usually a slow, indolent disease. So if the whole body, including the immune system, slows down and becomes a little less vital, so do the cancers themselves. This is perhaps the natural counterbalance to the immune decline of age.

A Look to the Future

Immunology is a wide-open field, with great potential for new understandings of disease and new, powerful therapies. In the area of molecular biology, we've learned so much; yet, we still don't understand the precise function of all the immune activities we can observe. But we may soon learn how to orchestrate the immune response and to selectively block or enhance different parts of the immune system in order to help with allergies, autoimmune disease, and organ transplants. Another key area is the mind–body connection: the whole field of psychoneuroimmunology. We're still finding new ways in which the nervous system, the immune system, and the endocrine system interact, and we can expect this knowledge to provide new approaches to modulating immune response. We're also learning more about impact of nutrition on the immune system, and this is offering an important "low-tech" approach to modulating immunity. I expect the next ten years to offer exciting new developments in supporting immune health for the baby boomer.

CHAPTER FIVE

Nerves and Brain:
Memory and the Energy Pathways

Everyone who is growing older is concerned about long-term heart health, arthritis, osteoporosis, and a few other prime risk areas. At the same time, I believe we should be paying more attention to the brain and nervous system. Some 50 million Americans are affected each year by disorders and disabilities involving the brain and nervous system, including mental diseases, inherited and degenerative disease, stroke, epilepsy, addictive disorders, environmental neurotoxins, trauma, and cognitive disorders. Treatment, rehabilitation, and the related costs of these disorders add up to over $300 billion annually.

Fortunately, researchers are beginning to identify genetic factors that affect brain activity and are mapping the parts of the brain that are involved in everyday functions such as sensory perception, movement, reading, and speaking and in dysfunctions such as epileptic seizures. We are now able to look into the brain and figure out what parts are involved in specific kinds of behavior.

A couple of hundred years ago, many people believed in the "science" of phrenology. Two German scientists proposed that you could feel the skull, map its surface, and identify bumps and shapes in different areas that would explain personality types and mental abilities. Phrenologists prepared elaborate charts with grids and diagrams superposed on the cranium to identify mental, emotional, and personality traits. Supposedly, the bumps would tell you whether someone was intelligent or passionate, or had a choleric temper. Of course, there was never any real experimental evidence to support this belief, and phrenology was ultimately condemned as a pseudoscience.

But strangely, we're coming full circle. While there's still no evidence that bumps on the skull can tell us anything about the personality, we are beginning to build a map of the *interior* of the brain and to identify specific areas that are related to memory, the emotions, seeing, hearing, speech, musical and visual activity, and movement. Even such complex and elusive traits as sexual orientation are tentatively being linked to specific structures in the brain—and this is all based on hard laboratory evidence.

Much of the research has come about through new imaging techniques, such as the MRI and the CAT scan, and functional scans such as the SPECT scan that enable us to watch the brain at work. We can ask patients to do arithmetic problems and watch specific parts of their brains literally "light up" with activity. We can also discern that the brains of people with different types of cognitive or emotional problems look different. For example, the brains of people with depression glow with less intensity under the SPECT scan than the brains of nondepressed people. The brains of patients with chronic fatigue syndrome show Swiss cheese–like "activity holes" where typical brain activity seems to have gone dead.

While our tools for monitoring brain activity are becoming ever more sophisticated, we are at the same time suffering from an increasing assault by environmental toxins on all body systems, including the nervous system. In the last hundred years, some sixty thousand new chemicals have been synthesized and released into the environment. There are many indications that the brain and nerves are the organs most sensitive to environmental toxins. Partly for this reason, we are seeing a baffling array of neurological syndromes that defy our attempts to treat them. It's a standard joke among physicians that neurologists are great on diagnosis but terrible on treatment. In fact, a physician who goes into neurology has to be able to deal with a tremendous degree of frustration. Though they can wonderfully characterize the problems of most patients, neurologists can often do very little to fix them. Part of the explanation has to do with the sheer complexity of the nervous system and its intricate interaction with other systems of the body.

Extending the Boundaries of the Nervous System

The old-fashioned, conventional image of the brain is that it's the control center—the central computer of an electrical system that reaches out through the nerves to control the body's functions and receive sensory input. But this model is too simple. Many of the big discoveries of the twentieth century have to do with the chemistry of the brain, with neurotransmitters like dopamine, serotonin, natural opiates, and the like—all of which enable the transmission of impulses between synapses in the brain and nerve cells. Now we're discovering that common chemicals like nitric oxide and carbon monoxide are also neurotransmitters. The brain is not just hard-wired electrical hardware; it's wetware—a chemical soup.

It turns out there is a deep-level interface between the nervous system and the endocrine system, which is responsible for the production of hormones in the body. Some hormones are neurotransmitters themselves. Others are released in response to activities of the brain and act on different organs. Conversely, hormones released by various glands in the body can have a direct impact on brain functions. In fact, we now have to look at certain glands and other organs as almost a kind of extension of the nervous system. New research into the neural system of the stomach, for example, shows that it is laden with neurons and has neurotransmitter activity that rivals that of the brain.

We are also discovering that the immune system interacts at a deep level with the nervous system. For example, we've found that the cells of the immune system have receptors for neurotransmitters, which apparently act directly on other kinds of cells besides nerve cells. In fact, the immune system acts in some ways like a complex sensory organ that feeds signals directly to the hypothalamus and the limbic system of the brain.

Our new understanding of the interface of the nervous system with other parts of the body resonates in an interesting way with the principles of traditional Chinese medicine, which suggest a close exchange between the mental and emotional and the somatic and physiological. For example, traditional Chinese medicine looks at excess anger as arising out of an unbalanced liver function. This allows "liver energy" to rise into the upper reaches of the body, where it is thought to cause eye problems and dry skin as well as emotional imbalance. The Chinese conception of "heart imbalance," to give another example, is associated with insomnia, depression, and feelings of hopelessness. In fact, new studies link hopelessness with a higher risk of heart attack. Now we are finding that depression may really be linked to physiological symptoms through the newly identified neurohormonal pathways defined by sophisticated Western medicine. The Western conceptual split between mind and body is crumbling in the face of new biological discoveries. The Chinese concept is much closer to the mark and may represent an ancient empirical understanding of health that we are just beginning to elucidate scientifically.

Oh, My Aching Head!

Headaches are among the most common causes of disability in the United States, necessitating 50 million doctor visits per year and costing $50 billion in lost productivity. Four billion dollars are expended annually on over-the-counter (OTC) pain relievers alone. Many OTC drugs are only minimally effective and — worse yet — have harmful side effects.

Aspirin and newer nonsteroidal anti-inflammatory drugs (NSAIDs) like ibuprofen and naprosyn carry the risk of gastrointestinal bleeding. Too great a dependence on these pain relievers can result — albeit rarely — in kidney failure. And acetaminophen burdens liver function and depletes the critical antioxidant glutathione.

What is worse than their side effects is that the temporary relief sometimes afforded by pain relievers obscures the discernible and treatable causes of headaches. Rather than palliating pain with drugs, intelligent medicine attempts to trace the origin of symptoms. Pain is seen as a wake-up call to address hitherto unrecognized problems. Since headaches arise from many causes, there is no one therapy that will solve everyone's headache problem.

One of my patients, Arthur, illustrates this. Arthur was a busy CPA with a thriving practice. He had had headaches starting in high school and had controlled them initially with OTC pain remedies. By the time he was forty, though, his headaches had taken a turn for the worse. As tax season neared each year, he began to be crippled by debilitating migraines. He consulted a neurologist, who offered a multidrug approach involving Prozac, antianxiety medications to take the edge off the Prozac, a sleep prescription, anti-inflammatory drugs, additional powerful pain medications to be used as needed, and a self-injection medication for true headache emergencies.

Arthur's headaches had subsided somewhat when he came to see me, but he admitted to experiencing some degree of mild to moderate discomfort every day. On some mornings he'd be tempted to take a pain medication on awakening, especially if he had a busy or challenging day planned.

But worst of all, Arthur was now suffering from fatigue as well as a troubling new symptom: he was having more and more trouble *concentrating*. "I can't crunch numbers the way I used to, doc," Arthur complained. "Sometimes I space out completely . . . it's embarrassing when I'm with clients."

Arthur's was a case of CDH (chronic daily headache). A recent study showed that CDH patients have multiple drug dependencies, and they suffer severe rebound headaches when they withdraw elements of their complex medical regimen. It may be that what were originally mild infrequent headaches are amplified by medication withdrawal. The body "asks" to be restored to its medicated state by manufacturing headache symptoms. This condition can begin to develop very innocently; for instance, someone discovers he has a headache if he doesn't drink a few cups of coffee every day, and gradually he adds a few acetaminophen tablets to his regimen. By the time he gets to Arthur's stage, the case is very difficult to unravel, since not much relief will be obtained at first until drugs are skillfully withdrawn and natural therapies substituted.

"Arthur," I said, "think of yourself as a house of cards. You've jerry-rigged yourself into this position by years of tinkering with ever more powerful drugs. When we reach in and try to eliminate even just one medication, the whole house of cards threatens to fall. So expect some withdrawal symptoms as we gradually detoxify you. We'll support you with proper nutrients and some natural therapy, but I'll tell you right now, it won't always be a picnic."

"But Dr. Hoffman," Arthur countered, "I'm a busy professional! I can't afford to be anything less than 100 percent! That's why I sometimes take my medication *before* I go into work."

"Yes, Arthur," I replied. "But as it is, you're already underperforming. How high do you think we can build that house of cards before it collapses?"

Frequently, patients with headaches — even intelligent, health-conscious ones — delay the inevitable day of reckoning with withdrawal symptoms by claiming that they must be at their peak at all times and that they can't take a chance on underperforming brought on by symptom recurrence. I explain that this is part of the "headache personality" — perfectionist, hard-driving, tending to internalize stress and censor emotions. Fundamentally, delaying detoxification until some perfect future date that never materializes is classic addictive behavior: "I'll quit, eventually, but I can't just now."

Arthur finally decided to take the plunge. "I know I'll have to sooner or later, and it won't get any easier if I keep putting this off." He scheduled a few weeks after tax season to kick things off.

I had already tested Arthur, finding him critically low in magnesium, a mineral essential to control of muscle spasm. Headache researchers have discovered that many migraineurs are low in magnesium and that magnesium injections help to gradually restore a normal mineral status, reducing instability of the smooth muscles that govern the caliber of blood vessels in the scalp. Additionally, while Arthur's conventional blood tests never showed abnormalities, a test designed to evaluate his liver's detoxification abilities showed poor scores. Burdened by years of processing drugs, his liver's efficiency was impaired, leading to symptoms of fatigue and brain fog.

So, to help Arthur with the initial phases of the program to eliminate his medication dependency, I prescribed a special detoxification diet with supplements designed to support his liver function. Our staff administered magnesium injections and acupuncture to lessen his pain. I also gave Arthur feverfew, a natural herbal treatment for headaches, which has been shown to reduce the number and intensity of severe and incapacitating headaches when taken prophylactically. The dose used in studies was two 25-milligram capsules of freeze-dried pulverized leaf daily. Natural supplements of valerian, kava, and hops, 170 milligrams each in the evening, helped Arthur adjust to going without sleep drugs or antianxiety medicine. We also used vitamin E and the essential fatty acids from borage oil as natural prostaglandin blockers, gently mimicking the anti-inflammatory action of NSAIDs.

After two weeks on this program, Arthur returned. "How are you doing?" I asked expectantly. "Well, pretty rocky at first," Arthur replied. "Those first few days I felt so bad, I was glad I took some time off from work. It wasn't so much the headaches—the acupuncture helped make them tolerable. It was the body aches and total exhaustion—it felt like I'd played tackle football while having the flu." I reassured Arthur that these sensations were frequent accompaniments of the initial phase of withdrawal. I asked how he was coming along now. "Well," replied Arthur, "I still feel a little weak, and occasionally that dull headache comes back, but for the first time in years, I feel *clear* again—I can think clearly."

Arthur recovered completely from his chronic daily headaches. He now uses biofeedback to better control the stress that originally prompted his headaches when they began during high school. He has not taken *any* medication for headaches in over a year, and he maintains a healthy natural foods diet with proper nutrient supplements, especially magnesium. Tests now show that his magnesium level and liver detoxification ability have returned to normal.

Of course, Arthur's story isn't everybody's, though it does represent a common pattern of overmedication and magnesium deficiency. Other underlying conditions that can contribute to headache include chronic sinus inflammation caused by allergies to food, dust, mold, and pollen; TMJ (temporomandibular joint) dysfunction, neck muscle tension, and spinal misalignment; unsuspected chronic dental infections; eye and neck strain from maladaptive posture during repetitive close work; sensitivities to perfumes, household cleaners, and natural gas; chronic hormonal imbalances, as in premenstrual migraine; and chronic *Candida* overgrowth in the gastrointestinal tract. All these factors can conspire to make someone headache prone. The best way to handle a headache problem may be to consult a nutritionally oriented physician who will have a sense of the range of possibilities. Since the causes of headaches are diverse, the methods for addressing them sometimes need to be multipronged in order to succeed. But the results are far more gratifying than with conventional approaches that rely on drugs as the first line of therapy.

INTELLIGENT MEDICINE TIP:

A good general magnesium supplement level would be 200 milligrams twice daily of magnesium citrate, though diarrhea is a possible side effect.

Panic Attacks and Anxiety Disorders

Marjorie, forty-two, suddenly felt "spacy" with tingling in her fingers, a crushing chest pain, and a sense of imminent death. She cried out to her husband, "Will, I can't breathe—I'm dying." Seeing that in fact she was unable to take in a full breath, Will rushed her to the emergency room of a nearby hospital. It certainly looked like a heart attack, but after examining Marjorie and performing an electrocardiogram, the physician told Will, "Nothing is wrong. The electrocardiogram is normal. This is an anxiety attack." Will and Marjorie couldn't quite accept this. She hadn't been feeling particularly anxious about anything, and the physiological symptoms had been overwhelming and terrifying. Yet, the doctor was trying to tell them that Marjorie's nervous system was out of kilter. For some reason, she had experienced a sudden neurological meltdown.

The kind of panic attack that Marjorie experienced seems to be fairly epidemic. Anxiety disorder is a modern phenomenon, and it may be related to the tremendous jarring stress of modern life and perhaps to some of our common but powerful dietary stresses, such as excess sugar and excess caffeine, which are often combined, as in cola beverages. Sugar and caffeine can't by themselves set off a panic attack, but what they may do is destabilize brain activity so that anxiety ultimately reaches meltdown proportions. I also suspect that the epidemic of panic attacks has a lot to do with our upbringing. Some people feel themselves under enormous pressures to achieve, and some parents load their children with heavy conditioning through punishments and negative incentives, overprogramming the control functions so that these people ultimately break down.

Marjorie's case was typical of panic attack in that she did not perceive her experience as panic or anxiety. No one goes to the doctor or the hospital and says, "I suddenly felt very scared." People do feel scared, but they experience this is a result of the symptoms, not the cause. A typical panic attack often involves strong sensations of chest pain and pressure, or heart palpitations, which leads people to think they're having a heart attack. Panic attack can take other forms: inability to concentrate, spaciness, a feeling of levitating, tingling in the hands, shortness of breath. A lot of patients come in and tell me, "Doctor, I can't catch my breath; I just can't take in a complete breath." I have to ask myself, is there a respiratory disease, is it asthma? Often I do a pulmonary function test, or use a peak flow meter, and find out that the person is actually breathing normally. Other patients tell me, "Doctor, I can't concentrate, I feel spacy all the time. Am I sick with something? Do I have mono?" They may complain of gastrointestinal symptoms, such as stomach pains, cramps, or diarrhea. I look for viruses, parasites, food allergies or intolerances, *Candida* infection, or peptic ulcers. If someone has chest pains or palpitations, I of course do an electrocardiogram. But the tests often come up negative, without a clear cause in the affected organ, so I have to rule out these physical causes. This leaves a diagnosis of acute anxiety.

I really go the limit to find causes in the organs, because all too often doctors ascribe vague symptoms to anxiety, which is often the byproduct of a real physical problem. On the other hand, a lot of young to middle-aged people are walking around with powerful anxiety disorders that often translate to physical sensations. This may be a sign of the times, an indicator of the increased environmental and behavioral assault on our nervous systems. This is a distinct modern syndrome, which is real and pervasive. Even for those who haven't experienced them, the prevalence of panic attacks should remind us not to take the health of the nervous system for granted.

People often resist or deny a diagnosis of panic attack. Some people cling to their physical symptoms, convinced that they are pointing to a heart problem or something similar. They have trouble believing that it's actually the nervous system that is causing the symptoms. They may feel that there's a stigma attached to the diagnosis of panic attack, as there often is to mental illness — that it's somehow humiliating or implies cowardice, moral failure, or weakness of character. They're afraid I'm telling them that it's all in their mind.

But it's not really like mental illness or delusion — it's as if your whole body were being jolted with electricity, with nervous impulses gone out of control in a kind of short circuit or feedback loop. It's like an involuntary discharge of the autonomic nervous system — a strictly physiological response that is not subject to your mental control or caused by your thinking process. In fact, people sometimes say that they were feeling very calm before an attack, or not thinking about anything particularly stressful or emotionally jarring. Sometimes they protest that it can't be "nerves" because they weren't really under stress that day. But it doesn't necessarily take a stressful incident to set off a panic attack. Rather, stress to the nervous system builds up gradually, over a long time, and finally reaches a limit and spills over in a sudden overload. A similar thing can happen in some people with heart problems — a nerve network in the heart muscle can suddenly start to generate amplified signals, in a kind of neurological feedback loop. This can go haywire and cause fibrillation: the heart stops beating rhythmically and just vibrates. Panic attack is a true physiological syndrome, which people should accept and take constructive steps to correct.

In fact, there are some indications that certain congenital conditions may predispose some people to having panic attacks. For example, some people have a fairly common congenital heart condition called mitral valve prolapse. This is a congenital anomaly in a heart valve that causes a heart murmur and sometimes causes palpitations that can trigger panic attack. These people's nervous systems may simply be wired in a more "hair-trigger" fashion, predisposing them to a whole array of physiological syndromes, including panic attacks, weird chest sensations, palpitations, irritable bowel syndrome, migraines, and others.

Treating Panic Syndrome

As panic syndrome has become more frequently diagnosed, the number of specialized hospital clinics and support groups devoted to the problem has grown. They publish informational brochures and propose conventional treatment protocols that include drug therapy and counseling. The first line of treatment may be the use of a tranquilizer just to reduce the immediate overactive nervous response so that more long-term therapy can begin. Antidepressants may be used if the physician believes that the anxiety may have its root in depression.

Unfortunately, some of the drugs used to treat anxiety have an addictive component, and this is one of the risks of conventional treatment. If judiciously used, these medications can be very helpful, but all too frequently doctors have overprescribed them to the point of inducing dependency or true addiction. The most popular antianxiety drugs—Xanax, Valium, Klonopin, and Ativan—all have addiction potential. It's not uncommon for patients to start taking them, find that their anxiety symptoms are reduced, and try to taper off only to find that the anxiety comes back. And Prozac, an effective antidepressant, actually leads to a slightly stimulated or hyped-up condition, sometimes causing sleeplessness or anxiety. Then antianxiety drugs are often prescribed to "take the edge off," setting up the patient for multiple-drug dependency. So in the long run, we really need to develop a nonpharmacological approach.

Since drug therapy is generally only a stopgap, we have to look at cognitive and behavior strategies and especially nutritional strategies. I do recommend some kind of behavioral practice, whether it's yoga, t'ai chi, meditation, or Dr. Herbert Benson's "relaxation response." In my own practice, I've found nutritional therapy an important aspect of treatment. This includes limiting the intake of sugar, alcohol, caffeine, and sometimes drugs and also providing the necessary vitamins and nutrients that may be undersupplied in the diet.

To treat panic syndrome, I first get my patients to cut out coffee, tea, and cola drinks and start a stress reduction program. I do a glucose tolerance test to check blood sugar levels and how they vary in response to eating. I sometimes measure blood levels of adrenaline. Sometimes there is a tremendous outpouring of adrenaline, precisely when blood sugar levels bottom out, and this is when patients have the symptoms of panic attack. It's normal for the body to release stimulating hormones like adrenaline when blood sugar is low—this prevents fainting and a dangerous drop in blood pressure.

Panic syndrome is especially common in people who have used cocaine or other stimulants. The jarring nature of the cocaine high seems to destabilize the nervous system and set the stage for neurological reverberations that continue even after withdrawal from the drug. But even milder stimulants can throw off the neurological balance in some individuals, especially with long-term use. The relationship is not one of simple cause and effect—you don't have a cup of coffee and become enraged or go into panic. But these stimulants can put the nervous system into a constant keyed-up state of alert. You can feel fine and enjoy being alert and active, but over weeks or months of steady use you can suddenly reach a threshold where continued use or an outside stimulus can make it all spill over and shift you into having psychological or neurological symptoms. And you wouldn't necessarily connect the symptoms with coffee because you've been drinking it for months or years.

Alan, one of my patients who taught in a university sociology department, told me he had gotten into a habit of drinking tea from a thermos throughout the long hours of his workday, which involved a long commute by car, teaching several classes, planning budgets, going to meetings, and advising students on special projects. One fall semester, he found himself getting into frequent hysterical rages over next to nothing—at other drivers on the highway and his wife, students and colleagues. Afterward, he'd be left shaking, hyped up, and easily set off again by another petty annoyance or frustration. He was very disturbed by this but thought it was due to his long hours and stresses at work. At about the same time, he started having chronic stomach pains. Fearing an ulcer, he stopped drinking tea and cut out all caffeine from his diet. He was amazed to discover that his mood changed completely—no more rages, no more constant impatience, no more hysterical responses. After a month or two of cold turkey, he found he could permit himself two to three cups of coffee or tea a day without serious side effects. But everyone's individual response is different. Some find that even a single cup a day winds them up too tight.

Nutrition therapy can also play an important role in treating panic disorder. Thiamine (vitamin B_1) and magnesium are especially useful. (See the section on nutrition at the end of this chapter.)

Treating Hyperventilation Syndrome

Hyperventilation syndrome—breathing in increasingly rapid, shallow breaths—is a pervasive medical problem, and many people throughout the population suffer from this bad breathing habit. It is also a common component of panic attacks. People who hyperventilate can get into a real state of panic, with the sensation that they just can't draw a deep breath and can't get enough oxygen.

When you hyperventilate, you feel short of breath. Ironically, the more you hyperventilate, the more short of breath you become. If you are hyperventilating, you feel that you must be short of oxygen, and logically you want to breath more, so you start to pant. What happens? You increase your production of stress hormones, and you also blow off carbon dioxide at an increased rate. When you blow off carbon dioxide, your blood becomes more alkaline—a condition called alkalosis, which creates symptoms such as tingling and numbness of the fingers, and makes you crave oxygen even more.

Hyperventilation also promotes magnesium deficiency, since this is an alkaline mineral that is excreted to compensate for the excess alkalinity in the blood. Magnesium supplements sometimes help relieve the symptoms.

The first line of treatment, however, is behavioral. Paradoxically, the way to break the hyperventilation cycle is to build up more carbon dioxide in the bloodstream. You can do this in a few minutes by breathing into a paper bag. Another way is to consciously breath with a slow outbreathing cycle: give yourself time to let your lungs empty after each inbreath.

Hyperventilators tend to breathe too quickly, up to fifteen or twenty times per minute, even when they are not having a full-fledged attack. A normal resting respiration rate is eight to twelve breaths per minute. This means that a complete cycle of inhalation and exhalation should last five to eight seconds. The meditation practice of counting while inhaling and exhaling is an excellent way of establishing a normal breathing rate.

One thing you can do to block hyperventilation is to follow a singing teacher's advice and breath from the abdomen and not from the chest. Breathing from the abdomen tends to trigger the relaxation response. No matter what you are feeling, you can mechanically make yourself relax just by breathing properly.

To make sure you are doing this, lie on your back, put one hand on your chest and the other on your stomach, and breathe so that you are moving the hand on your stomach and not the one on your chest. You can accentuate the effect by counting slowly as you breath in, feeling the pause between breaths, and counting slowly as you breath out.

Free-style swimming is an excellent exercise for breath control. To breath properly while swimming, you turn your head out of the water to quickly gulp a new supply of air, and then s-l-o-w-l-y exhale with your head face down in the water as you take the next stroke or two.

Other forms of gentle stretching exercise like yoga, which involves breath control, can be extremely valuable. In Hindu tradition and in yogic practice, the breath is the gateway to mind control. There are various types of breathing exercises, some simple and some elaborate, which are designed to produce a meditative state.

Growing Older and Memory

Isabel, a choreographer in her mid-forties, came into my office and said, "I don't know if something is happening to me. I can't remember the name of this step when I'm teaching; I use it all the time, but I start to say it in class and it just doesn't come. And yesterday in class I kept saying 'left' when I meant 'right.' Is something happening to my brain?" Well, Isabel was just tired and stressed that week, and the following week she had no trouble with names or directions in any of her classes. But many of us wonder sometimes, when we can't recall a name that is totally familiar to us, whether something is wrong with us. These worries take on a little more weight as we grow older, because we do know that there's some degree of memory loss with aging. Many have had the disturbing experience of talking to an aged, ill person who seems to have forgotten big chunks of what happened that morning, or even the names or faces of family members.

There is definitely a natural decline in short-term memory and learning ability with age, and it seems to be a slow, progressive decline. It has even earned a medical acronym: ARMI, for age-related memory impairment. There are also physiological changes in the nervous system with age — some of the neurons in the brain die off. On the other hand, studies suggest that older people may actually be able to improve in some areas of intelligence and mental ability, such as the ability to verbalize complex ideas, and global comprehension — the ability to synthesize meaning from a lot of data. Another word for this might be wisdom.

Human intelligence may adapt naturally to the accumulation of memories and experience. As data accumulate, the brain learns to make leaps or bridges to find the common ground, the means of integrating experience, so that we aren't simply submerged in the endless details of life. So maybe it's a mistake to talk about a decline in memory and intelligence with age, when what really happens is a qualitative change. It may be more difficult to go to law school or medical school and memorize a lot of minutiae at the age of fifty than at the age of twenty. On the other hand, it's no accident that world leaders and business executives in their fifties and sixties and seventies are able to make major decisions about complex issues and balance huge agendas every day. Clearly, they're not suffering from mental decline. And many artists from Pablo Picasso to Martha Graham to Henri Matisse have seemed to lose little of their creativity with age. Though neurons can deteriorate as the brain ages, intelligence and alertness can be compatible with very advanced age.

In fact, recent studies have shown that a global decline in mental function with age is not at all inevitable. About 25 percent of people in their eighties who volunteer for cognitive testing perform just as well as volunteers in their thirties and forties. So the moral is, for the brain as for the rest of the body, use it or lose it!

There are also nutritional aspects to brain function in older people. Vitamin B_{12} plays an especially important role. Many cases of Alzheimer's disease and senile dementia share a component of undiagnosed or borderline deficiency of vitamin B_{12} — a kind of selective malnutrition. I have given vitamin B_{12} supplements, or even injections, to some elderly patients and seen a sharp increase in general alertness and mental responsiveness.

Beyond stimulation and nutrition, there are unfortunately some pathological processes that affect memory. The two major ones are cerebrovascular disease and Alzheimer's disease, and many people are afflicted with several degenerative processes. Cerebrovascular disease, which affects the circulation of blood in the brain, can cause a progressive decline in memory. At the same time, someone who has changes in personality, memory, and understanding at an advanced age may be suffering from the degenerative features of both cerebrovascular disease and Alzheimer's. We do know quite a bit about cerebrovascular disease and how to prevent it, so let's look at that first.

Starving the Brain: Cerebrovascular Disease

The brain requires 20 percent of the body's oxygen and is extremely sensitive to a deficient blood supply. In fact, there is some speculation that most age-related senility may be linked to decreased blood flow in the brain rather than to degeneration of the tissues and nerves. Some striking research to support this has been done with a natural extract from leaves of the *Ginkgo biloba* tree, which increases blood flow in the brain and actually improves memory and attention in elderly patients as well as short-term memory in younger volunteers. Maintaining a healthy supply of blood to the brain is essential to normal mental function and may help prevent what we think of as age-related memory loss.

When blood flow to the brain is sharply reduced, usually through gradual degeneration of the blood vessels, some form of cerebrovascular disease is present. In fact, this is really an atherosclerosis of the brain, with hardening and narrowing of arteries caused by the buildup of fatty cholesterol deposits. The result of severe cerebrovascular disease is often a major blood-supply failure: a stroke. There are two types of stroke: those caused by a blood clot in narrowed arteries, which cuts off blood to portions of the brain, and those caused by rupture of a blood vessel and the hemorrhaging of blood into brain tissue, often called apoplexy or cerebral hemorrhage. Both kinds of stroke can "black out" major portions of the brain, such as speech centers and movement centers. They can cause partial paralysis, partial blindness, dizziness, slurred speech, mental confusion, and personality changes. The symptoms may strike immediately or worsen more slowly over hours or days. Sometimes persistent long-term therapy can lead to complete or partial recovery, but often the damage is permanent.

Not everyone who suffers from cerebrovascular disease will have a stroke, but many will have TIAs — transient ischemic attacks — which are short, passing ministrokes caused by temporary constriction of blood flow. They can cause temporary blackouts, dizziness, numbness, or slurring of speech. Real damage may be done, but not in such a dramatic way that you'd think to rush someone to a hospital. Many others will not experience even these symptoms, but with progressive reduction in blood flow to the brain will suffer a decline in thinking ability, balance, memory, emotional stability, sleep patterns, or any other functions regulated by the brain.

GINKGO — A SURVIVOR AND HEALER

Ginkgo biloba is the oldest living species of tree, nicknamed the "living fossil" by Darwin because this 200-million-year-old-tree survived the Ice Age. Its complex and unique chemistry has given it remarkable resistance to pests and disease as well as a storehouse of active nutrients. The green leaves were first used by the Chinese in 2800 B.C. to improve brain function and treat other ailments such as bronchitis, asthma, and cough, as well as certain parasites.

Ginkgo biloba has been well studied in Europe and is the best-selling natural product there. The plant extracts are used to treat heart disease, circulatory problems, asthma, bronchitis, senility (including loss of memory and attention), vision problems in the elderly, and accidents involving brain trauma. Ginkgo has helped patients suffering from Raynaud's disease, in which the hands and feet become painfully cold and white because of reduced circulation. Studies show that the plant contains not only bioflavonoids and beneficial acids but also chemicals unique to the ginkgo plant, called ginkgolides. It has marked effects on the central nervous system in humans.

Ginkgo biloba can help restore cerebral blood flow after a blockage, and one German study showed that *Ginkgo biloba* given to patients with chronic cerebrovascular disease reduced major symptoms, including vertigo, headache, ringing in the ears, and loss of short-term memory. Ginkgo not only increases blood flow in the brain but increases oxygen and glucose consumption and the rate of neuron activity. Studies in both healthy younger women and older people have demonstrated that *ginkgo* can produce improvements in memory and mental performance.[1] American researchers are beginning to take an interest in *Ginkgo biloba* and have conducted several studies that show improvements in memory and attention in elderly patients, and short-term memory improvements in healthy younger people. In European research, 120-milligram tablets of 24 percent standardized extract are given two or three times a day for three to six months minimum. Side effects are rare, but do include occasional stomach upset and, more rarely, headache or dizziness.

If we use sophisticated CAT scans or MRI to look at the brain of someone suffering from cerebrovascular disease, we may see little gaps or holes — a "Swiss cheese" look that neurologists call an *état lacunaire* (literally, the "condition of lacunae"). What we see are all the tiny portions of the brain that have simply died because of impaired circulation or ministrokes. The holes or lacunae represent dead tissue, and this kind of damage certainly affects brain function.

The good news is that the ongoing degenerative process of cerebrovascular disease can be prevented, and possibly even arrested once it's begun. Let's look at some of the risk factors.

Risk Factors for Cerebrovascular Disease

The effects of cerebrovascular disease usually don't show up until advanced age, but the stage is set much earlier. The risk factors are primarily the same as those for heart disease: a high-fat diet, smoking, poorly controlled blood pressure, and insufficient nutrients, especially antioxidants. In fact, we are now seeing cerebrovascular disease symptoms in younger people in their forties or fifties who smoke, are alcoholic, or have hypertension. It's interesting that the incidence of heart disease in Japan is very low because of a low-fat diet. But the incidence of strokes there is quite high, because the Japanese diet has a high level of salt, which causes high blood pressure and strokes. And frankly, cerebrovascular disease is also a disease of poverty. Many socioeconomically disadvantaged groups suffer from poor medical care and poor treatment for hypertension, eat poor-quality fast food or processed food that's laden with sodium or fat, and are more susceptible to alcohol and smoking problems because of life pressures and stresses. They can wind up on a fast track to cerebrovascular disease.

High blood pressure has been shown to lead to mental decline and may accelerate the pace of cerebrovascular disease. Studies have shown that people with chronic high blood pressure, especially over a period of years, have the greatest decline in mental tasks that involve short-term memory. In fact, the studies show a direct correlation between specific, measured rates of increase of blood pressure and scores on memory tests. There is some evidence that high blood pressure may reduce the oxygen supply to the brain, and increase tissue damage in the tiny arteries of the brain.[2]

Alcohol consumption is only a moderate risk factor for heart disease and can even have a protective effect at low levels. However, it seriously increases the risk of strokes and cerebrovascular disease, even at fairly low levels. Anything more than two drinks daily for men, and two or three weekly for women, is associated with higher risk of stroke.

Diagnosing Cerebrovascular Disease: Conventional Treatment

Since the damage from cerebrovascular disease builds up very slowly, the damage has already been done by the time someone has symptoms or a recognizable pattern on a CAT scan. However, some new tests can offer an early warning. The Doppler test does an ultrasound scan of the carotid artery, the biggest blood vessel that supplies the brain. If it shows signs of constriction, and the fatty deposits and hardening of artery walls we call atherosclerosis, it's a fair bet that there's pervasive atherosclerosis throughout the cerebral vascular system. A newer technology called MRA, magnetic resonance angiography, will enable us to visualize the soft tissue of the arteries and the flow characteristics of blood. This can directly reveal atherosclerosis in cerebral blood vessels.

As with cardiovascular disease, current treatments attempt to bypass portions of the diseased carotid artery or use the balloon angioplasty technique to loosen and expand a hardened artery. These are fairly risky procedures and can sometimes cause a stroke themselves. In fact, the guidelines for performing this type of surgery were recently made more stringent because the potential benefits were thought to not justify the risk. Worse, "fixing" the carotid artery does not help hardened and clogged arteries within the brain itself.

As for medication, there's some evidence that taking an aspirin a day can help prevent stroke as well as heart disease. A whole new generation of drugs, of the calcium channel blocker family, selectively dilate blood vessels in the brain but are not very satisfactory on the whole. Then there are various blood thinners, but they can be problematic; anything that thins the blood and therefore promotes bleeding may cause hemorrhagic or "bleeding" stroke.

Since none of the high-tech approaches for treating stroke or cerebrovascular disease are very safe or effective, this is one more case where we're led straight back to prevention as the best "treatment." Fortunately, this disease process can be prevented or arrested in most individuals if they start early enough. And the best way to start is by following the protocol for preventing heart disease, including a low-fat, low-sugar, low-sodium diet; regular exercise; avoidance of smoking and excess alcohol intake; and sufficient heart-healthy nutrients. See chapter 12 on the cardiovascular system for the complete protocol, and the section at the end of this chapter for more nutritional aids.

Alzheimer's Disease

We've all had the experience of forgetting the name of someone we met at a party, or where we put the car keys, or even where we parked the car. But Alzheimer's disease causes memory loss of a different order: forgetting a spouse's name, or what the car keys are *for*, or how to get home once you've found your car in the supermarket parking lot.

Alzheimer's begins with a subtle loss of initiative and energy, which is followed by forgetfulness and loss first of short-term, then of long-term memory. In later stages, the Alzheimer's patient becomes confused and disoriented and may wander and get lost if not confined. In advanced Alzheimer's, patients are really unable to care for themselves and require twenty-four-hour supervision. Unfortunately, we know much less about Alzheimer's right now than about AIDS — we don't know enough about risk factors, preventive factors, or effective treatments. The disease causes a great deal of suffering and high costs for patient care. While relatively rare when first described in 1906, Alzheimer's disease now affects about 10 percent of the United States population over the age of sixty-five and 20 percent of those over seventy-five, or about four million victims in all. More than half of all Americans in nursing homes are suffering from Alzheimer's, at tremendous cost to families and insurers.

Alzheimer's disease is not an extension of the normal decline with aging, though it can coexist with other forms of mental confusion or senility. It tends to strike people in their fifties and sixties, when we wouldn't expect severe memory problems, and is an actual degenerative disease of the brain, not part of any normal process of decline. Doctors call it presenile dementia because it can set in long before the age when senility might be expected. Alzheimer's disease is not always easy to diagnose, especially if there are other potential causes of mental impairment that could affect memory tests and word tests. The newest approach is to use PET (positive emission tomography) scanning of the brain to observe characteristic patterns of glucose metabolism, which can confirm a diagnosis with physical results.

Frankly, we don't know much about the causes of Alzheimer's disease. There may be a genetic predisposition, which may be triggered by environmental factors. Some types of Alzheimer's, but not all, seem to run in the family. Aluminum poisoning has been studied as a possible cause, since aluminum-containing plaques are found in the brains of Alzheimer's patients, but that now seems too simplistic an explanation. There is evidence of a type of aluminum-induced dementia that can strike workers in an aluminum smelting plant, or kidney dialysis patients because the dialysate solution that cleans the blood contains a lot of aluminum. So although aluminum poisoning can damage the brain, that doesn't seem to be the necessary single cause of Alzheimer's. High aluminum intake may be a cofactor for some or all Alzheimer's patients, but it's not a simple matter of coming down with Alzheimer's disease because you cook with aluminum pots and pans.

The typical senile plaques in the brains of Alzheimer's patients also contain a protein called amyloid, and some have suggested that Alzheimer's patients may not be able to properly metabolize or break down this protein.

Researchers are also looking at viral or bacterial infection, endocrine system failure, and cardiovascular problems as possible causes. One group of researchers has found that brain tissue can produce specialized immune proteins called complement and is investigating the possibility that an immune reaction gone awry may cause the brain damage in Alzheimer's patients. Nutritional deficiencies of antioxidants may play a role. To complicate matters, people with a certain type of blood protein called apo-E4 have a higher risk of getting Alzheimer's disease. (This is one of the apolipoproteins associated with the body's production of cholesterol particles.) Actually, one apolipoprotein-E variation is associated with increased risk for disease, and another variant is associated with reduced risk. However, the test for apo-E4 identifies only a minority of people with the predisposition and is not very reliable. This has raised a knotty ethical question: whether the patient should be told, at a time when we have no effective means of preventing or treating the disease.

At the time of this writing, the search for a cause is still on. In fact, we may not be able to trace Alzheimer's disease to one single cause. It may resemble a disease like arthritis, of an autoimmune character, where brain cells are the target. In fact, a preliminary study suggests that the drug ibuprofen, an over-the-counter anti-inflammatory, may slow progression of Alzheimer's. Like arthritis, too, it may have multiple distinct causes. A group of people may all have swollen, painful, arthritic joints, but one has the version caused by Lyme disease, one has the autoimmune syndrome rheumatoid arthritis, one has osteoarthritis, and a retired athlete has arthritis caused by excess wear and tear to the joints. Further, Alzheimer's disease progression may be slowed by estrogen replacement therapy, so we are often looking at a mixed disease syndrome.

Researchers are investigating several treatments for Alzheimer's disease; some look promising, while others haven't lived up to their original claims. The drug tacrine was recently hailed as a marvelous new remedy for Alzheimer's. It works by increasing the brain levels of acetylcholine, an important neurotransmitter that is depleted in Alzheimer's patients. Tacrine has been used for some time in England but has serious drawbacks. It helps slow the course of the disease, but not dramatically, and a dose high enough to slow Alzheimer's disease puts patients at a very high risk of liver damage. So it's a very imperfect drug. A new tacrinelike drug called Aricept promises to deliver the improvements without certain of the side effects. Lecithin and lecithin derivatives have also been touted for the treatment of Alzheimer's because they too increase acetylcholine levels.

Some studies have shown that removing heavy metals from the bloodstream through a procedure called chelation can help Alzheimer's patients. (For more on chelation, see chapter 12, page 323.) In particular, the use of desferoxamine, a chelator of aluminum and iron, has been shown in some studies to retard the progression of Alzheimer's disease. The implication is that the high level of industrial metals in our environment may be a cofactor for Alzheimer's disease. I do offer chelation therapy for patients with Alzheimer's disease and have seen some improvement in mental function, especially in patients who also have circulatory problems.

Some of the most promising treatments for Alzheimer's disease involve nutritional therapies, including treatment of thiamine deficiencies, and the use of acetyl-L-carnitine, a special form of the energy nutrient L-carnitine that easily traverses the blood-brain barrier, fueling neuronal activity. See the section at the end of this chapter for more on the nutritional aids. *Ginkgo biloba* extract has also been shown to improve mental function in some cases.

Dozens of other possible treatments are under investigation. One study, by a group of researchers led by Dr. Victor Henderson of the University of Southern California at Los Angeles, has suggested that estrogen may protect women against Alzheimer's. The researchers found that postmenopausal women who were given estrogen replacement therapy were less likely to get Alzheimer's than those who didn't, and their symptoms were not as severe. There's even some evidence that the "use it or lose it" approach to brain function in general may apply to Alzheimer's as well. Researchers at the University of Kentucky Chandler Medical Center studied a population of 678 elderly nuns and found that the most highly educated and intellectually active nuns not only lived longer and maintained brain function longer but seemed less likely to develop Alzheimer's.

Though we don't yet have an effective treatment, the good news is that some drugs and nutritional therapies have some effect, and we're starting to understand the neurochemistry. At some point, we may also be able to identify the gene for Alzheimer's and alter its effects to prevent expression of the disease.

INTELLIGENT MEDICINE TIP: _____

For information and referrals to support groups in your state, write to the Alzheimer's Association, P.O. Box 5675, Dept. P, Chicago, IL 60680, or call (800) 272-3900, twenty-four hours a day.

Nutrition and the Nervous System

Good nutrition is extremely important for the overall health of the nervous system. We are learning more and more about nutrient requirements for maintaining a stable, balanced, autonomic nervous system: the side of the nervous system that carries on reflex activities like breathing that don't require conscious direction, and is the pathway for panic attacks. Nutrient supplements can play a role in the treatment of panic disorder, cerebrovascular disease, and Alzheimer's disease as well as other neurological problems. Let's look at some of the key nutrients. (*Note:* For general supplemental dosages of these nutrients, and for good food sources, see the chart in chapter 16. For therapeutic nutritional dosages, consult a holistic or nutritionally oriented physician. Therapeutic dosages should not be taken without a doctor's supervision.)

Vitamin B_1 (Thiamine) Dr. Derek Lonsdale, a colleague of mine, has advanced the theory that certain people with neurological symptoms may have unrecognized borderline vitamin B_1 deficiencies. Lonsdale worked especially with children who had autonomic nervous system dysfunction — not specifically panic syndrome, but a syndrome of drastic swings between lethargy and hyperexcitability — and found that thiamine often helped stabilize them. Interestingly, it's been shown that vitamin B_1 is necessary for the metabolism of sugar. People who consume a lot of sugar and refined carbohydrates not only may deplete their vitamin B_1 by using large amounts to metabolize sugar but at the same time may not be getting enough vitamin B_1 because refined foods are notoriously low in this nutrient. In fact, the origin in Asia of the classic vitamin B_1 deficiency disease, beriberi, was the polishing of rice — stripping the husk off brown rice to make it into white rice. It's the husk that contains the vitamin. So if your diet contains a lot of white flour, sugar, and processed foods you may not get enough vitamin B_1.

Recent studies have shown that thiamine deficiency plays an important part in Alzheimer's disease because of a link to thiamine-dependent enzymes.[3] In fact, thiamine therapy has a safe and beneficial effect in a wide range of neurological disorders.

Folic Acid may help stave off neurodegenerative diseases by blocking formation of homocysteine, a toxic metabolite that contributes to arteriosclerosis. High levels of homocysteine are linked to stroke, mental retardation, and perhaps Alzheimer's disease. Folic acid must be teamed with B_6 and B_{12} to lower homocysteine. Protective doses range from 800 micrograms per day (obtainable over the counter) to 25 to 50 milligrams per day (which must be prescribed by a physician).

Vitamin B_6 (Pyridoxine) has been used to treat a variety of neurologic conditions, including carpal tunnel syndrome, nerve pain, seizures, and childhood autism. As with many nutritional therapies, there is usually a delay of as long as several months from the beginning of treatment to the first signs of improvement. Nevertheless, vitamin B_6 therapy is a highly valuable alternative treatment, especially because it significantly raises the pain threshold in several ailments, such as lower back pain. Carpal tunnel syndrome is a "pinching" of the median nerve in the wrist that strikes assembly-line workers, typists, and computer-terminal operators who suffer repetitive strain injuries. Vitamin B_6 treatment has been shown to be very effective in treating this condition and is far preferable to painful surgery, which does not always cure the problem. A dosage of 100 milligrams a day should be safe for most people, or up to 200 milligrams under the supervision of a nutritional physician.[4]

Vitamin B_{12} deficiency can cause fatigue and neurological symptoms such as balance problems and difficulty walking. Some people have an intrinsic malabsorption of vitamin B_{12}, a condition called pernicious anemia, which can cause odd neurologic symptoms. Most people who eat fish, chicken, eggs, and dairy foods will get sufficient vitamin B_{12} from their diet.

Calcium deficiencies are common in elderly people, and chronically low levels of calcium are often involved in disorders of memory and learning. Older memories, which are more widely "distributed" throughout the brain, are less vulnerable to disruption than more localized recent memories. Recent studies cited in the British medical journal *The Lancet* suggest that calcium deficiency may be a more important factor in the development of Alzheimer's disease than aluminum poisoning. The researchers recommend that more attention be paid to calcium levels and suggest that possibly supplementation may provide some protection against the decline of cognitive function in Alzheimer's patients.

Magnesium is depleted by production of the hormonal neurotransmitters called catecholamines, which stimulate the body into the kind of heightened readiness for activity we call the fight-or-flight response. When there is a perceived stress or danger, the brain releases these hormones, which very quickly speed up the heart rate, increase the blood pressure, and put the body in a state of readiness for physical action. This may have been useful for our ancestors, who needed to fight off a saber-toothed tiger, but it's not so helpful to have our heart rate soaring when someone cuts in front of us in high-speed traffic on the freeway. Cortisol, another stress hormone, also depletes magnesium. Some studies have shown that certain phobic disorders like agoraphobia are associated with lower levels of magnesium, and other kinds of nervous system instability may also be involved. One clear symptom of magnesium deficiency is *hyperreflexia*—a kind of heightened startle reflex marked by sensitivity to noise and exaggerated reflex responses. In fact, one of the symptoms of magnesium overdose is the suppression of normal reflexes. So the idea is to keep the body supplied with the ideal levels of magnesium—though deficiencies are the real concern. In our high-stress postindustrial environment, daily stresses and shocks may literally leach away the magnesium we need to maintain our neurological equilibrium.

Acetyl-L-Carnitine (ALC) is a bioavailable form of L-carnitine, a biological compound that plays a role in cellular metabolism and is found in high concentrations in the heart, brain, and skeletal muscle. Animal studies in Germany have shown that ALC can improve cognitive function in aged rats, improve age-dependent neurological damage, and actually delay the aging process of the central nervous system.

THE NEW NEUROPHARMACOLOGY

———— ∞ ————

Our new vision of the brain and nervous system may lead us to new treatments and therapies beyond the classic tranquilizers and antidepressants. Some clinicians who are beginning to think about ways to influence brain function in nonclassical ways, with other means than drugs. Drugs like Prozac may be all the rage, but researchers are also discovering the powerful effects of light therapy in curing depression. They are studying the use of hormones like testosterone, estrogen, and natural progesterone as psychoactive agents that can somehow modulate mood and mental processes. Whether or not these therapies turn out to be useful, they are all inspired by our new understanding of the complex interaction of mental and nervous function with other bodily processes.

Several studies on Alzheimer's patients have shown that ALC relieves many of the symptoms, enhancing attention and learning ability, temporal and spatial orientation, judgment and abstract reasoning, short- and long-term memory, and powers of personal recognition. Other trials are under way. The usual maintenance/preventive dosage is 120 milligrams three times daily. This should be taken between meals, as it is best absorbed by an empty stomach.

Phosphatidylserine (PS) is a natural constituent of the white matter of the brain and the nerve sheaths. A relative of phosphatidylcholine and derived from lecithin, PS has been shown to offer even more decisive benefits in forestalling memory impairment and may even play a role in myelin repair in neurodegenerative conditions like multiple sclerosis. Doses range from 50 to 100 milligrams taken two to three times daily.

Inositol, considered one of the B-complex vitamins, is vital to nerve function. It is an important building block for myelin. Recent Israeli research has highlighted a role for high-dose inositol in alleviating depression, obsessive-compulsive disorder, and panic attacks. Therapy can be pricey, since doses used range from twelve to eighteen *grams* daily.

The Energy Pathway—An Alternative View

In Western medicine we have typically concentrated on understanding organs and their metabolic functions. We have developed an exquisite physiological knowledge that reaches down to the biomolecular level and considers organ function as the workings of a marvelous living machine.

Yet, our culture-bound perspective may have overlooked important aspects of how the body and mind function. In fact, the very latest scientific discoveries are leading us to a more global, holistic view of health and life.

In the West we've mapped nerves and the brain. We've traced physiological functions and pathways. Yet, over five thousand years ago the Chinese began to develop an alternative view of what we call the nervous system, which encompasses much more than its anatomic structures. They postulated pathways of circulating energy, which they called *chi*, and traced and mapped meridians of energy flow that connected all the organs and parts of the body. They developed a system of understanding and healing disease in terms of energy ebb and flow, and interconnection between organs. This is the basis for acupuncture therapy, which stimulates specific energy nodes to affect distant parts of the body. Well, we are now beginning to find that many of the nodes of the autonomic nervous system correspond to the energy nodes of Chinese medicine.

The autonomic nervous system — our view of the body's energy control system — is the branch of the nervous system that governs involuntary body functions like breathing, heart rate, blood pressure, balance, temperature, the preferential flow of blood to organs and muscles, digestion, mucus secretions, and sexual functions, to name but a few. What can happen when the autonomic nervous system goes awry? Almost anything, including chronic pain syndrome, exhaustion, muscle aches, indigestion, asthma, high blood pressure, palpitations, panic episodes, vertigo, visual problems, skin rashes, allergies, headaches, menstrual cramps — a vast range of medical complaints. Sustained autonomic dysfunction can even cause permanent damage to organs, tissues, and joints, because malfunctioning autonomic nerves can literally deprive their target organs of life-giving blood circulation.

To give credit where it is due, this is a long-held tenet of chiropractic. D. D. Palmer, the originator of modern chiropractic, held that "subluxations" causing nerve interruptions in the spine interfere with autonomic messages to organs and limbs. Correcting these spinal misalignments with manipulation is the mainstay of chiropractic therapy. Acupuncture, too, aims at regulating bodily functions, but it targets nerve junctions and reference points mapped centuries ago. Researchers have even shown that laser light, directed at appropriate acupuncture points, can regulate energy flow. Similarly, massage techniques like shiatsu can act on energy pathways.

Disciplines such as yoga are also designed to influence energy flow in the body. The chakras of Ayurvedic medicine, a tradition of ancient India, correspond faithfully to our modern conception of autonomic ganglia: relay stations and control points for the autonomic nervous system. Yoga breathing exercises are intended to provide regulatory feedback to the autonomic nervous system.

On a recent trip to Germany, I learned about an alternative-medicine practice called neural therapy, based on the work of Ferdinand Huehneke, a German physician who discovered the healing power of strategic injections of local anesthetics into areas of disturbed energy in the body. Huehneke observed what he called lightning reactions — rapid reversals of pain, immobility, and dysfunction of various kinds. In Germany, holistic physicians use a series of neural therapy injections to alleviate long-standing conditions such as migraine headaches, sinus congestion, low back pain, period cramps, vertigo, tinnitus, and even Raynaud's syndrome. Even depression and anxiety are sometimes alleviated by neural therapy.

While German holistic physicians routinely practice neural therapy, only a handful of practitioners in the United States use this technique. It will become more widely known as news of its healing power spreads. Whether or not you ever have reason to turn to any of these traditional or alternative practices, we can expect medical research and practice to focus more and more on the subtle functioning of the autonomic nervous system and the flow of "nervous energy" through the body.

A Look to the Future

Knowledge about the brain and nervous system is expanding at an enormous rate. We are finding out more and more about risk factors and preventive measures against neurological illness, and discovering scientific justifications for some of the ancient traditional treatments of the East. While Alzheimer's disease remains a serious problem, we've made enormous gains in the past ten years, and the chances are good we'll come up with effective treatments or preventive measures. However, we do need an attitude shift in our approach to neurological illness. We need to develop a greater awareness of what we are doing to our autonomic nervous systems with poor diet, environmental pollution, high-stress habits, and self-inflicted poisons. We should stop accepting strokes as the scourge of the elderly when there are clear methods for preventing and slowing cerebrovascular disease. And we should no longer accept the notion of an inevitable decline of mental function with old age — we now have the knowledge and tools to arrest or slow many types of decline. We have to stop taking our mental function and autonomic nervous functions for granted and start treating them with the same proactive approach that we now use to prevent heart disease. *Mens sana in corpore sano* — the old slogan of "a sound mind in a sound body" — is an ideal that's not just for the young.

CHAPTER SIX

The Endocrine System: Key to Your Well-Being

Normally the various glands of the endocrine system do their work so smoothly and efficiently that they go unnoticed. In fact, most people can name only a few of the more than a hundred hormones that are secreted by the glands of the endocrine system. These hormones regulate the function of nearly all the organs and tissues of the body, so the endocrine system really is the ultimate regulator of our well-being. When this complex network of glands malfunctions, it can affect our overall health at a very basic level.

By the time a person enters midlife, the delicate balance of the hormonal system has been subjected to stress, a busy lifestyle, drugs, or nutritional deficiencies for so long that problems may start to appear. Sometimes the symptoms are subtle and may be overlooked as just "feeling older." But for many people this will be the first time in their lives they have had any inkling that the body needs regular maintenance to keep it in good working order and, even more importantly, to avoid bigger problems that may develop down the road.

In this chapter we'll take a look at some of these likely problems of the endocrine system. I'll also give the risk factors for these problems and show you what can be done both to prevent these disorders from developing and to treat them if they do occur.

You undoubtedly know by now that a healthy diet and regular exercise are important to maintaining your health, but another prudent step toward keeping healthy is to know your family health history — not just the cause of death of your maternal and paternal grandparents but also such facts as these: Did Grandpa Jones have diabetes? Was that medication that Grandmother Smith was always taking for her thyroid? It's worth asking your living relatives what they know about the health of their parents, grandparents, aunts, and uncles. A family health history can be very important in determining what genetic predispositions you may have and what might manifest in your own body. Ask your parents and your aunts and uncles whether anyone had diabetes or thyroid problems. If they're not around, try checking with a family doctor who has treated your relatives. With this information in hand, you are then prepared to assess, with your doctor, your risk factors for hormonal problems. Besides family or genetic history, they are weight (either overweight or serious underweight), lifestyle, stress (in all forms, including things like dieting, which can stress the delicate hormonal balance), past illness, drug use, and depression.

It is well known that depressed people are far more vulnerable then others to physical illnesses. The interaction of the endocrine system and the nervous system is so complex that many facets of their functioning are not fully understood. What we do know is that an endocrine problem can be projected as depression, and this can work the other way around, also. Small wonder that damage or shock to the adrenals or thyroid can be sustained through mental stress or depression, because these are organs that are ultimately triggered by the brain. The triggering mechanism works through the pituitary gland, which in turn is influenced by the limbic system of the brain, the seat of the emotions.

The pituitary gland is the "master gland" of the body. It is made up of two distinct organs: the anterior lobe, a typical endocrine gland, which secretes several hormones that regulate many processes of the body, and the posterior lobe, which is really a modified part of the nervous system. This close relationship between the brain (cerebral cortex) and the glands that regulate essential body functions means that emotions act on body processes. In fact, the thyroid, along with the adrenals, is probably the gland most susceptible to the stresses of our fast-paced modern life. Studies have shown that Graves' disease, a form of hyperthyroidism, is strongly linked to negative and stressful life events.

Thyroid disease is one of the more common problems that can occur in the endocrine system as a person approaches midlife. In fact, thyroid disease — including both hyperactive and underactive types — is so prevalent today that even by conservative estimates it may affect up to 15 percent of the adult population. We don't know why thyroid disease is on the rise, but one reason may be that the thyroid doesn't have built-in reserves like the kidneys or the liver. Even if 90 percent of the liver is removed in surgery, the remaining 10 percent can suffice and can even regenerate. But if thyroid capacity declines through the wear and tear of life itself, there is no possibility of regeneration, and the symptoms can be profound.

Women are particularly susceptible to thyroid disease, and it seems to run in families. Typically, I see women in their thirties and forties who aren't producing sufficient thyroid hormones and who will require thyroid medication. Unlike many medical interventions, thyroid hormone, correctly prescribed and monitored, is one of the least invasive drugs for the body. This drug is an exact copy of something that the body either isn't making any longer or isn't making in sufficient quantity. It's the ultimate in gentle medicine.

The increase in thyroid disease throughout the population may be linked to the prevalence of autoimmune disease today. Immunity in general is being assaulted by toxic chemicals in food, water, and air. Several forms of thyroid imbalance are the result of autoimmune problems, as a result of which the thyroid becomes inflamed, sometimes initially produces too much hormone, and then in exhaustion finally sputters out.

When the thyroid malfunctions, it can either produce excess thyroid hormone (hyperthyroidism) or degenerate and produce too little hormone (hypothyroidism). Answer the following questions to determine whether you might have either of these conditions:

Could You Be Hyperthyroid?

1. Do you feel wired but tired? Are you exhausted and yet jittery, as if you're perpetually drunk too much coffee?
2. Have you lost weight recently for no apparent reason?
3. Do you have trouble sleeping?
4. Do you suffer from heart palpitations?
5. Does your resting pulse race?
6. Do your hands shake? Extend your arms and hold a piece of paper. The fine hand tremor of a person with hyperthyroidism will be magnified.
7. Do your eyes bulge? This is symptomatic of one type of hyperthyroid condition, Graves' disease.
8. Do you feel heat-intolerant and sweat a lot?

Could You Be Hypothyroid?

In contrast, the hypothyroid patient produces too little thyroid hormone, and the symptoms are much different. Ask yourself the following questions:

1. Are you depressed, lethargic, and easily chilled? Are you the person who is always asking someone to close the window because you're cold?
2. Do you gain weight easily?
3. Do you suffer from chronic fatigue?
4. Do you have dry skin, hair loss, eczema, or adult acne?
5. Do you suffer from muscle aches, constipation, and hoarseness?
6. Do you have PMS or menstrual abnormalities? Is your libido low?
7. Are your feet and legs swollen and your nails brittle?

8. Do you get a lot of colds and flu? One cardinal "unseen" symptom of low thyroid is increased vulnerability to infection.

If you've answered "yes" to three or more of these questions for one of these conditions, and suspect that you may have a thyroid problem, you should ask your doctor to give you the thyroid function tests. But first make a list or mentally prepare a list of your symptoms. Include all your symptoms even if you don't think they are related to your possible thyroid malfunction. Thyroid specialist Stephen Langer, M.D., lists over one hundred known symptoms of thyroid deficiency in his book *Solved: The Riddle of Illness* (Keats Publishers). It has even been linked to susceptibility to cancer.

Suppose your doctor orders a thyroid test, and the result is in the normal range. Even if you have a "normal" thyroid test result, you may still have what is known as subclinical hypothyroidism. If you still believe that your symptoms and risk factors point to thyroid trouble, make sure your doctor has given you the TSH (thyroid-stimulating hormone) test. A person with low thyroid function usually has high levels of TSH — a product of the pituitary gland — in the blood. That's because the pituitary gland is desperately signaling the thyroid to pump out more thyroxin, the thyroid's "energy" hormone.

One test that I favor is the Barnes basal body temperature test. This is a simple at-home test that provides a valuable clue to thyroid disease. Simply shake down a thermometer before going to bed at night and leave it within easy reach. As soon as you awake in the morning, insert the thermometer snugly in your armpit for ten minutes while you lie quietly enjoying that time in bed. Do not get up (and of course, don't talk) until you have finished taking this measurement. Record your results for three consecutive mornings. Results averaging under 97.4°F suggest hypothyroidism. Women obtain the most accurate readings when they are not ovulating.

We really need more sensitive tests to assess the possibility of thyroid malfunction. Tests for sugar metabolism and insulin resistance have become more finely tuned, and I hope that in the near future the needed thyroid tests will be developed. One uncommon test that I sometimes use is the TRH (thyroid-releasing hormone) stimulation test. It's almost like a stress test for the thyroid, for it measures the pituitary gland's response to a hormone secreted by the hypothalamus. Ask your doctor about this test. It enables the dynamic interaction of the pituitary, hypothalamus, and thyroid glands to be studied.

Another useful test detects the presence of antibodies the body has manufactured against the thyroid gland itself. These autoantibodies tell you when you're headed for thyroid trouble, since they indicate an inflammatory condition of the thyroid. Sometimes patients with normal blood levels of thyroid hormone have significant levels of autoantibodies, which may indicate that the thyroid is under attack and is fighting to maintain adequate levels. Giving a little thyroid hormone can help the thyroid rest, and adding antiinflammatory nutrients such as essential fatty acids and vitamins may help soothe the inflamed gland.

Suppose you have a thyroid problem. Your doctor agrees and has established that your thyroid gland isn't functioning effectively or perhaps your body isn't absorbing the hormone properly. You need medication. What thyroid medication should you take? How much? Will you need to take it for life?

Thyroid medication can be given in many forms (See the sidebar on page 99). Prescribing thyroid medication is part of the art rather than the science of medicine. Some physicians shy away from using certain forms of thyroid because they have to be closely monitored. If you are experiencing any symptoms that may be related to your thyroid, you want to be able to choose a doctor whom you can trust to understand the complexities of thyroid production and utilization. By the time you finish this chapter, you will be able to do just that. Even the medical community itself has been very slow to understand these complexities.

Each person responds differently to thyroid medications, and tests often rely on the presence of thyroid hormone circulating in the blood. That is a little like deciding whether people with diabetes need insulin by measuring their insulin levels. Instead, we measure their blood sugar levels. In fact, the treatment of diabetes offers a profoundly important clue to the treatment of thyroid disease. One of the key concepts in diabetes is that of insulin resistance: a state in which, although insulin levels in the body are adequate or even excessive, insulin is not being utilized well at the tissue level.

Even though a lot of research is being conducted on insulin resistance, there is almost no open acknowledgment of the parallel phenomenon of thyroid hormone resistance. If receptors for thyroid hormone are not soaking it up properly, an individual will show the symptoms of hypothyroidism (low levels) despite adequate circulating levels of thyroid hormone. That is one big reason thyroid disease can be "hidden." Studies show that the use of small supplemental amounts of thyroid hormone — even in cases where blood tests show it to be adequate — can clear up symptoms. In one study of ten women with blood tests that indicated normal thyroid function and severe PMS, nine of the women reported dramatic improvement in their symptoms when they were given thyroid hormone.

Possibly, if a doctor prescribes thyroid medication for you, you may still have the same symptoms even after taking the medication. The doctor may be more tempted to believe the blood test, which says you have adequate levels of thyroid, than to believe your report of no improvement. If you are taking Synthroid, the synthetic thyroid most commonly prescribed, there may be another problem. Synthroid is an artificial version of T-4, one of the hormones secreted by the thyroid gland. However, the body normally converts some of the T-4 to T-3, a different form. If the conversion is incomplete or inefficient, symptoms of thyroid deficiency can persist. You may need supplements of T-3 as well. This is just one example of the subtlety needed to treat thyroid problems — it's as much an art as a science.

In borderline cases, I often add the TRH stimulation test. Half of the borderline patients so tested end up needing thyroid medications, and at least nine out of ten of them benefit hugely from the medication. One of my patients had a TSH test result that was at one end of the "normal" range. Most endocrinologists would stop at that test result, which technically was normal. But my patient's symptoms were so pronounced (she was draggy, tired, and stiff in the mornings, tended to gain weight) that I repeated the TSH test along with a TRH stimulation test. The next TSH result was borderline, but the real tie-breaker was the TRH test result. She clearly needed thyroid and felt much better once she began taking it.

As I said earlier, most people will have to continue taking thyroid medication, but there are some exceptions. In a few cases, taking thyroid can "jump-start" your metabolism. If you then start exercising and losing weight, the hormonal output of your own thyroid can become adequate for your new body weight, and medication is no longer needed. I've seen this happen in a few instances. But most people do take the medication for life. The benefits far outweigh the inconvenience.

Some people have trouble adjusting to this lifetime program and start to wonder what would happen if they were to take the medication for a while and then stop. The answer is that they'll revert to the way they were. The actual output of the thyroid might be somewhat worse, but it's unlikely that it will be better. In most cases, the thyroid medication cannot "repair" the thyroid so that it then produces its own hormone. Rather, it simply replaces the hormone that the thyroid once produced. When you take it, the symptoms disappear and energy returns. Because thyroid hormone, correctly administered, has no side effects, this is not a grim sentence; in fact, it's a new lease on life.

Unfortunately there has not been enough progress in how we treat problems of the endocrine system. Both conventional and holistic physicians theorize that there are many people, as yet untested, who have undetected thyroid disease. Innovative physicians may go one step further: They believe there are many people with *normal* test results who should be getting thyroid therapy. Frankly, I support this view. I've seen some patients who don't have stupendously low thyroid benefit tremendously from thyroid therapy. We actually enhance their health and well-being by giving them thyroid according to strong clinical criteria, rather than simply according to test levels alone.

Endocrinologists, however, are reluctant to embrace this view because they are afraid that they will open the floodgates to erroneous diagnoses and to unnecessary and even harmful use of medication. I can see their point, but on the other hand, their diagnoses shouldn't be so jealously guarded.

WHAT KIND OF THYROID MEDICATION SHOULD YOU TAKE?

L-thyroxin (Synthroid) is most utilized by conventional endocrinologists. It is a synthetic analog of thyroid hormone, containing the same amino acid sequence. Doctors like it because Synthroid levels in the blood can be measured accurately by current tests, and so precise doses can be prescribed and regularly monitored.

Synthetic T-3 (Cytomel) is another medication currently available. The results can sometimes be remarkable. I've seen patients who have taken huge doses of Synthroid, or T-4, with little effect have an immediate and pronounced response when T-3 is added.

Natural thyroid hormone, an extract of thyroid glands from beef or pork, is available by prescription only. Endocrinologists are critical of it because it is difficult to standardize levels of natural extracts, so the dose strength may vary minutely from batch to batch. It is also difficult to monitor response via blood levels. But clinically, my experience is that patients often respond best to this kind of supplementation, because the medication is in a natural form.

Glandulars, available in health food stores across the country, supposedly contain extracts of thyroid gland without the hormone. Patients often resort to self-prescribed glandulars, but I don't recommend them. A recent study found that glandulars are actually too efficacious in some cases. Although the FDA has tried to eliminate active thyroid from these preparations, some brands seem to have sneaked through with actual hormone. One woman took glandulars, overdosed on them, and became hyperthyroid. Some chiropractors and naturopaths who advocate glandulars contend that even though in most cases they do not contain active hormone, they provide the body with a subtle signal to make more thyroid. However, I've never seen any solid evidence to suggest this. In my mind the use of glandulars is akin to the use of brain extracts to boost flagging memory.

Conventional Treatments for an Overactive Thyroid

The overactive thyroid, hyperthyroidism, is the other side of the coin. There are three treatment options in conventional medicine: medication, radioactive iodine, and surgery. Medication (in the form of pills) can cause side effects, and its effect in slowing the thyroid down is usually only temporary. Eventually the thyroid may simply gun its motor even higher.

The second treatment option, radioactive iodine, is actually a medical cocktail that is swallowed. Because the thyroid instantly soaks up iodine, the radioactive material is concentrated there and does not circulate to other parts of the body. It kills some of the thyroid cells, leaving the gland producing thyroid hormone at a lower level. The problem is that it's very difficult to determine the precise dose of iodine that should be given. Often the patient is given too much and ends up hypothyroid — sometimes instantly, sometimes a year or two later.

The third and most invasive option, surgery, requires removing part of the gland with the patient under anesthesia in a hospital. This option may be chosen over radioactive iodine if the patient is pregnant. But if the surgeon may remove too much of the gland, the patient may then end up being hypothyroid!

Remember that these are the three options in *conventional* medicine. I don't always recommend one of these three options. I believe that borderline hyperthyroidism can sometimes be carefully watched, without the immediate use of treatments that destroy thyroid function. Sometimes patients can use the thyroid "crisis" as an opportunity to learn stress reduction through meditation and relaxation. I've found that this will often stabilize thyroid function in mild, borderline cases.

Take one of my patients, a forty-two-year old, hard-driving psychotherapist, who had moderately elevated thyroid levels. She had been told that she was hyperthyroid and that the best treatment would be radioactive iodine. After she came to me she cut back on her work hours; learned to meditate; switched to an organic, vegetarian diet; and normalized her thyroid in three months. She used the thyroid crisis as an opportunity to balance her life. At midlife she has now become proactive about her health; the changes she has made will help her to avoid some of the common health problems that her generation will encounter in the years ahead.

The Adrenal Glands: A Multisystem Regulator

While some thyroid disorders are more prevalent in women, adrenal gland problems occur in men and women about equally. And along with the thyroid, these glands are equally susceptible to the effects of a stressful lifestyle or real-life problems. My practice includes many patients who suffer from adrenal "exhaustion." These patients may have been born with smaller, weaker adrenal glands and tend to suffer from allergies, low blood pressure, low body temperature, and a feeling of malaise and exhaustion. Adrenal insufficiency can also affect sugar metabolism. An adrenal hormone, cortisol, counters the effects of insulin, so when cortisol is low, unrestrained insulin may lower blood sugar excessively, causing patients to crave sugar. By the time they reach midlife, these people with weaker adrenals may therefore suffer from blood sugar abnormalities and "sugar disease."

Conventional medicine recognizes three states of adrenal function. The first, of course, is normal adrenal function, the second is adrenal failure, and the third is the hyperadrenal condition, which is an excessive production of adrenal hormones. The ACTH (adrenocorticotropic hormone) stimulation test is the conventional test for adrenal weakness. ACTH is the pituitary hormone that signals the adrenal glands to release cortisol. A doctor can inject ACTH and measure the blood levels of cortisol both immediately and 30 minutes later. Weak adrenals fail the test.

In my experience, however, this test misses many cases of mild adrenal weakness. I prefer to make a clinical diagnosis based on symptoms, and then employ preventive medicine. In this way the patient and I can catch problems before they become acute.

With some of my patients, I measure blood and urine levels of DHEA (dehydroepiandrosterone), an adrenal hormone that enhances mood and immune response. DHEA has been found to help rheumatoid arthritis and lupus and is used widely in Europe to extend longevity, boost the immune system, and combat nervousness and exhaustion. If you suspect your adrenal function is low, you can ask your doctor to measure levels of DHEA. Since DHEA is now available over the counter, many individuals are now self-administering the hormone. Despite being "natural," DHEA is a potent hormone, and over-replacement might lead to as yet unanticipated side effects. Therapy should therefore be directed to the goal of restoring natural, youthful levels of DHEA. Beware of megadosing which might lead to mood changes, undesirable masculinization in women including excess body hair, scalp-hair recession or acne, or intensifying the activity of thyroid medication.

For patients with weak adrenals, I find the best approach to be a mixture of Chinese herbal medicine and nutrients that subtly mimic the effects of the adrenal glands. This may sound like pallid therapy at best, but these herbs can actually be quite potent. Every internist is aware of the danger of licorice tea consumption in patients with high blood pressure. This is because licorice has a powerful effect on the adrenal glands, slowing the breakdown of the mineralocorticoids and causing the body to retain sodium. One eighty-year-old patient drank so much licorice tea that her blood pressure soared from 90/60 to a dangerous 180/120 in a few months. Licorice is best taken under a doctor's supervision, and blood pressure should be regularly monitored. Licorice's active ingredient is glycyrrhizin, a plant hormone that enhances the action of the adrenal hormones. (Licorice candy typically uses only a small quantity of extract for flavor, so it's not a problem, though large amounts of old-fashioned authentic black licorice candy could have an effect.)

The adrenal glands, sitting just on top of the kidneys, are richly fed by nerves that connect to the spine, so acupuncture and chiropractic can sometimes give the adrenals a much-needed boost. By the releasing of blockages through these simple and effective techniques, the glands can be stimulated and strengthened.

A good diet low in simple carbohydrates can also help the adrenals to stay in good working order. In fact, the easiest way to exhaust and totally wear down the adrenals is a diet that puts you on a sugar roller coaster. Let's take a closer look at the effects of sugar.

Sugar Disease

One of the most common abuses, or perhaps *the* most common abuse of the body in America today, is the high-carbohydrate, sugar-laden diet that leads ultimately to some form of sugar disease, or — in its most damaging form — diabetes. You can get away with this kind of a diet for twenty or thirty years, or maybe even longer, but it will damage the system whether or not the damage shows up right away.

The principal organ involved is the pancreas, though the effects of sugar disease reach into many other systems. The islet cells of the pancreas produce insulin, a remarkable hormone that is a key element of health and energy. Given the alarming levels of consumption of sugar and other simple carbohydrates in this country, it is not surprising that many Americans suffer from insulin surges that ultimately damage their health and lead finally to hypoglycemia, diabetes, heart disease, and chronic fatigue. Keeping your blood sugar and your insulin levels balanced is an important part of maintaining good health in midlife and beyond.

If you've never paid attention to your sugar consumption, perhaps now is the time to begin. Remember that sugar in its refined form, sucrose (table sugar), is not a naturally occurring food. It has to be refined through a chemical process from plant material, much as cocaine is refined from coca leaves, or medicinal drugs are extracted from rain-forest plants. In fact, sugar is more potent in the body than many drugs.

Sugar (in the natural form the body uses, glucose) is an essential component of life. When blood sugar is low, the body's cells, particularly the brain cells, are starved. To maintain optimal health, your body needs to keep a constant balance between glucose and oxygen in the bloodstream. What happens when you eat refined sugar, known as sucrose, or even "healthy" sweets such as honey, maltose, and maple syrup? Unlike complex carbohydrates, which require time to be broken down, sucrose is quickly absorbed into the blood, where it is quickly converted to glucose, upsetting the balance between glucose and insulin. The body goes into crisis mode. Here is what happens next:

As blood glucose soars, you feel a temporary lift, but you are flooding the body with much higher amounts of glucose than result from any natural food. As a result, hormones pour out from the adrenal glands and sound the call to arms. Insulin bursts from the pancreas and helps hold down the glucose level in the blood. Usually, because this happens under "emergency" conditions, the blood glucose level soon crashes and a second crisis occurs. Now you feel exhausted, listless, and irritable. The cells of the brain, in particular, respond to moment-to-moment glucose nourishment, so the roller-coaster ride from sugar highs to lows leads directly to powerful mood swings. Now that blood sugar has been oversuppressed because of the massive release of insulin, the pancreas shuts down its insulin production, and new adrenal hormones pour out to help raise the blood glucose. This scenario can be repeated many times a day, every time you have a sweet or a simple-carbohydrate snack.

Accordingly, sugar and carbohydrate snacking take a tremendous toll on your body's metabolic machinery by triggering fatiguing surges of insulin and counterregulatory stress hormones. This is one reason I find it so amazing that sugar is so often equated with fuel, because it is a fuel that is in fact ill suited to the body and wears away at two of the body's key glands: the adrenals and the pancreas. These sugar highs followed by sugar lows can trigger a disease process that spans decades. This is a perfect example of what medical scientists now call a diathesis: an evolving disease pattern that is looked at in terms of its progression throughout an individual's life.

An individual may succumb to sugar cravings a million times in the course of a lifetime, generating a staggering overproduction of insulin over the years and leading to a condition now known as Syndrome X, which is a precursor of heart disease and diabetes. In fact, the term *sugar disease* is a catchall for a host of modern conditions that result from an unbridled intake of sugar or refined carbohydrates. We can look at sugar disease as passing through three general stages, from a milder form to more advanced and destructive forms. They are

1. Hypoglycemia
2. Syndrome X
3. Diabetes

Hypoglycemia

Americans love to "carbo-load." We are a society that is in love with carbohydrates — and it shows in our poor health standing versus the other industrialized nations of the world. In fact, the United States Surgeon General's office says that eating habits helped account for two-thirds of all deaths last year from five of the top ten killer disease — and diabetes is one of them! But Americans don't get their nutrition information from the government or even from their doctors — they get it from advertising. Though we talk up things like fiber, what is often palmed off as a high-fiber food is a highly refined commercial "brown" bread made of food coloring and white flour in a wrapper depicting a log cabin on the front — a far cry from the fiber intake of our stone-age ancestors: roots, shoots, foliage, and occasional berries.

In essence, hypoglycemia is low blood sugar, and it is increasingly prevalent in our society. Hypoglycemia can cause an array of symptoms, including spaciness, fatigue, mood changes, PMS, sugar craving, headaches, difficulty focusing the eyes, tremors, temperamental outbursts, depression, excessive sweating, hot flashes, palpitations, cold extremities, abdominal pain, and panic attacks.

If you have any of these symptoms, the next time you go to a doctor, try asking him or her if the symptoms you experience could be due to hypoglycemia. You may provoke a bemused or annoyed look, or perhaps your doctor will, in fact, suggest a glucose tolerance test. Don't bother. Glucose tolerance tests, as performed conventionally, are not designed to detect hypoglycemia until or unless it has reached a very extreme level.

The truth is that hypoglycemia is far more prevalent than we're led to believe. Studies show that even in its full-blown form it is often misdiagnosed. Consider this example: In one study, of thirty-nine patients who had tumors in the pancreas, a condition causing profound hypoglycemia, eight were first diagnosed with epilepsy or neurosis! Detection and diagnosis of hypoglycemia can lead to treatment that can totally correct this condition. Even if the symptoms are vague and seemingly subjective (which makes most doctors want to shy away from this diagnosis), if you're the one experiencing them, they can destroy the quality of your life.

Why so many different kinds of symptoms? To learn the answer to that, we have to explore the physiology of low blood sugar.

The body is designed to digest and assimilate three primary nutrients: proteins, fats, and carbohydrates. Proteins and fats can be used for energy, but their conversion to forms usable by the body is gradual, not immediate. By contrast, carbohydrates are all more or less readily digested into sugar. Their rate of conversion to sugar depends on their complexity. Complex carbohydrates like beans provide a slow time-release of the sugar they contain in their complex molecules of starch mixed with fiber. The presence of natural starch-blockers in beans further slows the sugar liberation process. This is why if you have bean soup for lunch you probably won't feel hungry till dinner.

On the other hand, sugars and refined carbohydrates provide a rapid sugar fix. This results in an immediate, pleasant sense of gratification, sometimes even a mild drowsiness. It's the familiar sugar high. But then, in response to so much sugar in the blood, the body calls upon its insulin reserves, generated in the pancreas, to lower the blood sugar. This often happens precipitously, sometimes with crashing rapidity.

Experiments have now confirmed what the hypoglycemic person experiences. Low blood sugar triggers hunger — especially carbo craving. In addition, the brain is starved for its preferred fuel: glucose. At rest, the brain consumes one-third of the body's total glucose requirement. The brain is a hungry, rapidly metabolizing organ, and fuel shortages in it create problems with concentration, memory, and mood. A recent study showed that individuals with low blood sugar scored poorly on tasks requiring memory, concentration, and reasoning.

But perhaps most important, low blood sugar triggers an outpouring of counterregulatory hormones (catecholamines) from the adrenals. These hormones oppose the action of insulin and push blood sugar levels back up. Unfortunately for the hypoglycemic person, these "rescue" hormones are the very same ones that produce the adrenaline rush of a fight-or-flight reaction. The results are symptoms like palpitations, sweaty palms, nervousness, tremor, and sometimes even severe panic attacks.

If you think you suffer from blood sugar swings, what can you do? The best idea is to test yourself by going off sugar completely. Ultimately, it's the way that works best. The results can seem quite disastrous at first. Many of my patients report a week of severe fatigue and almost supernatural cravings for sugar. Their concentration may be affected, and they may feel fidgety, irritable, and deeply depressed. I'm often inundated with phone calls in that first week. Some of them will be very resourceful in trying to sneak sugar into their diets. "Gee, Doc," a patient will say, "I just found something in the health food store called barley malt. And rice syrup. Those are O.K., aren't they?" Actually they're not. Along with honey, maple syrup, dextrin, maltose, succanat, fructose, corn syrup, sugar cane syrup, and molasses, they are simply alternative forms of sugar and should all be avoided when you are going off sugar completely. Note, too, that when manufacturers use the term sugar-free or sugarless, they generally mean that no sucrose is added, but other sugars may be.

I don't relish being a food policeman. We should all do our own self-policing if we are going to kick the sugar habit. This initial period of withdrawal is sometimes tough because sugar is as addictive as any drug. In fact, I have a hunch that the same hereditary susceptibility that leads to alcoholism may be involved in sugar addiction. Virtually all recovering alcoholics become carboholics. One study published in the *American Journal of Clinical Nutrition* found that alcoholics don't consume that much sugar until they withdraw from alcohol. And another study recently showed that alcoholics favor high-sugar beverages at three times the rate of nonalcoholics. Many of my patients who are "carboholics" have a family history of alcoholism. "I don't drink alcohol, Dr. Hoffman. We've had enough of that in our family." Yet, they are addicted to sugar.

According to remarkable studies by Judith and Richard Wurtman of MIT, sugar tends to change the way the blood–brain barrier selects the appropriate amino-acid building blocks of brain chemicals. Carbohydrate intake promotes uptake of the amino acid tryptophan, which is the building block for a brain chemical called serotonin. Serotonin is a proven tranquilizer. Certain individuals suffer major depression as a result of low levels of serotonin in the brain.

Because sugar may combat depression, some researchers suggest using sugary snacks to "feed" the brain as a therapy. I disagree. My belief is that sugar perpetuates a cycle of craving and bingeing. I would recommend tryptophan (which was formerly a treatment for depression, particularly in Great Britain), but because of a much-publicized incident of tryptophan contamination that resulted in tragic poisoning, this amino acid has been taken off the market. The subsequent popularity of the Prozac family of antidepressants attests to the primacy of serotonin in the biochemistry of well-being.

By far, the best answer is to switch to a diet emphasizing protein and complex carbohydrates, which provide the body with slowly released and steady levels of blood sugar.

Syndrome X

Physicians are becoming more aware of nutrition lately, but it often seems as if their only advice for preventing heart disease is to avoid cholesterol and saturated fat. The public's awareness of cholesterol without an accompanying familiarity with basic nutrition principles allows food manufacturers to use this buzz word to sell their products. Products like vegetable oils sit on the shelves of supermarkets with bold labels declaring "no cholesterol," and consumers snap up these products, never stopping to consider that vegetables don't ever contain cholesterol. Meanwhile, the same bottle of vegetable oil may contain a dangerously high amount of saturated fat, or the no-cholesterol spread may contain risky hydrogenated oil. (Hydrogenated oils are a completely synthetic form of fat, engineered to turn liquid oil into solid fat for margarine or baking. They have been linked with heart disease and may be incorporated into our cellular structures, with unknown results.)

Syndrome X, the next stage of sugar disease, demonstrates why physicians' advice about avoiding cholesterol and saturated fat may not be enough, and why some patients on a "prudent" diet then develop heart disease without apparent cause. Our national call to arms against cholesterol and fat should be matched with a call to arms against sugar and starch — and then we would truly see a remarkable drop in heart disease and other serious diseases, like diabetes and hypertension.

Syndrome X is a relatively new concept in medical research, as important as the understanding of cholesterol a decade or so ago, but its importance hasn't yet trickled down to the level of most front-line health care deliverers. In the Syndrome X model, not just excess fat and cholesterol but also plentiful carbohydrates — especially the refined ones — are seen as keys to the process of arteriosclerosis.

How could that be? Remember the insulin surge we get with sugar intake? Replicate that surge many thousands of times over the course of a lifetime, and you end up with an overly sensitive insulin trigger and chronically elevated insulin. Why is that bad?

Consider these adverse effects of too much insulin:

1. weight gain, especially around the midsection
2. elevated blood pressure
3. elevated cholesterol and triglycerides
4. increased deposits of plaque in the arterial walls
5. immune suppression
6. insulin resistance

It's the last item on this list, insulin resistance, that leads to the most common form of diabetes in the industrialized world: adult-onset diabetes. Some people may be surprised to learn that they can be diabetic even when they have high levels of insulin. In fact, this is a common occurrence in adult-onset noninsulin-dependent diabetes mellitus (NIDDM).* The insulin receptors, after years of being bombarded with signals from insulin, become less sensitive. More and more insulin is required to get the job done, until no amount will successfully lower blood sugar. Diabetes is induced by a diet high in sugar, and during the early stages there may be no detectable changes in blood sugar, although high levels of insulin may be discovered on a glucose tolerance test with insulin.

Syndrome X, which leads to diabetes and to heart disease, may be the most prevalent cause of degenerative disease and premature death in modern society.

How can you tell if you have Syndrome X? A variation on the standard glucose tolerance test, called the GTT with insulin, will confirm it, but there are easier ways to tell:

1. An elevation of your triglycerides on a fasting blood test should alert your doctor to the fact that you're prone to Syndrome X. Make sure

---

* Doctors have abandoned the old terms Type I and Type II diabetes, which used to refer to childhood onset vs. adult onset disease, in favor of the more precise terms identifying types of diabetes according to whether or not insulin is required to treat it. Some adult-onset diabetes is IDDM, and some is NIDDM, hence rendering the Type I and II type designations inadequate.

you fast starting the night before, and ask your doctor to inform you of your triglyceride levels.

2. An even simpler means of diagnosing Syndrome X is to take a quick tape measurement of waist and hips, which will yield a waist-to-hip ratio. Waist divided by hip circumference in men should be no greater than 1.0; in women, no greater than 0.8. If it's greater, you've got the "central adiposity" that's a hallmark of Syndrome X.

One patient of mine, Steven, was a stockbroker in his midthirties who had a family history of high cholesterol. He came to me complaining of fatigue and mentioned that his doctor was advocating a new cholesterol-lowering drug. He was a lean man but had a small abdominal pouch — a tip-off for Syndrome X. His father had suffered a heart attack at age fifty-eight, his mother had diabetes, and his brother had already undergone heart bypass surgery at forty-four. Steven was frankly worried. He was so tired every afternoon that he consumed several "energy" bars and kept a mini-refrigerator in his office stocked with orange and apple juice. His afternoon carbohydrate binges staved off episodes of exhaustion; sometimes, he just had to put his head on his desk and sleep.

When I asked about his diet, Steven told me proudly how he'd eliminated breakfasts of sausage and scrambled eggs and substituted healthful granola cereal with raisins. His midmorning snack was coffee and a "healthy" bran muffin, and lunch was a sandwich. Dinner was usually a pasta dish with generous helpings of whole wheat bread. After a typical pasta dinner he'd feel dopey and tired. "I have a love-hate relationship with bread. I can't put it down, but it makes me feel stoned." There weren't more than a few grams of cholesterol in his diet; yet, he couldn't keep his cholesterol down.

Steven seemed to be on a healthful diet — and he didn't even consume large amounts of refined sugar. What, then, was the problem? It had to do with something called the glycemic index.

A fascinating key to Syndrome X — and to sugar disease in general — is the glycemic index. Until recently we viewed carbohydrates as either simple or complex sugars. When calculating the carbohydrate content of foods, we relied on the old "calorie bomb" concept, whereby foods were literally placed in a calorie furnace and burned. A baked potato might be equivalent in calories to a large bowl of brown rice, or three tablespoons of table sugar, because they all produced the same calorie burnoff. But their effects on the body are quite different, for our own energy retrieval mechanisms are infinitely more complex and ultimately far more efficient than a furnace. Also, the effects vary remarkably from individual to individual. We now realize that there are factors that influence the speed with which carbohy-drates are digested and sugar released into the body. As long ago as 1937, researchers found that the carbohydrate content of a food did not always correspond to the blood sugar response it triggered. Dietary advice for anybody with a sugar problem must be based on this glycemic response: the actual change in blood sugar that occurs after a food is eaten.

Researchers at the University of Toronto and other centers have now established a glycemic index for foods, based on the blood glucose level caused by the food in comparison with pure glucose. The glycemic index is based on the concept that pure glucose has a 100 percent response — it is the ultimate, instantly usable sugar. A high glycemic index creates a characteristic high peak in a glucose tolerance test, while a low glycemic index creates a kind of gentle, rolling hill. Carbohydrate-free foods such as meat, fish, poultry, salad, eggs, oils, and butter have glycemic indexes of zero.

The results of the new glycemic index studies are shocking. Many foods we always thought were "good" carbohydrates may not be good for patients with sugar disease. Potatoes, for instance, have almost the same glycemic index as pure glucose, especially the instant mashed variety. So do carrots and corn flakes. Whole wheat bread has a very high glycemic index, as do millet and white rice. Bananas and raisins, gram for gram, are as high as a Mars candy bar. Sucrose (refined sugar) has a lower index than couscous — a North African semirefined grain product — and ice cream is even lower. The reason may be that in refined sugar the glucose is tightly bound to fructose, while the starch in couscous is easily broken down by digestive enzymes into pure glucose. Ice cream, while packing a caloric wallop, contains so much fat that its sugar content is time-released. Oddly enough, white flour in the form of spaghetti has a lower glycemic index than white flour in the form of bread. The form of a food has a great impact on the way it changes blood sugar levels: rice ground into flour creates a much higher glycemic response.

Juices, most fruits, breads, muffins (even the whole-grain, high-fiber kind), and even milk and yogurt (which contain milk sugar) have relatively high glycemic GIs. Surprising to some is the fact that dried fruit, despite its "naturalness," has a glycemic index virtually identical with that of commercial candy.

The message is that not all that emanates from the health food store is beneficial for patients with sugar disease. No wonder my patient Steven, with his family history of diabetes and heart disease, and his morning granola, raisins, and apple juice and his evening pasta and bread, was suffering from Syndrome X. His diet was "healthy" by popular standards but was making his blood sugar problem even worse.

What are the alternative carbohydrates? Legumes and whole grains in their unmilled form, like brown rice, barley, bulgur, rolled oats, teff (an Ethiopian grain), and amaranth and quinoa (South American grains). A cardinal rule is to live as if the flour mill had never been invented. The milling process makes the starch inside grains more susceptible to digestion and rapid absorption of its sugar content, and it actually raises the glycemic index of a grain.

Research on the glycemic index has provided some fascinating clues to diet and blood sugar. For instance, raw foods seem to be processed more slowly — and produce a flatter glycemic "curve" or response — than their cooked counterparts. Another amazing tidbit: the carbohydrate in one meal affects the digestion of the carbohydrate in the next meal. Slowly digested carbohydrates improve a person's carbohydrate tolerance of the next meal. A breakfast containing lentils (which have a very low glycemic index) will cause a flatter glycemic response to a standard lunch than a breakfast of bread. In fact, I often tell my sugar disease patients to have split-pea or lentil soup for breakfast. It's an uncommon breakfast, but it starts the day off with a stable blood sugar curve, thus reducing sugar cravings.

Another interesting fact: foods eaten slowly and continuously in small, divided portions produce a much flatter glycemic index. Although it has a higher glycemic index, bread eaten in small doses over four hours causes the same blood sugar changes as lentils eaten in twenty minutes. Accordingly, one way to help keep blood sugar fluctuations to a minimum and

GLYCEMIC INDEX OF SOME COMMON CARBOHYDRATE FOODS

FOOD GROUP	PERCENT
Glucose (also known as dextrose)	100
Corn flakes, carrots, parsnips, potatoes (instant mashed), maltose, honey	0–90
Bread (white), millet, rice (white), potatoes	70–79
Bread (whole meal), rice (brown), muesli, shredded wheat, bananas, raisins, Mars bar	60–69
Buckwheat, spaghetti (white), sweet corn, peas, yams, sucrose (table sugar), potato chips	50–59
Spaghetti (whole-wheat), oatmeal, sweet potatoes, beans, oranges, orange juice	40–49
Butter beans, black-eyed peas, chick-peas, apples, ice cream, milk (skim and whole), plain yogurt	30–39
Kidney beans, lentils	20–29
Soybeans, peanuts	10–19

conserve insulin is to eat more frequent, smaller meals. Tracking the effects of foods with a high glycemic index suggests not a simple arithmetical effect, like the difference between 100 and 500 calories. Rather, as you pass certain thresholds you may get a geometrically destabilizing effect on the body's insulin system. This supports the concept of grazing — eating little snacks here and there — rather than sitting down to a big plate of pasta that will most likely overload the system.

Some have proposed that people with variants of sugar disease follow a diet that rigidly excludes carbohydrates, concentrating instead on meat, oils, and leafy vegetables. In my opinion this is rarely necessary and results in dietary imbalance, inviting other degenerative conditions engendered by protein, cholesterol, and fat excess. It's better to keep an overall dietary balance, emphasizing foods low in glycemic response, and avoiding those with high GIs.

You don't need to worry too much about the details of glycemic index numbers or get into counting them the way people count calories. The point is to be aware of high-carbohydrate, high-sugar foods, whether processed or natural (read those nutrition labels!), and limit them in the diet. Especially limit the amount in any one meal to avoid overload demands for insulin. These guidelines and others are embodied in the Salad and Salmon Diet, which I have designed for patients with sugar disease. See chapter 16 for more on this diet and on the glycemic index.

Diabetes

Premature heart attacks, blindness, impotence, limb amputation, kidney dialysis — these are but part of the deadly legacy of our national epidemic of diabetes. Thomas Willis, a brilliant anatomist and physician, first wrote about and named a new and extraordinary sweetness in the urine of his ill — and mostly wealthy — patients. That was in 1674. He described this symptom of disease as diabetes (from the Greek word meaning "inordinate passage of urine") mellitus (from the Latin word meaning "honey"). About the time of his discovery, sugar consumption in England had soared to 16 million pounds a year.

Diabetes comes in two varieties: insulin-dependent (IDDM), and noninsulin-dependent (NIDDM). (See note on page 107.) The former results from the body's failure to produce insulin; the latter usually from an overabundance of insulin. The final common endpoint of both types of diabetes is high blood sugar. Paradoxically, the sugar level inside the body cells of people with diabetes remains low. Fuel is unavailable for metabolic work, and power failure results — a degenerative process resulting in cellular deterioration and finally death.

The miraculous substance that allows sugar from the bloodstream to be metabolized into energy (or stored as fat in the cells) is insulin. Most people are aware that in insulin-dependent diabetes, the problem is with low insulin. But few are aware that in noninsulin-dependent diabetes, insulin levels are usually elevated.

Both types of diabetes respond well to the measures I've outlined for controlling sugar disease in general. But although patients with IDDM can reduce their insulin requirements, they can never do without it entirely. Those with NIDDM, on the other hand, often require no medication if they follow a rigorous dietary and exercise program.

In my opinion, treating NIDDM with drugs before trying diet and exercise modifications is totally unnecessary, unless, of course, the patient just refuses to take an active role in his or her own healing. Hypoglycemic agents are only for people who really have no interest in following any kind of recommendations for diet, exercise, and supplements. Drug therapy can lower blood sugar, but some risk is associated with taking these agents, especially cardiovascular risk. These drugs allow us to fix a number, just as with cholesterol, but we may not be affecting the bottom line: length of life and mortality.

Maria was an overweight patient who came to me with recently diagnosed early-stage diabetes, high triglycerides, and high cholesterol. Her physician, one of the top diabetes specialists in the city, did recommend diet changes: the limited calorie diet prescribed by the American Diabetes Association. He also prescribed oral medication, which would stimulate the pancreas to produce more insulin. Unfortunately, this can ultimately worsen the cycle of insulin resistance and lead to full-blown diabetes requiring daily injections.

I explained to Maria that the 1200-calorie diet recommended by the ADA was based on the old concept of calories and not on the state-of-the-art glycemic index. I asked her to get on the scale, and she refused, bursting into tears and explaining that her mother had always made a tremendous issue about her weight problem, so she did not want to weigh herself. I offered her an alternative.

"Maria," I told her, "I'll never weigh you here. But this is a serious disease that threatens your life, and it has nothing to do with a mother trying to get her daughter to lose weight. As an alternative, I'll check your blood sugar with you on each visit. As long as that's improving, your body weight is okay with me." I explained the glycemic index, gave her the Salad and Salmon Diet, and got her started on a very simple exercise program. I prescribed nutritional supplements (see later in this chapter for specific recommendations) and encouraged her to check her blood sugar levels using home tests. (The "finger-stick" glucose test involves placing a drop of blood on a strip of paper that is inserted into a reader with a photometric cell. The reader provides an instantaneous glucose determination.)

Often, people with noninsulin-dependent diabetes are told not to bother checking their blood sugar, since it's not essential in calculating the dose of their medicine. I find, however, that it is a profoundly important part of controlling any diabetes. A patient gains immediate and continuous feedback about blood sugar levels and about how different foods affect them. It's almost as if each meal becomes a mini–glucose tolerance test, and the patient learns to correlate symptoms with actual blood sugar levels.

The benefit to Maria was enormous. She now takes no medications. She also has lost weight (although she doesn't want to know how much)! While she may not conform to her mother's ideal fashion-plate image, she's healthy and active, and at sixty-five she contemplates opening her own word-processing business.

Determining Whether You Have Sugar Disease

As mentioned before, the glucose tolerance test (GTT), even if performed for five consecutive hours, may sometimes provide the mistaken reassurance that a patient does not suffer from sugar disease. Even patients who feel devastated by the sugar challenge used in the GTT are often told not to worry, that they have no problem, that their symptoms have no real basis. The answer lies in designing a better, more sensitive GTT.

How is this accomplished? At my office, we measure not only blood sugar at each of several designated times but also the body's insulin response as well as the production of adrenaline at the crucial instant when blood sugar "bottoms out" and symptoms occur. This assures that even when glucose levels are normal, any abnormality in metabolism will be recognized. A hypoglycemia index can be calculated, also, by applying a mathematical formula to the glucose results obtained. The index takes into account not just how low blood sugar dips but also how rapidly it occurs. The result: more accurate testing for hypoglycemia, Syndrome X, and unsuspected diabetic tendency.

If you are interested in getting a reading of your insulin response and your hypoglycemic index, suggest it to your doctor.

Preventing and Treating Sugar Disease

Diet and dietary supplements play a principal role in preventing and treating sugar disease. Behavioral factors such as exercise also play an important part. Let's look at some of the key areas of prevention.

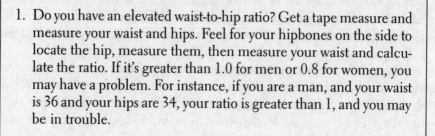

DO YOU HAVE SUGAR DISEASE?

1. Do you have an elevated waist-to-hip ratio? Get a tape measure and measure your waist and hips. Feel for your hipbones on the side to locate the hip, measure them, then measure your waist and calculate the ratio. If it's greater than 1.0 for men or 0.8 for women, you may have a problem. For instance, if you are a man, and your waist is 36 and your hips are 34, your ratio is greater than 1, and you may be in trouble.

2. Do you have a love-hate relationship with pasta and breads? Do you crave them but find that after eating them you feel tired?

3. When you're depressed, do you eat sweets?

4. During the winter months, do you eat more sweets? Studies show that some people suffer from a form of depression, seasonal affective disorder (SAD), that occurs only during the winter months when they aren't exposed to much sunlight. A concomitant of SAD is craving for sugar.

5. Do you sometimes get weak, irritable, and shaky and find that these symptoms are relieved by eating sweets?

6. Do you wake in the middle of the night feeling hungry?
   Score one point for each yes answer. Rate yourself as follows:
       0 points: you're fine
      1–2 points: mild sugar disease
      3–4 points: moderate sugar disease
      4–6 points: serious sugar disease

Good Fats

While all fats get a bad rap because of their high calorie content, in the treatment of sugar disease there are "good fats" and "bad fats." Saturated fats, such as those found in modern feedlot-raised livestock, hasten the development of sugar disease. In addition, altered fats like margarine and hydrogenated oils may impair the body's carbohydrate metabolism while adding unwanted pounds.

Conversely, omega-3 oils — such as those found in flaxseed oil; cold-water fish like salmon, trout, and tuna; and the wild game our ancestors ate — help cure insulin resistance. Monounsaturated fats, found in olive oil and canola oil, also help adjust blood sugar. A recent study turned the diabetes world upside down by demonstrating improved blood sugar control and better cholesterol levels in diabetic patients eating a Mediterranean diet, in which *40 percent* of all calories were derived from mostly monounsaturated fat, especially olive oil, compared with diabetic patients following the American Diabetes Association low-fat, high–complex-carbohydrate regimen. Of course, fats should be limited in terms of their total calorie payload.

Supplements

A key supplement for treating various forms of sugar disease is chromium. I'm frequently asked, "If chromium is helpful in diabetes, a disease of excess blood sugar, how can it be helpful for the opposite condition — hypoglycemia?" The answer lies in the unique ability of chromium to enhance the action of insulin, allowing the body to step down its production of the critical hormone. This results in fewer of the roller-coaster highs and lows.

RECOMMENDED DOSAGE: Chromium picolinate or poly-nicotinate, 200 micrograms three times daily, one-half hour before meals.

Vitamin E and magnesium also potentiate insulin action, so that the body has to produce less of it. Eicosapentaenoic acid from fish oil reduces insulin resistance, thus reducing the demand.

RECOMMENDED DOSAGES: Vitamin E, 400–800 International Units daily; magnesium, 400 milligrams daily. Fish oil: from diet, or two to three 1000-milligram capsules twice daily.

Several herbs help maintain blood sugar and even attenuate the craving for sugar: *gymnema sylvestre*, the ancient Ayurvedic "sugar destroyer"; stevia, an Amazonian herb, which is a noncaloric sweet sugar equivalent; and fenugreek, a mild, natural blood-sugar lowerer. Garlic, too, helps lower blood sugar and has a lipid regulating effect.

Diet

It's not uncommon for many of my diabetic patients to reduce or eliminate their medication. This is due in part to the Salad and Salmon Diet, described in chapter 16. The diet emphasizes low–glycemic-index foods and is weighted toward omega-3 and monounsaturated fats.

Exercise

Exercise is a great leveler for persons with sugar disease. Studies show that mild, regular aerobic exercise of short duration, like power walking twenty minutes a day, can forestall the development of diabetes in susceptible individuals or reverse it when it has already occurred. I've found aerobic exercise helpful, too, for people with hypoglycemia — it makes them more resilient and helps stabilize troublesome autonomic nervous system symptoms. Exercise is certainly an antidote to the abdominal weight gain that is a hallmark of Syndrome X.

How much exercise is required to achieve these benefits? While more is better, not much exertion is required to raise the bottom line. As little as thirty minutes of brisk walking five times weekly, or one fifteen-minute aerobic session daily, will reduce blood sugar levels by an average of twenty percent. Remember, to avoid hypoglycemia, take that walk or do some mild exercise *after* meals.

Exercise is the most important lifestyle change that people with diabetes can make. It helps diabetics in several ways. By burning calories and speeding metabolism, it helps reduce insulin resistance. It also promotes better circulation, safeguarding against heart disease and reduced blood flow to the extremities, and it improves the lipid profiles. People with diabetes should always exercise *after* eating to avoid hypoglycemic reactions.

Give Up Smoking

Smokers may sometimes have hidden sugar disease. They often pick up a cigarette instead of sweets, not because there is sugar in tobacco smoke but because the nicotine in tobacco has a powerful effect on the metabolism. In particular, nicotine causes glucose that is stored in the liver as glycogen to be released into the bloodstream. This may be one reason that some people who quit smoking gain weight — they crave foods that will make up for the drop in blood sugar. Efforts should be made before quitting to address an individual's sugar craving and possible hypoglycemia by adopting a proper diet, rich in foods that have a low glycemic index. According to studies, although smoking helps some people keep thin, even lean smokers have higher waist-to-hip ratios than their nonsmoking counterparts. The good news, according to the latest findings, is that quitting smoking reduces insulin resistance, so the pancreas won't have to work so hard to produce enough insulin.

One question you may have after reading so much about the dangers of sugar is this: Why do we crave a substance so seemingly harmful? Did nature go awry?

Not really. There was once a profound survival mechanism in our sweet tooth, for in the plant kingdom many of the foods with a sugary taste are also the most beneficial and nutritious — from fruits to squash and carrots. In contrast, many poisonous foods contain toxic alkaloids that have a bitter taste, and it was a general rule of thumb that sweet was nutritious and bitter was toxic. We had a tremendous drive to seek out the sweet foods, but they were seasonal and, in spite of their sweet taste, not nearly as abundant in sugar as a typical modern dessert, like apple pie à la mode. Finding pure

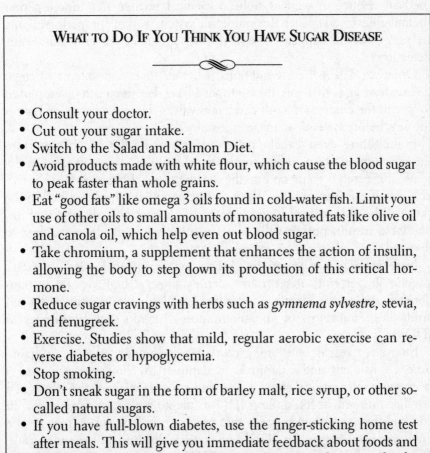

WHAT TO DO IF YOU THINK YOU HAVE SUGAR DISEASE

- Consult your doctor.
- Cut out your sugar intake.
- Switch to the Salad and Salmon Diet.
- Avoid products made with white flour, which cause the blood sugar to peak faster than whole grains.
- Eat "good fats" like omega 3 oils found in cold-water fish. Limit your use of other oils to small amounts of monosaturated fats like olive oil and canola oil, which help even out blood sugar.
- Take chromium, a supplement that enhances the action of insulin, allowing the body to step down its production of this critical hormone.
- Reduce sugar cravings with herbs such as *gymnema sylvestre*, stevia, and fenugreek.
- Exercise. Studies show that mild, regular aerobic exercise can reverse diabetes or hypoglycemia.
- Stop smoking.
- Don't sneak sugar in the form of barley malt, rice syrup, or other so-called natural sugars.
- If you have full-blown diabetes, use the finger-sticking home test after meals. This will give you immediate feedback about foods and your blood sugar levels and help you adjust your diet accordingly.

sugar was an extremely arduous process. American Indians, for instance, spent long hours tapping sap-laden trees in early spring and laboriously cooking the syrup in wooden bins to distill and purify it. This was hardly akin to driving to the supermarket and picking up a six-pack of sweet soft drinks.

Sugar can affect mood profoundly. Over many years, sugar consumption can cause constant, stressful insulin surges that seriously damage your health. If you can cut refined sugars from your diet, you may find yourself both more energized and calmer. This simple change could alter your life.

A Look to the Future

What's ahead?

Some of us who are now in our thirties to fifties can anticipate that medical science as well as holistic medical science may develop new therapies designed to keep the endocrine system working properly well into old age. Until that happens, our watchwords should be prevention and early detection.

Once we detect these conditions, whether thyroid problems or sugar disease leading to diabetes, the methods I have described can be employed to give us the chance for a full and healthy life — but early detection here is the key, before systemic damage is sustained.

In the future, even diabetic patients requiring insulin may benefit from the development of pancreas implants, which will release insulin on demand. Research is going on into the development of treatments like inhalable insulin or insulin pills. We can anticipate that sensors applied to the skin will be able to read blood glucose levels continuously, and that implantable insulin pumps will deliver insulin automatically, according to demand.

New techniques in genetics will soon enable doctors to read a person's genetic "fingerprint" at birth and identify those at high risk for insulin-dependent diabetes. Already, methods are available for detecting "islet cell antibodies," indicators of an autoimmune reaction that contributes to IDDM.

Innovative researchers are exploring nondrug approaches, utilizing omega-3 fish oils and vitamin E to dampen the immune response. A fascinating international study is now under way to evaluate the effects of a familiar nutrient in forestalling IDDM: nicotinamide, or vitamin B_3. In addition, new evidence suggests that protein from cow's milk may be the environmental trigger for IDDM in genetically susceptible individuals. The way is open to the prevention of IDDM in our time. Also, in recognition of the importance of Syndrome X in the causation of not just diabetes, but also hypertension, high cholesterol, and consequent heart disease, new drugs designed to combat it are being devised. One such drug, Glucophage, has long been used for NIDDM with relative safety in Europe; another, called Rezulin, is the first of a new generation of medications targeted specifically to insulin resistance.

Still, no matter how much we can benefit from innovative research or new technologies, people must be willing, especially when they are approaching midlife, to participate in their own health choices and to insist on getting sufficient information from their doctors and other sources to help them make those choices.

CHAPTER SEVEN

Muscles, Bones, and Joints

I call it "the rusty suit of armor syndrome," and baby boomers are prime targets. This joint or that one is a little achy, your neck is stiff in the morning, you have lower back pain that's worse when you're tired, or a shoulder that acts up. Those of us who jog, do aerobics, engage in sports, or work out with a vengeance suddenly discover we're nursing a chronic sore knee or tennis elbow.

This is the age of soreness. Even if you're basically healthy, with no serious ailments, you may be plagued by a shifting collection of nagging aches and pains that just never seem to completely go away. And you're just not as flexible. You used to pop in and out of little sports cars and compacts, and now you like the tall, roomy sport utility vehicles. You notice you're shopping for orthopedically correct chairs instead of futons and pillows for the floor. For many, a chronic ache or pain is the first initiation into the realities of aging, the first intimation that they're not indestructible.

When confronting accidental injuries, or even just the aches and pains of this period of life, whether they're "natural" or self-induced, many react with impatience and dismay. They look for a sure-fire solution, a quick fix. They start consuming medications daily, or go for the operation, but often without achieving real relief from pain. Our preferred model for healing is the "magic bullet" model: find a bug and zap it with a drug, or find the broken body part and fix it up with surgery. Unfortunately, many of the ailments of the musculoskeletal system are slow to develop and slow to correct. Often, gentle physical therapy or nutritional support can help correct problems of the musculoskeletal system, but it doesn't happen overnight.

Chronic neck pain or stiffness or tingling in the fingers can signal the onset of arthritis, a degenerative process that affects joints and the spine and can develop slowly, over the years. This is not something that happens just to old people — it can strike people in their thirties and even their twenties. The first symptoms in midlife are generally not very troubling, but they can become painful and debilitating in old age. Treatment is complicated by the fact that arthritis is not a single, clear-cut disease with a single, clear-cut cause. Doctors divide arthritis into two major types: osteoarthritis, which affects the bones, and rheumatoid arthritis, which has an immune component. But in fact, a long list of factors — from diet to infections — can initiate or complicate arthritis, and at this time we still don't know the whole story. Fortunately, we are finding new ways to treat or possibly prevent this problem.

People often suffer mysterious aches and pains in muscles or joints that are difficult to diagnose or treat. They just don't find much relief from the standard medical therapies. They may be suffering from an infectious disease that affects the system, such as Lyme disease, or they may be victims of the vastly underdiagnosed ailment called fibromyalgia. Others suffer from trigger point pain, which may be caused by blockage of nodes of the autonomic nervous system. In this chapter we'll look at some of these lesser-known problems that can affect the musculoskeletal system, as well as exercise patterns, chronic aches and pains, and arthritis.

If we give these problems proper attention now, we can avert many of the syndromes that we think of as typical ailments of the elderly. It is possible to keep the body strong and flexible well into old age.

Exercise—But Don't Kill Yourself

More and more studies show that regular moderate exercise is one of the most powerful ways of maintaining the strength, flexibility, and health of the musculoskeletal system as well as benefiting almost every other organic function of the body, from cardiovascular health to a strong immune system. It's also a means of stretching out or delaying the aging process. Regular exercise can slow the normal loss of lean body mass that comes with aging and allow a person to maintain a higher degree of strength, flexibility, and vigor. It's almost never too late to start gaining these benefits. A recent study of effects of moderate weight-lifting exercise among nursing home residents found that even those of advanced age and feebleness significantly improved in flexibility, energy, freedom from pain, and the ability to get around.

Exercise is also positive for the bones. It helps keep them mineralized and, along with sufficient calcium intake, should be part of any program to prevent osteoporosis. The effects of exercise, or the lack of it, on our bone structure can be startling. When astronauts are on long voyages with sustained weightlessness, their muscles tend to atrophy because they are not pushing against the pull of gravity. But there's an effect on bone mass as well. Astronauts lose a tangible percentage of bone mass on longer space flights — and this happens to healthy, middle-aged men and women who work out regularly as part of their training. It's remarkable that this change can be measured over a period of just days or weeks.

We think of creaky, inflexible joints as a sign of aging, but it may really be a sign of insufficient use. Joints are really amazing mechanisms. What other machinery do we know of in the physical world that can move flexibly and carry weight for decade after decade without breaking down? And joints are a very complex kind of machinery — a system of interface between muscles, bones, tendons, and the blood supply. All of these components benefit from safe exercise and can decline if they don't get it. Joints also contain specialized tissue, cartilage, which cushions the bones, and synovial fluid, which lubricates the joints and keeps them slippery. There is a decline in synovial fluid with age and a concomitant risk of arthritis, which involves damage to the cartilage. Twenty years ago, arthritis sufferers were advised to avoid moving painful joints, but we now know that moderate, gentle exercise can help keep joints flexible and reduce pain, even in advanced arthritis.

Though there are still far too many people who don't get enough regular exercise, the 1970s and 1980s witnessed an explosion of interest in sports and exercise, reflected in the jogging phenomenon, the marathon craze, aerobic exercise classes and videos, and coed urban gyms filled with businessmen and businesswomen wearing Spandex and doing their repetitions, or "reps," on space-age exercise machines. While organized sports were not so common at the beginning of the century, they've become an increasingly important part of high school and college life as well as a big entertainment industry. As a spin-off, amateur athletes now engage very intensely in all kinds of sports, from skiing to handball to triathlons.

It's perhaps ironic that the exercise explosion has engendered a whole new category of physicians — the sports medicine specialists, who deal with syndromes as common as tennis elbow and as arcane as "stair-stepper's feet" a repetitive strain injury caused by excessive use of stair-stepping machines at the gym. In fact, doctors are seeing more and more frustrated, impatient baby boomers who suffer from a bewildering array of strain injuries and chronic pain syndromes caused by obsessive or inappropriate forms of exercise.

The wrong kind of exercise can be dangerous. The *New England Journal of Medicine* recently devoted almost an entire issue to the question of whether exercise is good for the heart. One study showed that people who normally exercised less than once a week were about fifty times more likely to have a heart attack after exercise than people who exercised four or more times a week! This is why couch potatoes who decide to get out and clear the driveway during the first big snowstorm of the year are putting themselves at tremendous risk.

The same risks apply to musculoskeletal injuries, from tendinitis to muscle spasm to joint injury. Someone who feels guilty about not having exercised for years and suddenly starts training for the marathon is running the same risk. Someone who spends most of his time behind a desk and then goes out once a week to run around a tennis court and whack the tennis ball with a good strong serve is really asking for trouble. Sporadic exercise puts enormous strain on muscles, joints, and tendons that haven't been built up to handle this kind of physical force and stress. Sure, you can physically propel yourself around the court, but you're unleashing forces that your body just may not be able to handle safely. If you have a basically sedentary lifestyle but go out once a month for a touch football game, or go skiing two weekends during the winter, you're putting yourself at risk. The consequences are worse if you engage in a sport like tennis or skiing that challenges unusually specific muscle groups.

A Sane Approach to Exercise

I've seen many of my patients get into an exercise program and, after a few months or a year, seem effectively born again. Sometimes their stories are truly astounding, like that of Julie, a 32-year-old young woman with chronic fatigue syndrome who now enters triathlons regularly and has gained tremendous self-esteem because of it.

Let's look at some of the keys to safe, beneficial exercise.

• *Make exercise a regular habit — avoid intermittent bouts of intense activity.*

We've already looked at the dangers of intermittent paroxysmal exercise in an otherwise sedentary lifestyle. The most beneficial exercise pattern is to do something three to four times a week, even if none of the sessions are terribly long or intense. This is much better for you, and safer, than doing one big workout or sports session on the weekend. Consider three or four short running sessions, or even long walks, if you have trouble scheduling anything else.

• *If you haven't been physically active for a long time, start very gradually.*

If you're not used to exercise, you won't have a good internal gauge of just how much you're pushing yourself. The first couple of times you go jogging or take a dance class, you may find the experience so new and exhilarating that you seriously overdo it. But if you're limp and sore for a week after you start a new activity, this is a sign that you did too much. Give yourself a time limit or activity limit when you start an exercise program, so that you stop long before you're exhausted and sore.

• *If you're starting a specialized sport or activity, find out whether you're going to be stressing specific muscle groups, and deal with this appropriately.*

There are two ways to deal with this. One is to gradually build up the specialized muscle groups *before* you start to stress them with the sport you're interested in. This is the theory behind the specialized exercise machines that work the muscles used for skiing. But be careful not to plunge into a sport while at the same time trying to build the specialized muscles — this is just doubling the strain.

The other approach is cross-training. Simply vary your exercise patterns: switch between two or three different activities — a little swimming, a little running, a little tennis. Realize that you're not going to build up the speed or skill level in any one activity that you would if you were to specialize.

A patient of mine told me he'd once decided to take up modern dance for the exercise and the fun of it. Mark was using the Graham technique, which is based on the energy and the kind of movement that comes from contracting and releasing the muscles of the lower back. He really got into it and was going to classes several times a week but not doing any other exercise. One day he went to class pretty tired, was doing those lower back movements, and later that evening found himself totally immobilized with a very painful spasm of the muscles in his lower back. One side of his back was in spasm, so he was all twisted up, and he couldn't walk or even sit up without severe, shooting pain. He was on his back for two weeks and hobbled around with a cane for a month after that. When he tried to go back to dance classes he felt he was on the verge of another spasm. It took a very long period of rest and physical therapy before his back completely healed.

It's not hard to see where Mark went wrong. He'd basically been leading a sedentary lifestyle, and while the Graham technique was a good overall workout, with stretching and aerobic exercise, it was placing an especially heavy strain on back muscles that were weak from lack of use. Mark was enjoying the classes and the energy boost so much that he wasn't really aware of this weak link in the system until it caught up with him. Unfortunately, this is an all-too-common pattern.

- *Listen to your body — don't ignore chronic pain.*

Because exercise makes you feel better, and because sports or other physical activities can be really enjoyable, they can be habit forming. This is all to the good, right? What could be wrong with a good habit like exercise? Well, the downside is an exercise habit that becomes a psychological addiction, so that you want to keep doing it even if you've suffered an injury or strain. This is a syndrome professional athletes get into. They suffer a strain or injury, push themselves to get back on the field before they're completely healed, and suffer a reinjury. This can lead to chronic pain and debilitation that are even harder to treat and take longer to cure. Amateurs get into this too — they want to keep on running on that sore knee and then drive it farther and farther into trauma.

There's a physical process that plays into this syndrome. Exercise causes the release of neurotransmitters called endorphins, which mask pain and produce a kind of natural euphoria. Runners are always talking about the "runner's high." Dancers know about this too. They may be hobbling around with all kinds of aches and pains, but once they start moving they feel fine — until later. This experience can be very deceptive — if your knee doesn't hurt while you're running, you figure it can't be a serious problem. Well, that's just wrong.

The moral is that if you've got a chronically sore knee or a bad foot, but it doesn't really bother you "that much" when you're exercising, stop and take this seriously. Try switching to an alternative exercise that doesn't stress that particular joint or muscle group. Have an orthopedist or chiropractor look at the painful area and tell you what is going on. No matter how enjoyable your activity is, it's better to pull back a little and have the possibility of continuing later, perhaps at a less intense level, than to keep driving on until you have to stop anyway, permanently, because of irreversible damage that may affect even your normal daily activities.

• *Consider an orthopedic or chiropractic checkup to see whether you have any quirks in your musculoskeletal system that might predispose you to strain or injury.*

This is advisable if you plan to take up a heavy sports or exercise program. Find an orthopedist who will take time with you or less surgically oriented health care professionals, such as chiropractors or physiatrists (physicians who practice rehabilitative medicine), who will give you a more prevention-oriented check-up.

If you're beginning to run or take up related sports, you might want to visit a good sports podiatrist who can analyze the wear patterns on your shoes, check your footfalls, and offer corrective exercises or shoe inserts called orthotics to reduce stress on your feet, ankles, or knees. This could also help you prevent serious injury. One of my patients took up flamenco dancing for recreation until she began to experience pain in the ball of one foot. She eventually consulted a podiatrist, who told her she had a dropped metatarsal: the ball of the injured foot was congenitally lower than normal. It turned out she'd actually mashed the bone there, and had to wear orthotics to walk without pain. Needless to say, she gave up the flamenco dancing. If she'd known about this quirk in her bone structure before she started, she might have worn orthotics and done exercises to prevent the injury.

• *If you develop chronic pain, consult with a trainer or professional to see if you need movement retraining.*

Ergonomics, the study of safe, efficient movement, began with scientists looking at movement patterns in factory workers and has since been extended to sports. An athlete may adopt a nonergonomic movement pattern, such as a faulty gait as a runner or a faulty swing as a tennis player, that could induce chronic injury. A sports medicine doctor or a good trainer should be able to analyze your movement patterns and recommend changes. This can apply to musicians and dancers, as well. In fact, there is a specialized clinic at Roosevelt–St. Luke's, a major New York teaching hospital, where the staff will take videotapes of your movements as a musician, a dancer, or an athlete and help you analyze them so you can learn to make necessary adjustments.

Alternative Exercise: The Wisdom of the East

As a medical student, I once attended a lecture by Michio Kushi, the founder of the macrobiotic movement. At that time he was in his sixties, a seemingly ageless, slender gentleman. At one point, talking about physical flexibility as an indicator of biological aging, he proceeded to do a series of stretching and floor exercises. He got into positions that absolutely defied any of the younger people in the audience to match. It was almost embarrassing — we were in our twenties and couldn't begin to stretch our bodies the way he was doing. And this was a time when I was swimming and running heroically and thought I was in terrific shape. In his quiet way, Kushi was illustrating the alternative approach to exercise and conditioning, which is to maintain suppleness and flexibility. In fact, Michio Kushi's exercises come out of a long tradition of preventive therapy in East Asia, one that embraces hatha yoga, t'ai chi, and others. All these practices work against the stiffness of aging, the rusty-suit-of-armor syndrome, the loss of flexibility that means you can't touch your toes anymore.

Most strikingly, these are gentle, "friendly" exercises that people can maintain for many years, well into old age. In China, people of all ages are up at dawn in the parks and public squares, going through the simple stretching movements of t'ai chi. Men and women of ninety do these light, lithe movements, which keep the joints flexible and stretch the muscles.

Our Western concept of the body has led to forceful, energetic, high-speed, high-impact, competitive sports and exercises. Yoga and t'ai chi take a completely different approach. They are the "yin" to our Western "yang," and they represent a different concept of the body from ours. They are not competitive, though they can be done either alone or sociably in groups. They induce peacefulness and relaxation rather than tension and excitement. They promote flexibility rather than strength, range of motion rather than dexterity, flow of energy through the whole body rather than concentration of energy in individual muscles and joints. The stretching and gentle movements of yoga and t'ai chi can also "massage" the lymphatic system, promoting the removal of toxins and metabolic wastes from the body. There are good reasons for making one or both of these practices part of your overall exercise plan. They are certainly in keeping with one motto of the medical profession: "First, do no harm." If you take up yoga, observe this caution: do not zealously force yourself into extreme positions too soon. This can cause injury. A good teacher will show you how to start small and gradually work your way up.

Aches and Pains—The Garden Varieties

Patrick is a college teacher plagued by lower back pain. He can swim with no problem but can't sit at a desk for more than an hour without having to lie down on the floor and pull his knees up to his chin to relax his back. Melissa sits for long hours every day writing at her personal computer. Now her wrists are starting to feel sore and her hands seem weak, so that it's hard to pick up a glass of water. Marty owns his own retail business and has started to feel strange tingling sensations in the fingers of his right hand after a few hours on the job. He wakes up every morning with his neck so stiff and sore that he has trouble lifting his head. Beyond the rusty armor syndrome and the athletic injury, many people in their thirties and forties find themselves dealing with constant chronic pain that seems to have no apparent cause. These pains often strike the back, the neck, the shoulder, the hands, and the wrists.

Scores of books have been written on back pain alone, and it's beyond the scope of this book to deal with each of these problems in detail. But we can take a quick look at some of the more common musculoskeletal ailments, which can be upsetting when they come on without warning, and at the preventive measures and alternative treatments that can help relieve much of this type of pain and suffering.

Neck and Back Pain

Though most people have one or the other, both are caused by conditions that affect the spine. The spine is built from a series of bones called vertebrae, which are separated by disks of cartilage that keep the bones from grinding together. When a disk herniates, or "slips," a small bulge of cartilage pushes out from within the disk and can press against and pinch one of the nerves that extends out from between the vertebrae, or even press into one of the nerves that run down the center of the spinal column. This can cause local pain and inflammation but can also project pain along the length of the nerve as it branches out from the spinal column. A herniated disk in the neck can cause shoulder pain, pain in the arm, and tingling or numbness in the fingers. This very common syndrome usually seems worse on awakening, after the neck has stiffened or twisted in sleep. A herniated disk in the lumbar spine, or lower back, can cause back pain, tingling or numbness in the foot, or sciatica: a shooting pain that runs along the length of one of the nerves extending through the buttocks and down into the leg. Whether in the neck or the back, this condition can be extremely painful and debilitating and can prevent normal work and activity. Over time, pressure on a nerve can cause a state of chronic inflammation, which is difficult to treat.

The standard treatments for this condition include anti-inflammatory medications, bed rest, traction, and microsurgery to remove the herniated portion of the disk. In extreme conditions, the entire disk of cartilage is sometimes removed, and a "splint" of bone from elsewhere in the body is used to fuse the two vertebrae together so that they can't move and grind against each other. Surgery is not always effective, however, and the problem persists in some people even after surgery. Alternative treatments include chiropractic, physical therapy, and acupuncture, which we'll discuss later.

It's worth mentioning, too, that disk abnormalities may not always be the cause of the pain. In one study, MRI scans were used to examine the spines of people with no back pain. Two thirds of them had spinal abnormalities, including herniated and degenerated disks. If these problems had been seen in someone with back pain, they probably would have led to surgery. The researchers suggested that it may be sheer coincidence when a person with back pain is found to have a disk abnormality and that physicians may do surgery simply because they have a bias toward *doing* something.

Muscle Spasms

Athletes are familiar with the charley horse, or muscle spasm, that can cause a calf muscle to tighten up like a rock—a painful rock. This is caused by a kind of feedback loop in the autonomic nervous system that causes nerve signals to amplify repeatedly, cueing a muscle to contract over and over again, and blocking the signals that permit it to release. If you're exercising, this can happen to a muscle that is weakened or tired, that's been pushed too far. But it can happen in equal or lesser degree to muscles in the back, the shoulders, and the neck that are constantly and unconsciously contracted or stressed. Many people express emotional tension in the body, unconsciously pulling their shoulders tight or tensing other muscle groups. We're usually unaware of the tremendous force and strength that muscles exert just to hold the body and the neck erect and in place. Muscles of flexion and extension are pulling against each other even when we're sitting at rest. Large muscles of the leg may be gently and rhythmically pulsing in response to autonomic signals from the brain in order to maintain the venous circulation that keeps blood flowing back to the heart.

After days or weeks or months of extended stress, these muscles can go into mild spasm, remaining constantly contracted, or extreme spasm of the kind that can really immobilize you. The muscle spasm itself is painful, and if it pulls on the spine it can contribute to problems like herniated disks. Muscle spasms can be caused by circulatory problems, and they especially plague athletes who are cross-training, when they switch from running to swimming and cool down warm muscles too quickly. Deficiencies in calcium, magnesium, and potassium can all make someone prone to muscle spasms.

Muscle spasm can be treated by massage, gentle stretching and, if it becomes chronic, by physical therapy. There are exquisitely sensitive stretch receptors called Golgi receptors in muscle tissue that send signals to the brain, indicating whether a muscle is relaxed or tensed. A trick used by massage therapists and chiropractors is to put extreme pressure on a muscle even to the point of pain for a few seconds, which will send a signal to the brain that the muscle should be relaxed. One of the best ways of preventing or treating chronic muscle spasm is a practice of gentle stretching, such as yoga. A physical therapist or movement therapist can help you become aware of unconscious habits of muscle tension that you can then consciously work against.

Repetitive Strain Injury

Factory and industrial workers have long suffered from injuries caused by working at an assembly line or machine and repeating the same motion, in the same way, day after day after day. With the advent of personal computers, office workers, writers, and information managers now suffer from this type of injury. Sitting for long hours at a computer terminal working a keyboard can set people up for carpal tunnel syndrome, a painful condition in which nerves are compressed in the narrow carpal tunnel within the wrist joint, causing numbness, tingling, pain, and weakness of the hand and fingers. A rather painful test for this is the EMG, or electromyelogram, which involves sending electric currents through the arm and fingers. Writers and other computer users can wind up with multiple strain syndrome, with pain in the neck, shoulders, back, and/or wrists, caused by sitting for long hours hunched in an unnatural position at a computer, typing away.

There is a surgical procedure for carpal tunnel syndrome, which involves cutting into the wrists and enlarging the passageway for the nerves. This procedure is painful, has a long recovery time, and does not always give 100 percent improvement. As an alternative, I first prescribe complete rest accompanied by vitamin B_6 supplements, which act as a pain blocker and are especially helpful with this condition. B_6 can also act as a natural diuretic, relieving some pressure caused by water retention.

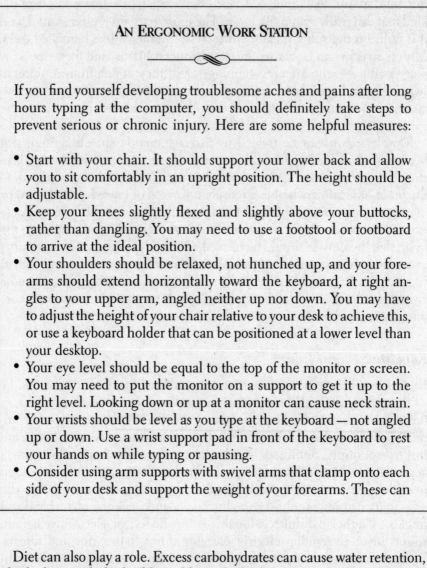

AN ERGONOMIC WORK STATION

If you find yourself developing troublesome aches and pains after long hours typing at the computer, you should definitely take steps to prevent serious or chronic injury. Here are some helpful measures:

- Start with your chair. It should support your lower back and allow you to sit comfortably in an upright position. The height should be adjustable.
- Keep your knees slightly flexed and slightly above your buttocks, rather than dangling. You may need to use a footstool or footboard to arrive at the ideal position.
- Your shoulders should be relaxed, not hunched up, and your forearms should extend horizontally toward the keyboard, at right angles to your upper arm, angled neither up nor down. You may have to adjust the height of your chair relative to your desk to achieve this, or use a keyboard holder that can be positioned at a lower level than your desktop.
- Your eye level should be equal to the top of the monitor or screen. You may need to put the monitor on a support to get it up to the right level. Looking down or up at a monitor can cause neck strain.
- Your wrists should be level as you type at the keyboard — not angled up or down. Use a wrist support pad in front of the keyboard to rest your hands on while typing or pausing.
- Consider using arm supports with swivel arms that clamp onto each side of your desk and support the weight of your forearms. These can

Diet can also play a role. Excess carbohydrates can cause water retention, which along with the buildup of fat in the body tissue can cause additional pressure in the wrist area.

Also, many who suffer from carpal tunnel syndrome have hidden hypothyroidism, especially if they have other symptoms such as low body temperature, susceptibility to colds, dry skin, or lethargy. We can then use natural thyroid medication and make a medical end run around the need for surgery.

So carpal tunnel syndrome can often indicate some kind of metabolic imbalance that needs to be addressed. The exception, of course, is when it is caused by repeated physical strain and stress, in which case we're dealing with musculoskeletal injury and can apply the same treatment strategies of be especially helpful. They completely relieve your shoulders of the need to support several pounds of the dead weight of your extended forearms for hour after hour. They're available at most big office supply outlets.

- Typing at a keyboard forces you to hold your hands unnaturally together, bent outward at the wrists, and rotated downward so that the backs of the hands are flat. Consider an ergonomic keyboard, which is split and even angled upward in the middle, so that the wrists don't have to be twisted.

- Make sure there's no glare or reflection coming off the screen that can cause eyestrain. Use a hood or shield for the monitor to cut off glare, if necessary.

- Stay at least eighteen inches from the face of the monitor, and use a low-emission monitor to avoid potential hazards from electromagnetic radiation.

- If possible, use a high-resolution monitor to avoid eyestrain from reading fuzzy letters and figures. Use a noninterlaced monitor to reduce monitor flicker.

- Don't forget to breathe! Some people go into a kind of suspended animation in front of a computer, holding their bodies in a tensed, frozen position and almost holding their breath. Put up a note or other physical memory jogger to remind you to breathe deeply and keep your body relaxed.

- Most important of all, take regular breaks. Get up and move around a little every fifteen or twenty minutes. Stand up, stretch, touch your toes, and shake out your hands and arms and shoulders. Keep a clock on your desk so you don't forget to stretch, or use a timer if you have to.

extended rest, physical therapy, and behavioral adjustments that we would with skier's knee or tennis elbow.

Patients also respond well to acupuncture, chiropractic, and a new form of therapy called cold laser. But the best approach to carpal tunnel syndrome and other repetitive stress injuries is preventive: setting up an ergonomic work environment and avoiding sustained, uninterrupted movement patterns. See the box for tips on preventive measures.

Bad Movement Habits

Jeanne came to me with a history of knee problems. She'd had persistent, chronic pain and had received cortisone injections and, finally, underwent knee surgery, which hadn't really helped. Yet, I didn't see signs of classic arthritis, or Lyme disease, or the other conditions that could cause this joint pain. As we were doing a workup, I noticed that there was something odd about her gait. At first I ascribed it to her pain itself, but then I began to wonder. I asked her to see a podiatrist, who identified an aberration in the bone structure of her foot and prescribed orthotic inserts for her shoes to correct it. Shortly thereafter, her knee pain began to abate, and within a few months it had nearly vanished. Her manner of walking had been placing unusual stress on the knee joint.

This was not an isolated case. I've seen it with several patients with knee problems and even with hip or back problems. Jeanne had a structural abnormality in her foot, but some people will unconsciously develop an awkward gait that causes them to stress or grind their other joints. Retraining by a physical therapist can often alleviate this problem. Athletes and musicians, too, can fall into bad movement habits that can cause chronic pain or even injury. A tennis player may have a faulty swing; a violinist may be forcing the shoulder into an unnatural position. Sports medicine specialists are often able to help them retrain their movement patterns to relieve the problem.

CAN FOODS CAUSE BACK PAIN?

Though it's not well known, there is evidence that some kinds of chronic muscle pain, the "achy body syndrome," may actually be caused by food allergies. We do know that an allergic reaction can manifest itself in many ways, from classic inflammation and congestion of the respiratory system to more subtle symptoms, including stomach upset, recurring headaches, tiredness, and achy body. (See chapter 4 on the immune system for more on allergies.) Inflammation is a frequent symptom of the allergic reaction and can affect muscles and joints as well as sinuses. Environmental physician Sherry Rogers has told of how she was plagued by chronic lower back pain until she was able to identify her own food and chemical allergies. If you suffer from muscle or back pain with no otherwise evident cause, you might consider trying an elimination diet, under the supervision of a holistic doctor or allergist, to try to identify inflammation-causing allergies.

Fibromyalgia

This troubling but little-known ailment is one of the most commonly underdiagnosed or misdiagnosed diseases in the United States today. It strikes predominantly women, typically develops when they are in their thirties or forties, and is characterized by achy body, muscle pain, and sleep disturbances. It can lead to insomnia, irritable bowel syndrome, and depression and is a real source of misery. A typical patient is someone who falls asleep with relative ease but sleeps lightly with frequent awakenings and wakes up exhausted. There are very specific symptoms, so it can be diagnosed if a doctor takes the care to look for it. But the causes and disease process are not well understood. Fibromyalgia seems closely related to chronic fatigue syndrome, and some researchers see it as a specific variant of CFS. It's thought not just to be a condition of muscle inflammation but to involve a feedback loop in the nervous system that originates in the brain and repeatedly amplifies and transmits pain symptoms to specific points in the body. In fact, there are seventeen specific pairs of trigger points of pain that confirm the diagnosis. Some people may suffer additionally from "leaky gut" syndrome — a disruption of intestinal flora causing inflammatory immune reactions that can contribute to symptoms of fibromyalgia. Fibromyalgia is one of a newly identified range of ailments, from CFS to some autoimmune diseases, that seem to operate in a subtle cross-systemic way and are difficult to resolve.

Rheumatologists are familiar with fibromyalgia and diagnose it frequently by ruling out other typical causes of muscle pain: inflammation, arthritis, and more obscure autoimmune problems. To make a more specific diagnosis, the physician will palpate the specific trigger points that have been mapped across the body, including points on the shoulder blades and the forearms. Normally everyone will feel some tenderness when these points are pressed, but someone who has fibromyalgia will really squawk. Despite the pressure points, this can be tricky to diagnose even by a qualified rheumatologist, so it's not likely you can self-diagnose by pressing your arms and shoulders. Not everybody who has aches and pains is suffering from fibromyalgia, but a specialist can recognize some of the patterns.

How is it treated? Conventionally with antidepressants, such as Elavil or Pamelor, which are thought to disrupt the neurological feedback pattern and enable normal sleep. Magnesium supplements, either taken orally or injected, sometimes help, and the condition sometimes responds to acupuncture or chiropractic. Some fibromyalgia patients benefit from supplementation with DHEA, an adrenal hormone, particularly if their blood levels of this hormone are found to be low. Those with "leaky gut" syndrome can additionally be aided by detoxification regimens.

Troubleshooting and Treating Your Aches and Pains

I believe there's a strong psychological component to all pain syndromes and that a reassuring, healing ministration from a doctor can work wonders.

It's important to talk about stress level, and how the pain is making the patient feel, and what impact it's having on his or her life. In any pain syndrome, the autonomic nervous system is involved, as well as the parts of the brain that involve emotion and mood. It's all too easy for chronic pain to trigger depression and anxiety that in turn amplifies and increases the pain.

Surgery can produce wonderful results. I once worked with an acupuncturist who had a knee problem, which he had had treated by acupuncture in vain for many years. I finally suggested arthroscopic surgery, and he was better within a week, walking without pain and playing basketball a month later. But we shouldn't start out by thinking of surgery as a panacea. If there is an obvious physical finding, a clear-cut injury, we still need to offer something beyond a ticket to the operating theater. Physical therapy, stretching, gentle exercise, acupuncture, hydrotherapy — all can offer some relief. If we try the conservative therapies, starting with rest, physical therapy, perhaps acupuncture, and they don't really seem to help, then it's time to start thinking about surgery. Right now, let's take a closer look at some nonsurgical therapies, both conventional and alternative.

Pain-Killers

When you first see your doctor about joint pain, back pain, or muscle spasm, unless it's unusually severe, nine times out of ten you'll get a recommendation to try aspirin or another of the family of medications called nonsteroidal anti-inflammatory drugs, or NSAIDs, for short. These drugs reduce pain sensations and also block the release of prostaglandins, a group of hormonelike substances that can promote inflammation. Some are prescription only; others, like aspirin and ibuprofen, can be found on drugstore and supermarket shelves in various brand names and dosages, all the way up to the high-dosage "arthritis formulas." They are effective in the temporary treatment of moderate pain but have the potential for causing stomach disorders as well as other long-term side effects. Long-term use may also cause kidney disorders and tend to induce high blood pressure. There's also some evidence from a study of people with arthritis of the hip that while these drugs may ameliorate pain, they certainly don't change the course of joint disease. Over the long term they may even accelerate the course of joint degeneration.

The NSAIDs typically cause some stomach upset, which is why we take aspirin in buffered form, as well as some degree of ulceration and bleeding in the stomach. They can also cause tiny pinpoint perforations in the surface of the small intestine, and this has troubling implications. The small intestine has a semipermeable surface that permits nutrients to pass into the bloodstream, but it presents a protective barrier against other food components that need to be kept out of the bloodstream, to avoid setting off

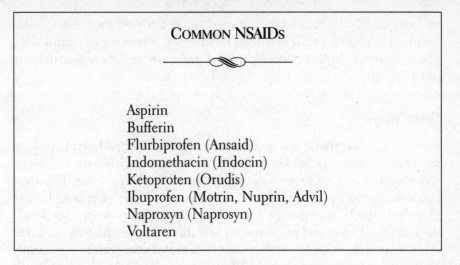

COMMON NSAIDs

Aspirin
Bufferin
Flurbiprofen (Ansaid)
Indomethacin (Indocin)
Ketoproten (Orudis)
Ibuprofen (Motrin, Nuprin, Advil)
Naproxyn (Naprosyn)
Voltaren

an allergic immune reaction. If you damage the integrity of the intestinal wall, you can induce "leaky gut syndrome," which is thought to be part of the mechanism of allergy, autoimmune disease, and even arthritis itself! Long-term use of NSAIDs may weaken the intestinal barrier and thus allow allergenic substances to pass that may actually promote inflammation in the joints.

INTELLIGENT MEDICINE TIP:

As an alternative to oral NSAIDs, ask your doctor about a prescription for ketoprofen organogel or ibuprofen organogel, topical ointments containing one of these two NSAIDs, which are then absorbed directly through the skin. These avoid the problems of stomach upset and gastrointestinal bleeding.

Other medications sometimes used for joint pain are the steroids themselves, which block inflammation in a different way. Orthopedists often use steroid injections to treat bursitis, a chronic inflammation of the bursae, which are small cushioning sacs found in several joints including the shoulder joint. Steroid injections work quite well in the short term; they can relieve pain quickly and completely. Unfortunately, the effect wears off, and the second injection is a little less helpful, the third a little less than that, and so on. You can only give a limited number of steroid injections to a joint, after which you run the risk of actually killing off tissue and weakening bones.

Some doctors give out prescriptions for a codeine/Tylenol combination that certainly blocks pain, but does nothing for the underlying causes of chronic pain. It also has all the characteristics of a powerful narcotic: people build up a tolerance to it and require a higher dosage for the painkilling effect, there is a dulling effect on mental processes, and there is a high risk of addiction.

Back Surgery

Here's a typical scenario that leads to back surgery. You bend over to pick up something — a box of books, a TV — and as you straighten up you feel a shooting pain in your lower back. It's sore for the rest of the day, but when you wake up the next morning it's more than sore. There's a painful knot of clenched muscle in your back, you can't sit up except by propping yourself up with your hands, and when you try to walk your whole body is twisted to one side, and stepping on one leg makes it feel as if your bones are painfully grinding against each other. You call your general care physician, who tells you to get complete bed rest for a few days. But that doesn't seem to help, so your doctor orders an MRI and sends you to an orthopedic specialist. The specialist prescribes bed rest and muscle relaxants, but your MRI shows evidence of some abnormalities — maybe something that looks like a compressed disk. And you find yourself on the way to the operating room for back surgery that may or may not cure your pain.

A look at some of the statistics for back surgery makes you wonder how rational these decisions for surgery are. To begin with, the United States has the highest rate of back surgery in the world, the South has the highest rate of any region in the country, and Boston has five times the rate of that in New Haven, Connecticut. Do Bostonians really suffer more from back pain than New Havenites? Or does Boston just have a large contingent of aggressive orthopedic surgeons and a good selection of hospitals? I think it's the latter.

In fact, even the standard recommendation of bed rest may not be so effective. A recent Finnish study divided people suffering from back pain into three different treatment groups. One group had complete bed rest, the second group had physical therapy to try to release knotted back muscles, and the third group was told to just try to go about their daily activities as well as they could. Guess which group had the shortest recovery time? The people who just tried to go about their business! In light of studies like this, the government has recently issued new guidelines recommending less reliance on MRIs — which are likely to show some kind of abnormality in almost anyone — and less back surgery. This is all to the good, since there are powerful forces, such as the demands of malpractice insurance companies, that tend to push doctors to prescribe more and more expensive tests. Of course, some people can be helped by back surgery, but they are a lot fewer than are currently getting the surgery. A colleague who does this type of surgery says his main job is to determine who can really benefit from it and to rule out the numerous people who won't.

Knee Surgery

Professional athletes often seem to have knee surgery the way most people have a haircut. This may be part of the price they pay for success in a physically punishing career. These highly paid professionals are used to dealing with high pain levels and will fearlessly undergo repeated surgery or have repeated steroid injections because these procedures support their very good livelihood. They can make their millions and then retire and just coast. Unfortunately, the passion for knee surgery seems to be filtering into the growing ranks of amateur athletes. These weekend warriors — joggers, skiers, tennis players — are delivering unusual forms of physical stress to their knees in the form of pounding on pavement, twisting on skis, the sudden stops and turns of tennis, the concussions of contact sports. What's worse, they usually load this extreme physical stress onto bodies that have not been built up, strengthened, and kept flexible through the sort of daily physical training that athletes engage in.

It's no wonder these people have knee problems. And when they do, they're despondent because they can't jog or can't ski, since it may be their major recreation and source of unadulterated pleasure in life. Postinjury depression is a common, recognized phenomenon in sports medicine. People get fixated on performing at a certain level, perhaps because they get "addicted" to those feel-good hormones, the endorphins, that are generated during exercise. They want a quick fix that will let them immediately resume their full level of punishing physical activity, without pain. So they're increasingly turning to surgeons, looking for miracle procedures that will patch them up and get them back on the jogging track or the slopes. And many surgeons are only too happy to oblige, whether or not this is really appropriate for an amateur athlete.

I counseled a woman like this, an avid skier who was on the slopes every single winter weekend. She developed a lot of pain in one knee and was devastated because it was grounding her at the height of the ski season. A surgeon told her, "You have a very, very slight tear in one of your tendons, and we can repair it, or you can just wait it out with rest and physical therapy." She came to me for advice and I said, "Don't do the surgery. It's sometimes remarkably effective, but not always, and some people are left with pain that just won't go away." I told her, "You may be able to beat this but you'll have to take a completely different approach. You'll need to get into physical therapy, build up the muscles that keep your knee in place, and gradually prepare yourself for your next ski season — which will not be this winter, but next winter." She was crushed, so I said, "Make it a fun thing, get a kayak, develop your aerobic ability by rowing this summer, do the upper body exercises you've neglected, and meanwhile strengthen your knees." To her delight, she began gradually getting back into skiing the next season. Starting off gently, she was skiing at top form by the end of the season and had avoided an unnecessary operation.

The watchword here is patience. People need to think more conservatively and rationally about these kinds of injuries and resist the irrational need to continue a pleasurable activity at whatever cost. They may need to step back from the activity that caused the injury so as to avoid a succession of operations and chronic pain. Rest for the injured body part, physical therapy, and strengthening exercises require patience and discipline, but the chances of long-term payoff are much greater.

Nutritional Therapies

Inflammation is a natural process that actually has a protective function in case of injury. Blood vessels are dilated and immune cells are rushed to the injured area in order to clean up and remove toxins and damaged cells. Certain foods and nutrients can modulate the complex cellular metabolism that sustains chronic inflammation. They will not relieve pain quickly in the way that conventional medications do but generally have to be used over a period of weeks and months before they take effect. But they will affect the underlying physiological mechanisms of inflammation and degeneration, which the NSAIDs do not.

First among these nutrients are the *antioxidants* and the *antioxidant precursors* and *cofactors*. Whenever there is an inflammatory reaction in the body, toxic substances called free radicals are released. These free radicals can cause further damage to tissue, which again increases the inflammation in a kind of vicious circle. Enhancing the antioxidant reaction in the body can help relieve symptoms caused by inflammation. (See chapter 16 for food sources for some of these nutrients.)

• *Vitamin C.* This is an essential antioxidant, which can support healing of musculoskeletal injuries and relieve chronic pain. Ester-C and buffered C are both more easily tolerated in the gastrointestinal tract. Recommended dosage: up to 2000–3000 milligrams per day.

• *Bioflavonoids* such as quercetin and catechin are often utilized as companion nutrients with vitamin C. They have an antioxidant effect and also diminish capillary permeability, which can directly reduce joint inflammation and swelling.

• *Vitamin E* has both an anti-inflammatory and an immune regulating effect. Recommended dosage: up to 800 International Units per day.

• *Zinc, copper, and manganese* are cofactors for the activity of superoxide dismutase (SOD), the body's premier naturally produced anti-inflammatory enzyme. SOD is used in injectable form in Europe, in which form it acts as a relatively weak anti-inflammatory. Augmenting the body's own SOD with manganese, zinc, and copper, provides a stronger antioxidant effect. Recommended dosage: copper, 2 milligrams twice daily; zinc, 30 milligrams twice daily; manganese, 50 milligrams twice daily. Zinc and manganese also function directly as antioxidants. Excess zinc can create copper deficiency and depress immune function, so it's important not to consume more than 90 milligrams per day.

• *N-acetyl-cysteine* is an amino acid and *selenium* is a mineral that together function as precursors for glutathione peroxidase, another of the body's own natural antioxidants. Recommended dosage: N-acetyl-cysteine, 600-milligram capsule three times daily; selenium, 200-microgram tablet twice daily.

• *Carotenoids* make up an important family of antioxidants from which the body can also synthesize vitamin A, an important immune-enhancing nutrient, which is also essential for tissue repair. Recommended dosage: 25,000 International Units daily.

• *Vitamin A* assists with cellular repair and regeneration. Recommended dosage: 10,000 International Units daily.

Many health food stores offer special antioxidant tablets or capsules that combine all of the above factors. It may be necessary to boost them with additional vitamin C and vitamin E.

• *Essential fatty acids*, including EPA (eicosapentaenoic acid), GLA (gamma-linolenic acid), and linolenic acid, have been shown to help in treating arthritis, and particularly rheumatoid arthritis, which is immune-mediated. These oils work together through different pathways to reduce inflammatory prostaglandins. Linolenic acid is found in flaxseed oil and in cold-water fish such as tuna, salmon, herring, trout, mackerel, sardines, and cod liver. GLA is found in vegetable sources, including primrose oil, borage oil, and black currant seed oil. (See dosages below.)

• *Borage oil* is a source of GLA, or gamma-linolenic acid. It has been shown to improve symptoms of rheumatoid arthritis as well as other types of musculoskeletal pain. Recent studies have shown that a 1.5-grams (1500-milligrams) daily dose of GLA over a period of twenty-four weeks provides benefits in the treatment of rheumatoid arthritis. This is contrary to prior studies in which GLA did not produce that effect. In those studies, however, a much lower amount was given, and the source was evening primrose oil, which delivers less GLA. Recommended dosage: six 240-milligram capsules of GLA per day. It may be necessary to build up the dosage gradually to establish tolerance.

• *Fish oil* is a source of EPA, or eicosapentaenoic acid, an omega-3 oil, which has similar effects to those of GLA through a related but different metabolic pathway. Recommended dosage: two to three 1000- or 1200-milligram capsules three times daily. Flaxseed oil in the same amounts provides a vegetarian alternative.

Other nutrients are able to relieve pain and slow degenerative processes through different means.

• *Vitamin B$_6$* has been shown to reduce neurological pain and may help with pain caused by pinched nerves, such as carpal tunnel syndrome. It may also help with arthritic symptoms. Recommended dosage: 50–200 milligrams daily. **Warning:** higher doses of vitamin B$_6$ may cause toxic neurological side effects, especially when it is taken alone without complementary B vitamins and magnesium.

• *Bromelain*, an anti-inflammatory enzyme derived from the pinapple plant, has been shown to reduce joint swelling and impairment of mobility. Recommended dosage: 500–1500 milligrams, two or three times daily.

• *Glucosamine sulfate* is naturally present in joint cartilage and has been proposed as a therapy for arthritis and possibly disk problems. Dosage: 500–1000 milligrams two or three times daily.

Physical Therapy

The term *physical therapy* is a bit of a catchall for a group of healing practices that include massage, stretching, ultrasound, electrostimulation, heat and cold applications, and muscle strengthening. A physical therapist will know which tendons, bones, and specific muscle groups are involved in a pain syndrome and can massage muscles and teach stretching exercises to release spasms and "knots." The therapist will also teach specific exercises designed to strengthen muscles that are causing misalignment or joint pain because they're underdeveloped. For example, weak stomach muscles can put extra stress on the lower back, and a weak quadriceps muscle in the leg can put strain on the knee. Since muscles usually work in opposing groups — one contracts while the opposing one extends — it's sometimes helpful to strengthen the muscles that pull against a muscle that's in chronic spasm. Cold applications can reduce inflammation; heat can relax a muscle group and increase healing circulation. Ultrasound can relax deep muscle tissue; electrostimulation can relax muscle spasms by overloading them with neural messages.

Chiropractic

Some people may wonder why a medical doctor would recommend chiropractors, but the truth is that they can play a key role in our health care system. Chiropractors can be especially helpful in dealing with low back pain, sciatica, neck pain, and other syndromes related to the spine. If you have back pain, it's reasonable to make a chiropractor's office your first stop. A responsible chiropractor will make a diagnosis, may take X-rays, and will suggest whether or not you might benefit from a trial of chiropractic manipulation of the spine. If it helps, so much the better. If not, it's a harmless therapy and you can go ahead and see an orthopedist. It's interesting that while American orthopedists generally offer drug therapy or surgery or appliances, or will recommend a physical therapist, English orthopedists are also trained to manipulate the spine. Many of them become quite adept at manipulation and perform some of the services that chiropractors do here.

The word *chiropractic* comes from the Greek, meaning "work of the hands." There is some evidence suggesting that Greek and Roman physicians applied this kind of therapy. (In medieval Europe doctors were sometimes called "chirurgeons.") In the nineteenth century, an American named Daniel David Palmer developed the principles of modern chiropractic. Palmer maintained that many health problems, not just musculoskeletal problems, are caused by a misalignment of vertebrae in the spine, which in turn puts pressure on nerves that run through the spine and out between the vertebrae to all parts of the body. He called such a misalignment a subluxation, which is the medical term for a partial dislocation of a joint. Some people feel he was visionary; others think he was a little fanatical. We do know that a slipped or herniated disk between two vertebrae can definitely pinch nerves and cause pain extending through a leg or an arm. But while the autonomic nervous system contributes to virtually every physical problem in the body, it's clear that merely manipulating the spine doesn't provide relief for every kind of physical ailment.

Still, the so-called straight chiropractors, who confine their practice to dealing with the bony structures of the body, can provide a great deal of relief and a healing touch for many musculoskeletal problems. They don't claim to be able to "adjust" your spine to reduce the intensity of your flu symptoms and are very conservative about getting involved with other areas like nutrition or treating other kinds of diseases. They are trained to recognize what they should treat and what they shouldn't treat. In fact, some of my best referrals have been from chiropractors who have said, "I'm not happy with what I know about your condition. I don't want to treat you, but I'd like you to see Dr. Hoffman to find out what's going on." Such patients have turned out to have everything from prostate problems to cancer to severe inflammatory disease and, in one memorable case, a rare tuberculosis of the spine. A chiropractor had recognized that there was a problem when another physician might have just said, "Go home and take some aspirin."

So, contrary to the belief of many, chiropractors are not wreaking havoc and turning the nation into paraplegics by twisting the necks of unsuspecting victims. Many physicians have been more or less indoctrinated in medical school to denounce chiropractors as quacks and charlatans. It's curious that this attitude persists. Chiropractic therapy is generally quite safe. There is a standardized four-year training program for chiropractors in the United States, and a small number of accredited chiropractic schools. While there may be differences in quality of the schools, it's one of the better regulated systems in the world. A medical doctor who warns people off all chiropractors is really denying them a valuable therapy. But this remains an entrenched position in the medical profession.

That said, there are some chiropractors who step over the bounds and overreach their capabilities, as do physicians in every area (for example, the occasional orthopedic surgeon who will sign you up for the operating room when disk surgery may or may not help your back problem). Chiropractors tend to overreach, too. Some will ascribe every physical problem, from sore throats to heart murmurs, to subluxations. Others peddle cures for autism or manic-depressive illness. As in any profession, some chiropractors are aggressive marketers and will make exaggerated claims.

Chiropractors tend to use X-rays more extensively as a diagnostic tool than do orthopedists and to read the X-rays more closely. An orthopedist will say, "This is a basically normal-looking X-ray," whereas a chiropractor will say, "Aha! Notice the compressed joint space here; notice the subluxation at this point in the spine." They are mentally comparing the appearance of your neck or spine with the ideal. The orthopedist is likely to say you're fine unless there's a gross deformity. In other words, you're fine until you are really in serious trouble. The chiropractors will tend to use the X-ray as a way of telling you there are subtle imbalances in the curvature of your spine, or in the space between your joints, or your way of standing or leaning — imbalances that may now or later cause problems. This is another source of controversy, of course. Chiropractors say that orthopedists are too casual in reading X-rays, and orthopedists say that chiropractors read X-rays as if they were tea leaves. I say, let's focus on the results. If a chiropractor spots something on an X-ray and uses that guidance to manipulate your spine in such a way as to relieve pain, this looks like a successful approach to me.

Acupuncture

Most people have heard of acupuncture, a traditional Chinese medical therapy, and know it has something to do with sticking "needles" into the body. The needles are long, thin, and flexible, much thinner than a sewing needle or a hypodermic needle, and don't cause the kind of pain you'd feel from a pinprick or puncture. According to traditional practice, they are placed at specific nodes along long lines called meridians that are carefully mapped on the body. In Chinese medical theory, the meridians represent paths of energy flow, but Western science has discovered that the nodes are physiologically located at junctures of the autonomic nervous system. Stimulation of the nodes thus affects the nervous system and can cause effects at some distance from the actual point of stimulation. There is documented research that supports the physiological and therapeutic effect of acupuncture. It has a wide variety of medical uses that include regulating menstruation, reducing the cramps of irritable bowel syndrome, treating tinnitus (ringing in the ears), stimulating immune cells, and inducing anesthesia for surgery. It can be especially helpful in dealing with musculoskeletal problems, such as arthritic symptoms, bursitis, neck pain, and joint pain.

It's not always easy to find a qualified acupuncturist, since it's still not an approved alternative therapy in some states. Actually many superb acupuncturists are not registered with the National Association of Non-Physician Acupuncturists. "Lay" acupuncturists may be certified, however, by the National Commission for the Certification of Acupuncturists, and they are registered as such in many states. Their training and examination requirements are considered by many to be far more rigorous than those applied to physicians — and many Asian lay acupuncturists have had the added benefit of initial training in traditional Chinese medicine. (See the Resources section at the end of this book for more information.)

Trigger Point Therapy

Trigger point therapy first came into the public eye when Dr. Janet Travell used it to treat President John F. Kennedy for his chronic back pain. In this country, trigger point therapy is performed by some physicians and by physician specialists called physiatrists. It's based on the phenomenon of painful trigger points that develop in the muscle, whether as a result of muscle spasm or as tangled knots of normally smooth muscle fibers. Trigger points are often associated with junctions of the autonomic nervous system. When you touch these points in someone who is suffering from muscular aches and pains, you'll find knotted muscles and a painful, tender spot. Painful in itself, a trigger point can radiate pain and sensation through nerves to other places on the body.

The treatment involves injecting a small amount of local anesthetic into the trigger point. The anesthetic seems to "defuse" the disturbed nerve reaction by scrambling the electrical signals that prompt pain sensation in the nerves, and switching the nerve-muscle complex back to a state of rest. Relief is at first temporary, but a series of treatments can cause the pathologically disturbed nerve and muscle to realign normally, resulting in long-term improvement.

Trigger point therapy can be especially useful when there has been an injury to muscles and nerves, whether caused by a traumatic incident or simply by repeated strain and tension.

Neural Therapy

Neural therapy, practiced widely in Europe and South America, is a treatment for chronic pain that's little known in the United States. Like trigger point therapy, it involves injection of small amounts of a local anesthetic into strategic points. However, the results can be even more dramatic. In 1940, the German physician Ferdinand Hueneke examined a patient with a painful, immobilized right shoulder that had resisted treatment. He injected an anesthetic (Novocain) without results. Several days later, though, the patient complained of severe itching in a scar on her left lower leg. Huneke then injected Novocain into the scar, with the amazing results that within seconds the patient was able to freely, painlessly move *her right shoulder joint*. It turned out that the patient had once had surgery on the lower left leg, apparently successfully, but after the surgery her right shoulder began to freeze up. Huneke continued to explore this phenomenon, which he called neural therapy, and found that the "lightning reaction" he'd observed was not at all uncommon.

European researchers theorize that injuries, surgical procedures, and scars can create local disturbances in the autonomic nervous system that actually change the electrical fields of the body, often causing pain or dysfunction at remote sites. Injecting a local anesthetic at the original place of disruption seems to neutralize or depolarize the local disturbance and relieve the pain in the distant affected area. A series of treatments may break the aberrant neurological pattern. The trick is to find the scar, the gland, or the trigger point that's causing the symptoms — it could be as ordinary as an appendix scar.

Just Forget About Your Pain?

We shouldn't leave the subject of chronic pain without mentioning another perspective, which several doctors and researchers have explored: the connection between chronic pain and chronic attention to pain. The idea is that if you adopt your pain as your own, make it an important part of your life, and go from doctor to doctor and therapy to therapy trying to "solve the pain problem," you may feed into the pain process and actually contribute to its longevity.

In this problem-oriented society, we love to focus on solving problems.

But when we try to apply the same approach to the body, it doesn't always work. We keep asking, "Why isn't the shoulder working? Why can't I make the pain stop? Do I need a better diagnosis, a different treatment? What am I doing wrong?" The idea persists that if you finally work hard enough on this problem it will go away.

Unfortunately, we put a lot of mental energy into getting rid of pain and end up making matters worse. A certain aspect of pain is actually learned; it's a conditioned response. A pain syndrome can become an ingrained pattern of the autonomic nervous system that we get comfortable with, the way a baseball player develops a habit of swinging badly, or a golfer keeps hooking the ball. Painkillers can strongly reinforce a pain habit because they themselves can make you feel good, in a way. So if you want to elicit that good feeling, you reenact your pain — perhaps unconsciously — and then you "get to" take a painkiller. Self-ministration of medications like aspirin, ibuprofren, and the antispasmodic painkillers, even though some are not highly addictive, can induce a spiraling pattern of pain-sensation, medication-response, more pain, more response. In the end, some of us may need to learn to live with a certain amount of chronic or recurring soreness and turn our attention elsewhere. Relaxation techniques can often help. We may find that some aches and pains come and go over time, as a natural part of shifts in the musculoskeletal system as we age.

Arthritis: Not for Seniors Only

What can you get from an injury, from a tick bite, from sex, from the food you eat, from lead poisoning, or from a bacterial infection of the gut? Arthritis. What is it exactly? Well, the term is used pretty loosely to describe any kind of pain or dysfunction in a joint. It can be caused by dozens of factors that we know about and probably by others we're still unaware of. In fact, it remains one of the less explored territories in modern medical science and may be just the common degenerative pathway for a whole array of different medical problems. It's been with us for millenia — researchers have seen evidence of arthritic degeneration in the bones of Paleolithic men and women.

It can start with pain and stiffness in the neck when you get up in the morning, or a sore knee that you notice when you're climbing stairs, or a gradually creaky shoulder that doesn't seem to move freely, or soreness in the finger joints. Yet, you may not have suffered any injury; you don't have a slipped disk; you didn't do anything to stress the joint unduly. Well, you might be joining the ranks of the thirty-eight million Americans who currently suffer from arthritis. In a few years you'll probably have even more company — it's estimated that by the year 2020 some sixty million people in the United States, or one in five, will have symptoms of arthritis. Even now, it's the leading disability in people over sixty-five and costs us $50 billion a year in lost wages and medical costs, including joint surgery.

In most cases of arthritis, there's inflammation and swelling of one or more joints; a simultaneous thinning of long, supportive bone shafts; and proliferation of extra bone material in the form of little spurs or protuberances in the joint itself. The bone spurs and the disease process start to damage the cartilage that cushions the two bone surfaces in a joint. As a result, the cartilage wears away, and bone starts to grind against bone, causing pain, stiff joints, and loss of range of motion. While cartilage and other tissue in the joints have normally few blood vessels, the arthritic disease process starts to infuse the area unnaturally with blood vessels, which carry in white blood cells, which in turn release immune factors called cytokines into the surrounding tissue, causing chronic inflammation.

This is the most common variety of arthritis, called osteoarthritis. It generally affects older people, though it can come in on midlife, especially after strain or trauma to the joints. This is the kind that affects an older person struggling to walk with painful hip or knee joints, or someone who is unable to hold a pen for writing or twist open a jar lid. Rheumatoid arthritis (RA), in distinction to osteoarthritis, can strike young and middle-aged individuals, especially women. In this condition, the joints become swollen, hot, and tender, including joints of the feet, shoulders, elbows, wrists, hips, neck, and lower back. Fatigue and anemia can accompany severe RA. It is primarily a disease of immune disregulation, a kind of autoimmune disease, as if the body is attacking its own joints. (Though the factors are different, there is an immune component to osteoarthritis as well, since it's an aberrant immune reaction that causes the inflammation to spiral out of control.) We don't really know what causes rheumatoid arthritis, but it's more common in the industrialized countries, so there may be something about our Western diet or physical environment that increases the risk. (I personally suspect that the transsaturated fats or hydrogenated fats found in margarine and other foods may play a significant role in immune disregulation, by becoming incorporated into cell walls and interfering with the exquisitely delicate cell-to-cell communication that the immune system relies on.)

We can diagnose osteoarthritis by looking at X-rays and seeing bone spurs, or at MRIs and seeing subtle changes in cartilage and joint fluid. We diagnose RA with sensitive blood tests that pick up levels of circulating proteins, called rheumatoid factors, that are associated with the disease. As in any medical syndrome, there are classic examples of each type and then individuals who seem to have a blending of symptoms and diagnostic factors. The disease doesn't always match the paradigm. Classic rheumatoid arthritis is distinctive and is shown by the blood test, but then there are some puzzling cases of seronegative arthritis and palindromic arthritis that mimic RA but aren't detected by the blood test.

What Causes Arthritis?

A better question might be, what doesn't? Ten to one, if you ask why you have arthritis, your doctor will say, "Well, you're not as young as you used to be. These things can happen when you get to be your age." We simply don't know what causes most cases of arthritis. At the same time, we do know of a long list of factors that can cause the disease in some individuals. They include trauma or injury, overweight, genetic and environmental factors, allergic reactions, and even some infectious diseases. Let's look at some of these more closely.

• *Genetic factors.* Genetic research is just beginning to identify faulty genes that may set someone up for arthritis. For example, researchers have found one altered gene sequence that can cause a weakened component of cartilage. This occurs in only 3 to 5 percent of arthritis patients, but there are indications that five, ten, or more genes may be involved in arthritis, and the hunt is on to identify them. A better understanding of genetic factors may lead us to a genetic fix through gene splicing or by supplying metabolic factors to make up for inherited weakness.

• *Infectious diseases.* Lyme disease, carried by the deer tick, typically causes arthritic symptoms, which can become chronic. In fact, Long Island residents gave the name "Montauk knee" to the arthritic symptom of Lyme disease. Anyone who lives in the East Coast or Upper Middle West regions, where Lyme disease is endemic, should consider it as a possible cause of sudden-onset arthritis. *Chlamydia*, a sexually transmitted microorganism, can also induce certain types of arthritic symptoms. Researchers have also looked at certain viral infectious agents, including human parvovirus, as possible instigators of arthritis. It's thought that Epstein-Barr virus, which is ubiquitous in the human population, may be implicated in rheumatoid arthritis. There may be many pathogens not yet identified that can cause chronic disease, including arthritis. (The Lyme disease bacteria, for example, were discovered only a few decades ago.) This possibility is supported by the fact that some people with arthritis respond to treatment with tetracycline, for reasons we don't really understand. Also, the antibiotic ceftriaxone, used to treat Lyme disease, also seems to help some cases of chronic inflammatory arthritis in people unlikely to have been exposed to Lyme disease.

• *Bacteria-induced immune reactions.* It's also been shown that some infectious organisms may not directly induce arthritis but can set off an immune reaction in the body that produces arthritic symptoms of inflammation in the joints. The *Klebsiella* bacteria, for example, make up part of the normal intestinal flora that inhabit the gut, usually without any adverse effects. But in a certain genetically defined section of the population, *Klebsiella* activates an autoimmune reaction called ankylosing spondylitis, which involves inflamed, arthritic joints. There are no bacteria in the joints themselves, but the immune response triggers the symptoms.

• *Environmental insults.* Lead poisoning in adults can produce arthritic symptoms, and "saturnine gout" was common among ancient Romans who deliberately leaded their wine. It's likely that other environmental poisons can have this effect. One rather controversial school of thought concerns fluoride, which is normally used to prevent tooth cavities, but which may affect bone metabolism. Some researchers have looked at the changes in bone caused by excess fluoride, which are visible in X-rays, and compared them with the growth of bone spurs in people with osteoarthritis. They've suggested that our epidemic of osteoarthritis may be partly due to the addition of fluoride to drinking water. This is really sheer speculation at this point, but the possibility is intriguing.

• *Obesity.* We're not completely sure why, but obesity definitely increases the risk of osteoarthritis, certainly by putting extra strain on joints and definitely through other yet-unknown metabolic processes. Obese people, while not inclined to walk on their knuckles like our primate ancestors, nevertheless show an exaggerated tendency toward arthritis of the hands, knees, wrists, and fingers.

• *Dietary factors.* Gout, which can affect the knees or the big toe, is probably the most notorious form of food-induced arthritis. Rich foods with too many of the proteins called purines, and organ meats containing high levels of DNA and RNA, can induce gout, as can excessive amounts of alcohol. Certain individuals may have trouble digesting or tolerating other types of foods, including wheat, corn, and dairy products, and may develop chronic aches that resemble arthritis. The condition may not be a classic allergy but a kind of intolerance in which digestive fragments of certain foods may induce an immune response or mimic other metabolic components of the body, causing chronic illness.

Even this brief list of causative factors, still laced with unknowns, is enough to suggest that we should not simply accept arthritis as a common or even inevitable aspect of aging. Much research remains to be done, but even with this much to go on, we have begun to identify alternative treatments, which can improve on the relatively ineffective conventional treatments for both osteoarthritis and rheumatoid arthritis.

Treating Arthritis: The Conventional and Natural Approaches

Nowhere in medicine do we see sharper distinctions between conventional and alternative therapies than in the case of arthritis, especially RA. Comparing the way orthodox and nutritionally oriented physicians treat these conditions underscores the difference in philosophy between these two medical approaches. The high prevalence of poor outcomes and undesirable side effects in patients receiving conventional therapy and the beneficial results obtained by patients using alternative therapies suggests that the latter should be given greater attention than they are getting.

Even by the admission of many arthritis experts, conventional therapy for arthritis, especially for RA, is far less than optimal. The first step is often palliative therapy with aspirin or other nonsteroidal anti-inflammatory drugs (NSAIDs) such as Motrin, Naprosyn, Voltaren, Clinoril, and, most recently, Ansaid and Relafen. These first-line drugs quench pain and stop inflammation to a certain extent, but they have little if any beneficial effect on the ultimate clinical course of arthritis. Some studies show that they may actually hasten joint damage. They possess several other unfortunate side effects, especially the tendency to cause stomach irritation and even severe gastrointestinal bleeding.

Steroid injections for arthritis and bursitis are another favorite tool of orthopedists. As we've noted, they are progressively less effective, and repeated injections can damage joints and induce osteoporosis.

In the case of RA, doctors often prescribe more powerful second-line drugs. These are the so-called DMARDs (disease-modifying antirheumatic drugs). These agents are designed not just to control symptoms but actually to delay progression of the disease. Unfortunately, many of them can cause severe adverse effects. They include such drugs as hydroxychloroquine sulfate, gold, penicillamine, sulfasalazine, prednisone, azathioprine, and methotrexate. The last-named is a powerful chemotherapy drug used in the treatment of cancer. Some of these drugs possess potent immunosuppressive effects.

There is one positive "new think" in conventional treatment, though, which is the idea that gentle exercise can help arthritis symptoms. Many arthritis clinics now offer water therapy. Patients undergo gentle stretching and exercise in a swimming pool, which helps take the weight off painful knee and hip joints. It's been shown that gentle exercise like swimming and walking can help maintain flexibility in joints so that patients require less care.

In contrast to the conventional drug treatments, a holistic approach to either kind of arthritis is to identify the causative factors and detoxify the body as a means of controlling and reversing the disease. Natural products and nondrug therapies are used whenever possible to avoid the toxicity of "designer drugs." I remember a patient in her sixties who came in absolutely racked with osteoarthritis, leaning on a cane and positively creaking when she slowly settled into a chair in my office. She had diffuse osteoarthritis in the shoulders, the knees, and the feet that seemed fairly well advanced. I was concerned that she might have so much destruction of

TRADE NEW BODY PARTS FOR OLD?

Replacement of hip and knee joints has become a common treatment for advanced osteoarthritis when the bone has been significantly worn away. We may expect procedures to replace other kinds of joints when better prosthetic devices have been developed. In the hip, for example, a new metal and plastic ball and socket joint can be grafted into the thigh and hip bones. This is usually done as a last resort, since the artificial joints do have a limited functional span, of ten to fifteen years, and the operation cannot be repeated more than once or twice.

joint tissue that even if we could reduce the inflammation she'd still be left with creaky, deformed joints. We treated her with diet changes, acupuncture, and specific oral nutrients, and she had an incredible turnaround within six months. At this point she needs only occasional maintenance acupuncture treatments, once every month. By no means do all patients respond as magnificently as she did, but I usually have an even more optimistic prognosis for patients who have only mild or localized arthritis. Let's take a closer look at some alternative treatments.

DIET MODIFICATION

Monolithic groups like the Arthritis Foundation long held the position that dietary cures for arthritis were quackery. But they have recently been forced to soften their position in light of scientific evidence that dietary approaches do make a difference. Dietary "cures" for RA, and even osteoarthritis, have long been touted by folk medicine. Researchers began to compile scientific confirmation as early as 1911, with studies showing that restricted diet programs could produce remission of arthritis. The subject is a difficult one because different patients respond in different ways to various dietary manipulations. In truth, arthritis can be considered the final common end point of a variety of factors. This may explain why not all patients respond to dietary intervention alone.

Patients who are obese must make permanent dietary changes. Experimental trials have shown that if arthritis patients go on a hypoallergenic diet in which common food allergens are eliminated and substituted by a neutral synthetic food supplement like Vivonex, their symptom scores improve markedly. Some studies have demonstrated the value of specific allergy testing of the skin or the blood to predict which food should be eliminated. Other studies have underscored the value of a low-fat diet based largely on fresh fruits, vegetables, cereal grains, and legumes. Some trials have produced benefits when patients eliminate cereal grains altogether and emphasize proteins rich in polyunsaturated fat, such as fish and nuts. These low-carbohydrate diets may help because they suppress growth of harmful or immune-active intestinal bacteria.

One diet that works with some people is to eliminate the nightshade foods, which include tomatoes, potatoes, eggplant, peppers, paprika, and cayenne. Tobacco is also a nightshade. In fact, there's an animal model for arthritis: if cows are mistakenly given fodder that is heavily laced with wild-growing nightshade family plants, they actually develop a type of osteoarthritis. Anyone who suffers from arthritis could try avoiding these foods for a month and then gradually reintroducing them to see whether they affect the symptoms.

Fasting has been shown to be therapeutic in some cases for both osteoarthritis and RA. Fasting allows the body to detoxify and offers a break from the onslaught of food antigens that may trigger joint inflammation. This traditional therapy seems to work in many cases — you go on a fast and your arthritis gets better. It may help because of food intolerances, or it may allow your gut to stop supporting the growth of certain harmful bacteria or fungi that produce toxic byproducts that somehow trigger the arthritis. In the "leaky gut syndrome," discussed earlier, a stressed intestinal tract may become permeable to microscopic food protein particles, allowing them to enter the bloodstream and set up an immune reaction in the tissue. An overgrowth of harmful intestinal bacteria or yeast, otherwise known as dysbiosis, may compound the problem. Detoxification regimens sometimes use fibers like psyllium or absorbent clays like bentonite, with or without the assistance of colonic irrigations or enemas. It may also help to replace harmful intestinal flora with cultures of benign bacteria like *Lactobacillus acidophilus* from yogurt or supplements.

DIETARY SUPPLEMENTS

Several nutrients affect arthritic symptoms, some by reducing inflammation and others by retarding the degeneration of cartilage or normalizing immune reactions. They have been listed earlier in this chapter, in the section on nutritional therapies for general aches and pains.

The omega-3 oils, present in flaxseed oil and in cold-water fish, such as tuna, salmon, herring, trout, mackerel, sardines, and cod liver, are especially helpful in relieving morning stiffness and tender joints. GLA (gamma-linolenic acid), an omega-6 oil that is present in primrose oil, borage oil, and black currant seed oil, has been shown to augment the anti-inflammatory effect of the omega-3 oils.

CARTILAGE AND COLLAGEN

Collagen is a living fibrous protein that is found in bone and is also a major component of cartilage, the cushioning substance that gets "worn away" by bone spurs in osteoarthritis and that simply degenerates in RA. For decades, holistic physicians have prescribed collagen, in the form of bovine cartilage or, more recently, shark cartilage, as a dietary supplement in the treatment of both kinds of arthritis. Just recently, mainstream scientific studies have begun to confirm the efficacy of this approach.

In one study, processed collagen was fed to a group of volunteers at Beth Israel Hospital in Boston, and their arthritic symptoms improved. Collagen feeding helps people who suffer from osteoarthritis, too, which suggests that there is also an autoimmune component to osteoarthritis as well.

Shark cartilage seems to have an additional effect: it slows the proliferation of blood vessels, called angiogenesis, which is a phase in arthritis. Cartilage normally contains inhibitors that keep it free of blood vessels, but when blood vessels start to invade the cartilage in advanced arthritis, they bring in more inflammatory mediators that escalate inflammation.

Some studies have shown beneficial effects from feeding patients with a cartilage extract of green-lipped mussel. This contains organic compounds called mucopolysaccharides, which may be biochemically similar to human collagen and may thereby induce some degree of immune tolerance. These compounds have also been extracted from cartilage of cows' tracheas. Most recently, shark cartilage has been shown to have specific antiarthritis effects that are probably due to the same compounds. A brand new addition to this genre of antiarthritic nutrients is glucosamine sulfate, also a mucopolysaccharide, which is now available in health food stores and natural pharmacies. The effect of all these supplements is subtle — it's not usually an immediate and spectacular relief of pain, but more of a gradual reduction of inflammation.

HERBAL REMEDIES

Many Western herbs are beneficial in the treatment of arthritis. It's worth remembering that the discovery of aspirin was predicated on the traditional folk wisdom that the bark of the white willow could reduce aches and pains. White willow bark is high in salicylate acid, the active ingredient of aspirin. Herbs that can play an important role in treating arthritis include curcumin (extracted from the spice turmeric), Jamaican dogwood, feverfew, devil's claw, licorice, ginger, and yucca. Many are available in easy-to-use alcohol or glycerine tinctures or in an encapsulated freeze-dried form. Capsaicin, an extract of cayenne pepper, is a topical counterirritant cream that provides relief from joint pain. It's an alternative to the traditional menthol-containing ointments and may be slightly more effective for some.

OTHER ALTERNATIVE THERAPIES

Acupuncture is helpful for several musculoskeletal problems and pain syndromes and is particularly effective in treating arthritis in some individuals. It can reduce dependency on harmful medications and reduce the degree of medication needed.

Another therapy that's relatively rare in the United States, though more common in Europe, is the use of bee venom to treat arthritis. It may work as a counterirritant, but it may also stimulate or recalibrate the immune system in some way. While most people have a painful reaction to a bee sting, with redness and swelling, I've spoken with European holistic practitioners who tell me that their severely arthritic patients typically have a very dulled response to bee venom and can take twenty or thirty bee stings to arthritic joints with barely visible redness or swelling, and little sensation other than moderate itching.

A Look to the Future

It may take some time, but I expect that eventually even the medical establishment will grant that using natural substances — such as vitamins and nutrients, herbs, and antigen feeding — may be beneficial in treating and preventing musculoskeletal ailments.

At present, arthritis remains a big unknown. We are still not clear about exactly what causes it, and we may not yet be looking in the right places. For now, if you want a quick fix, you can take the NSAIDs and other drugs, but at the risk of actually worsening the underlying physiology of joint degeneration. Natural therapies like antioxidants, the omega-3 and omega-6 oils, and the others I've mentioned don't provide instantaneous pain relief, but they do gradually alter the underlying physiology of inflammation and are safer in the long run. Again, this highlights the fundamental divergence between the conventional medical approach and the holistic approach. Since alternative therapies don't ameliorate pain so quickly, you have to tough it out for a while, but the results are ultimately more gratifying.

Though doctors and patients alike show a lot of enthusiasm for high-tech surgeries and imaging techniques, there are some good low-tech therapies that are probably being underutilized. Methods like the Alexander technique can be very helpful for developing a heightened body awareness and for overcoming habits of body posture that may create physical stress and even chronic pain. Chiropractors could do more useful preventive work against the degenerative processes of aging that work on the spine, and which may not only affect spinal health but the flow of neurological energy throughout the body.

One promising new high-tech tool is biomagnetic therapy, and it is already in use in several centers in the Northeast to help treat fractures and osteoarthritis. The technique was pioneered in the treatment of bone fractures, because it's been shown that applying an electromagnetic field to fractured bones that don't knit well tends to align the regenerating cells and promote normal growth. By the same principle, researchers theorize, properly applied electromagnetic fields might also help heal the physiology of joints in people suffering from arthritis. Biomagnetic therapy is now undergoing clinical trials supervised by the National Institutes of Health.

We are undergoing a sea change in our attitudes toward both osteoarthritis and rheumatoid arthritis, in admitting that there may be a nutritional component, an allergic component, and an infectious component to the disease and in recognizing that the use of natural substances such as vitamins, nutrients, and antigen feeding can be used to treat it. Probably the future breakthrough in the treatment of arthritis will be an immune-modulating therapy that will break the inflammatory cascade at the source, at the cellular level, and bring the immune response back into balance.

CHAPTER EIGHT

Keeping Bones Vital

When I scheduled a show on osteoporosis for my radio program, the people at the station got nervous. They asked me, "What kind of demographics are you reaching for here? You're only going to get elderly people with this topic." "Absolutely not!" I told them. I led off the show with the recent studies demonstrating that children who are given calcium supplements through their teenage years can build up their bone density by a few percentage points, and that those few percentage points may be crucial in averting osteoporosis in later life.

Even in adulthood, there's still time to enhance your resistance to osteoporosis. And it's worth doing, since fractures due to weakened, brittle bones are a leading cause of disability in old age. Ten to twenty percent of elderly people who fracture a hip die within six months, and by the age of seventy fully one-half of women will have developed spinal compression due to loss of bone mass. Osteoporosis is an especially insidious disease because you don't "feel" that anything is wrong with you. Many people first discover they have a problem when they actually have a serious fracture. One typical scenario is for someone to fall forward and reach out to break the fall only to have the wrist snap like a twig. Or someone may fracture a hip or leg just from stepping off a curb. Spinal pain may be another warning sign. Fortunately, we can take preventive action to keep bones stronger and more flexible well into old age, but we need to do this long before we experience any symptoms.

Many people forget that bone is *alive* — it's living, changing, regenerating tissue, not a dead, inorganic support structure. Blood flows actively through bone, and living bone marrow plays a key role in the immune system. Bone acts as a storage depot for nutrients such as calcium, magnesium, phosphorous, and manganese, which can later be mobilized in response to the body's needs. In fact, bone tissue exists in a state of rapid and dynamic flux — a constant process of building up and breaking down. You could think of bone as a kind of active bank account, with deposits and withdrawals, which hopefully show a net positive balance and not a progressive deficit. From about the age of twenty-five, your body becomes less efficient at absorbing the minerals in the food you eat and may start to borrow on the minerals stored in your bones. Eventually, these "accounts" become overdrawn and your bones become depleted, porous, and brittle. At this stage, what might have been a minor tumble fifteen years ago becomes a major fracture of the back or hip or wrist.

Furthermore, bone strength is not just a simple matter of density, the amount of bone mass. Bones have a degree of flexibility, which is also important in enabling them to resist fractures. Some older people may be more prone to fractures because they have reduced flexibility — hard, brittle bones that are more susceptible to fracture, even without actual bone thinning.

Inadequate nutrition and a sedentary lifestyle can profoundly affect the health of bone tissue. Yet, while exercise is generally a positive way of building bone tissue, dancers and athletes who put themselves under extreme physical stress, burning the candle at both ends, can actually increase the risk of osteoporosis.

We have it in our power as adults to maintain and support healthy bones and stave off osteoporosis, but we have to play an active part in doing this. The current flurry of books and articles about menopause has raised our consciousness about this issue, since estrogen replacement in women has a protective effect against osteoporosis. But the issue is not that simple — we can't simply prescribe estrogen replacement for all women entering menopause. And men should take note: while osteoporosis is statistically a "women's problem," men can also suffer significant bone loss in old age. For whatever reason, the human male has evolved with a heavier skeleton, of greater bone mass and density, which may also be increased by weight-bearing physical labor. This provides some added protection, but it's not absolute. Statistically, osteoporosis occurs in 25 percent of aging women but also in 11 percent of aging men.

What Causes Osteoporosis?

Well, it's not as simple as just losing calcium from the bones, though lack of sufficient calcium in the diet can play a part. It's a natural, progressive process to lose some bone mass, but this is normally balanced by factors that build new bone. In people with osteoporosis, some combination of nutritional and possibly immunological factors seems to set off a pathological process, creating an imbalance in the system. In severe cases, the imbalance is so advanced that bone can be losing density at the same time that the body is building up excess deposits of the weakened bone, causing arthritis.

Diet plays a key role. Almost everybody knows about the importance of having sufficient calcium (and it's almost impossible to get this from our current food sources without taking a calcium supplement). Vitamin D is important, and so are other minerals, especially magnesium and manganese. There was the well-publicized case of the basketball player Bill Walton, of the Portland Trailblazers, who had turned to an extreme vegetarian diet. Suddenly he began to have debilitating injuries and stress fractures. It turned out that he was suffering from osteoporosis in his feet. A nutritional analysis showed that he was very deficient in manganese, which is commonly found in the kinds of animal protein foods that he had given up. At the same time, excessive protein in the diet can favor a metabolic process called acidosis, which causes a more rapid leaching of calcium from the bone.

We actually have to ingest about seven times more calcium than our bones need, so that enough can be absorbed through the digestive system. The body tends to absorb the calcium according to need, but this is dependent on two other factors: the presence of vitamin D, and the presence of hydrochloric acid in the stomach. The body produces its own vitamin D during exposure to sunlight, so as you would guess, women in northern climes tend to have a greater risk of osteoporosis than women who live in tropical climates.

We also have to have sufficient hydrochloric acid in the stomach to enable the body to absorb calcium. An interesting genetic factor relates to this. Some women have a condition called hypochlorhydria, which means they have a reduced amount of hydrochloric acid in the stomach and therefore don't absorb calcium as efficiently. Their problem is that they can take all the calcium they like, but it doesn't get into the bloodstream and doesn't get to their bones. Mainstream medicine tends to discount the importance of hypochlorhydria, because it's considered rare, but it can actually be induced by regular consumption of antacids, which interfere with stomach acidity.

Dr. Mildred Seelig, a world-renowned researcher on magnesium, suggests that an imbalance between calcium and magnesium in the diet is also a significant factor for osteoporosis. She points out that a long-term deficiency of magnesium in the diet can induce a condition called hyperparathyroidism, which favors the breaking down of bone through the transformation of bone calcium into blood calcium. This happens to be a fairly common but relatively little-recognized condition. The American diet is in fact particularly magnesium-depleted, especially in refined foods.

Evaluating Osteoporosis Risk

Other factors can contribute to osteoporosis, including hormonal imbalance and hereditary predispositions, so women, especially, need to have their individual risk factors evaluated and compiled. When I evaluate a new patient for osteoporosis, I look at the family history, exercise history, dietary factors such as possible excess animal protein, and history of drug use, especially steroids. Steroid drugs are commonly used to treat inflammatory diseases such as asthma, rheumatoid arthritis, ulcerative colitis, and severe allergies, but they definitely cause bone thinning. Extremes of alcohol intake may produce osteoporosis. So can excess coffee consumption, though having milk with your coffee may offset the risk.

Interestingly, if you are referred to a specialist for osteoporosis, you'll probably see not an orthopedist but an endocrinologist specializing in bone metabolism, since hormonal balance is so significant in this disease. Menstrual history is a factor, since in general the longer you menstruate the less likely you are to suffer osteoporosis because of the protective effect of the female hormones. So I ask about eating disorders that may have caused loss of periods and also about smoking history. Smoking becomes a risk factor because it tends to reduce the amount of estrogen in the body and because smokers generally have an earlier onset of menopause.

Hormonal factors can be significant for men as well as women, especially if they experience a significant lowering of testosterone levels at andropause, or "male menopause." For more on this, see chapter 11.

In evaluating someone for osteoporosis, I also consider body type and race. People of thin or frail body stature are more prone; and Caucasians are more prone to osteoporosis than Africans or African Americans, with Asians falling in between.

To further evaluate the risk of osteoporosis, I do a series of tests, including a basic bone densitometry test, which is commonly available at most university hospitals and is technically called photon beam absorptiometry. In this test, an X-ray quantifies the thickness of bone in three key locations: the hip, the lumbar spine, and the wrist — the major sites of osteoporotic fractures. But this test, while helpful, only provides a static "snapshot" of bone status. Unless performed several years in succession, it doesn't yield information about the *rate* at which bone is being lost. For this you need to perform the cross-links test, a newly developed analysis that reflects the rate of progression of osteoporosis. Based on a sophisticated analysis of a single urine sample, the cross-links test measures levels of a crucial bone protein matrix building block. High levels of this substance in the urine means a rapid turnover of bone with resultant risk of osteoporosis. Together with information from the bone densitometry snapshot, the clinician can gauge not only the current extent of bone thinning but the future prognosis. Corrective measures can be undertaken and their effectiveness checked with further cross-links tests.

There is a big debate in the medical community about whether bone density analysis should be extended to women as a routine part of health screening. I personally think it is very important, especially near the time of menopause, to establish whether you really might be advised to use estrogen replacement therapy or whether you might comfortably avoid it. Right now there's a tendency to advise most women to take estrogen, but for some women there is a downside to this, and bone density testing can provide valuable support for making an informed decision. Ideally, you should have two bone densitometry readings, eighteen to twenty-four months apart, to establish whether there's a trend. The test uses a small amount of radiation, many factors less than that of a normal chest X-ray.

Another useful test is to measure levels of usable vitamin D, which is needed for the bone-building process. A fairly high percentage of older people suffer from a vicious circle of osteoporosis that actually contributes to further vitamin D deficiency and thus to further osteoporosis. We need sunlight for the body to manufacture vitamin D, and if you're immobilized by osteoporosis, you're less likely to get out into the sun, which means you're more likely to have a vitamin D deficiency, which in turn promotes osteoporosis. Also, elderly folks have less of the vitamin D–forming elements in their skin than do young people, so they won't make as much vitamin D in a given amount of sunlight as a young or middle-aged person.

For these reasons, and because of the risk of skin cancers from exposure to ultraviolet light, vitamin D supplements may seem like a good bet. However, we should note that vitamin D is one of the vitamins you can overdose on. While milk inherently contains vitamin D, it is often additionally fortified with this vitamin, sometimes to excess. Some studies of the milk industry have reported tremendously haphazard practices in the way vitamin D is added to milk. It may be safer to avoid fortified milk and milk products if you can, and stick to supplements. A safe range for supplementation is 400 to 1000 International Units per day.

When someone appears to have a risk of osteoporosis, imaging tests like MRI and X-rays are sometimes used to assess the condition. However, the standard X-ray can be misleading and is not a good screening tool because it will reveal osteoporosis only after a 30 percent bone loss! A regular X-ray may give you false reassurance. The radiologist may say, "Hey, your bones look O.K.," but you may actually have osteoporosis. On the other hand, if you first learn you have osteoporosis from a conventional X-ray, that's a bad sign because it's already fairly advanced.

Treating Osteoporosis

Most doctors typically recommend hormone replacement therapy for postmenopausal women who appear to have some risk for osteoporosis. But this isn't always appropriate, and there are alternatives. I treated one patient who was a perfect example of this. Sarah was postmenopausal, and a bone

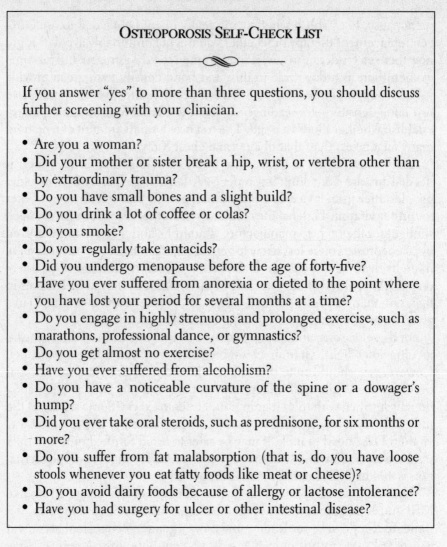

OSTEOPOROSIS SELF-CHECK LIST

If you answer "yes" to more than three questions, you should discuss further screening with your clinician.

- Are you a woman?
- Did your mother or sister break a hip, wrist, or vertebra other than by extraordinary trauma?
- Do you have small bones and a slight build?
- Do you drink a lot of coffee or colas?
- Do you smoke?
- Do you regularly take antacids?
- Did you undergo menopause before the age of forty-five?
- Have you ever suffered from anorexia or dieted to the point where you have lost your period for several months at a time?
- Do you engage in highly strenuous and prolonged exercise, such as marathons, professional dance, or gymnastics?
- Do you get almost no exercise?
- Have you ever suffered from alcoholism?
- Do you have a noticeable curvature of the spine or a dowager's hump?
- Did you ever take oral steroids, such as prednisone, for six months or more?
- Do you suffer from fat malabsorption (that is, do you have loose stools whenever you eat fatty foods like meat or cheese)?
- Do you avoid dairy foods because of allergy or lactose intolerance?
- Have you had surgery for ulcer or other intestinal disease?

density test suggested that she had some degree of osteoporosis. However, she had had a precancerous breast nodule that had been removed, and we were concerned that giving her estrogen could stimulate other latent precancerous nodules to become cancerous. She was clearly not a good candidate for estrogen replacement therapy. We also gave her a Heidelberg capsule test to see whether her stomach was making adequate levels of hydrochloric acid, which is needed to absorb calcium well. We determined that she did have low levels of hydrochloric acid and gave her betaine hydrochloride to assist with her absorption of calcium. We set up an exercise program and gave her high-dosage supplements of calcium, magnesium, manganese, silica, boron, and zinc — all the components of bone — in easily absorbable form, and, of course, vitamin D. We also prescribed natural progesterone in the form of progesterone cream. This is an extract of wild yam, has a demonstrable anti-osteoporosis effect, and is not cancer-inducing. (When women *are* taking estrogen, progesterone can help balance the effects of that hormone.) We also gave her Chinese ginseng, a traditional treatment for menopause in Chinese medicine.

Eighteen months later we sent Sarah for another bone density test. The radiologist sent back a query to me, commenting that I'd neglected to mention what amount of estrogen this woman was taking. When I told him she was not on hormone replacement or any drugs, he said, "This is the darnedest thing, because Sarah has had about a six to eight percent enhancement of her bone density, and that's a sizable amount for such a short period of time. We usually don't see this without some form of hormonal therapy." And he asked me again, "Are you sure she wasn't on hormonal therapy?" I told him, "No, her therapy has been nutritional." This was an exciting example of the potential for other approaches than estrogen therapy in treating osteoporosis. It shows that bone loss from osteoporosis can not only be slowed or arrested but actually be reversed. It's really possible to rebuild bone if the osteoporosis hasn't progressed too far. Really substantial bone loss is very hard to recoup, but that's why this is a disease that should be prevented.

I should say that exercise was an especially important part of Sarah's treatment, since the right type of exercise can make a big contribution toward building bone mass, as long as it's not a straining type of exercise.

As for estrogen replacement therapy, there is no simple rule of thumb for all women. This really has to be determined on a case-by-case basis, taking into account family history of breast cancer, a woman's desire to maintain "hormonal youthfulness," and so on. Doctors tend to preempt women's choice by simply making the decision for them, but of course not every woman is informed or in a position to evaluate all the issues, including current research.

Preventing Osteoporosis

Diet and supplements play the key role in preventing osteoporosis, along with weight-bearing exercise.

- Increase calcium intake by eating calcium-rich foods such as yogurt, low-fat cheese, broccoli, sardines, and tahini.
- Take a dietary calcium supplement. Recommended: 1000 to 1500 milligrams daily of dietary calcium plus supplementary calcium.
- Use other natural bone-builders and cofactors for bone mineralization to support bone strength. The following can be useful:

- Vitamin D, 800 International Units per day
- Magnesium, 500 to 600 milligrams per day
- Manganese, 50 milligrams per day
- Zinc, 45 milligrams per day
- L-lysine, an amino acid, 500 milligrams per day
- Vitamin C, 1000 milligrams per day
- Boron, 6 milligrams per day
- Perform some sort of weight-bearing exercise, such as walking, jogging, racket sports, or weight-lifting, or use an exercise machine.
- Stop smoking.
- Get some regular exposure to sunlight to promote vitamin D production. Avoid total reliance on highly protective sunscreens, allowing a few minutes of nonburning exposure before applying them.
- Consider hormonal supplements.

Testosterone is one of the hormones that contribute to increased bone mass in men. Theoretically, we could give testosterone to enhance bone mass, but the side effects would be unpleasant and unwanted by most. In some women and men, low levels of the adrenal hormone DHEA may contribute to osteoporosis. Because of its androgenic characteristics, DHEA acts as a bone builder. Replacing DHEA in DHEA-deficient older individuals may be an alternative to testosterone's bone-enhancing but masculinizing effects.

Treatment by Medication

The few drugs for treating osteoporosis have only recently been refined enough to show real promise. One, a natural substance called salmon calcitonin, prevents the reabsorption of bone calcium into the bloodstream. In its initial development, it had to be delivered by injection and was so expensive that it wasn't reimbursed by Medicare. A new nasal spray version of salmon calcitonin called Miacalcin was introduced in Scandinavia and is now available here in the United States.

Diphosphonates are drugs that signal the bone to absorb calcium. A new diphosphonate, alendronate (Fosamax), has recently been introduced for women who can't or won't take estrogen. The *New England Journal of Medicine* published a report at the end of 1995 of nearly a thousand women who used alendronate for five years, along with 500 milligrams of calcium daily. Not only did the drug stave off bone loss, it enhanced bone density slightly but significantly. And it proved effective in precisely the target group most in need of help: women over sixty-five with moderately severe osteoporosis. Best of all, the side effects were few and were limited to some

CIRCULATION FOR THE BONES

Most of us know that circulation problems can cause angina or heart attacks, but they can just as easily cause degeneration in brain function or in hip joints. A very common problem in older people is degeneration of the hip joint. As a result, many older people suffer hip fractures or find themselves getting a series of hip-replacement operations. This is partly a byproduct of osteoporosis: the bones of the ball-and-socket hip joint just start to wear away. But there's also a circulatory component of this condition. Healthy bone is constantly infused with blood through the circulatory system, and if the blood supply is reduced below a certain level, the bone dies! This condition is called avascular necrosis, and makes the person prone to hip fractures and to the simple wearing-away of the hip joint. This is just one of the many ways by which problems of the circulatory system can induce a degenerative process.

gastrointestinal disturbance. The advent of Fosamax, along with the recent introduction of an easier-to-administer nasal form of calcitonin, heralds an exciting new era in which early detection *and reversal* of osteoporosis will become routine.

A Look to the Future

Researchers are looking for better drugs that will more effectively increase bone mass, and there are some current candidates. But the big issue with osteoporosis is how to predict it effectively in order to begin early preventive efforts. Right now, there's controversy over whether or not extensive screening with fairly intensive tests like bone densitometry should be routinely performed. At $300 or more per test, it would be very expensive to offer it to every eligible patient. We'd love to have a simple and easy blood or urine test to accurately pinpoint the rate of bone loss and identify individuals at risk, and we hope the cross-links test will be just that. In the meantime, we should continue to evaluate for high-risk cases, starting with family and hormonal factors, and pursue the further testing when it seems warranted. Most of us can continue to optimize bone health by getting sufficient calcium and vitamin D and engaging in regular weight-bearing exercise.

CHAPTER NINE

Basic Plumbing:
The Gastrointestinal Tract

Nothing can make life more unpleasant than chronic stomach pains or intestinal troubles — they can literally stop us in our tracks. Too many Americans suffer from these ailments, popping antacids like candy and making regular stops at the drugstore to buy over-the-counter cure-alls for different problems of the GI (gastrointestinal) tract. Many try to grit their teeth and get on with life, treating intermittent GI problems as unavoidable annoyances and forgetting about them when they pass. Many others suffer nagging discomfort every day. It was the omnipresence of GI problems, and the way they undermine the quality of life, that compelled me to author a whole book on this subject: *Seven Weeks to a Settled Stomach*. Gastrointestinal disturbances needn't be an everyday affair, and they should be taken seriously as warning signs of possible long-term debilitating processes. To live healthily into our forties, fifties, and beyond, we need to take preventive care of our basic plumbing, and we'll gain the side benefits of increased vitality, energy and well-being. In fact, new medical thinking suggests that the GI tract plays a primary role in a variety of seemingly unrelated conditions, from eczema to arthritis.

We typically think of the GI tract as a kind of reverse assembly line that disassembles food, extracts nutrients at each stage, and finally excretes waste products. Strictly speaking, this is a useful mechanical model of the gut. However, new research is emerging that shows it to have a different function: We are realizing that the gut is an important buffer zone between our internal selves and the external environment. It is a selectively permeable organ that allows us to absorb beneficial nutrients while at the same time posing a barrier against external toxins and shielding our system from foreign proteins. As such, it is an immune organ of tremendous sophistication.

Moreover, the gut as buffer zone is also a symbiotic home to millions and millions of "fellow travelers" — bacteria, yeasts, and fungi. It's a little like a border area that processes immigrants, keeps some out, lets others in, and builds up its own native population. The gut is really designed to be properly colonized, and the process begins in infancy, when ideally it's primed with antibodies from mother's milk, and colonized by friendly flora from the mother's skin. We live in true symbiosis with the native flora of the gut, which not only help process nutrients for us that we cannot, but actually manufactures important nutrients for us from scratch, such as vitamin K. This relationship has evolved over centuries of evolution and is really much more primal to human existence than our reliance on food from agriculture or domesticated animals.

Accordingly, we can look at the gut as both a protective buffer zone and as a valuable and productive agricultural region that provides many important constituents for our bodies. As such it deserves more respect. When we take the strictly mechanical view, we tend to say, "Let's stop the acid production, let's kill the bacteria, let's speed up or slow down the assembly line." But in so doing we're failing to recognize the gut's importance as an immune organ and as a home to trillions of organisms that are as important to our survival as bees are to flowering shrubs and trees.

If we don't recognize how crucial this symbiosis is to our body, we risk destroying our health. The key risk factors are all around us: the chlorination and fluoridation of water, the synthesis of foods that do different things in our gut than foods ever evolved to do, the use of antacids that disrupt normal digestive function, the use of antibiotics that kill off beneficial bacteria, and the incredible proliferation of virulent drug-resistant bacteria that we're exposed to whenever we have to go to a hospital.

Most GI problems are problems of lifestyle or of civilization. They're a simple biological response to the substances we pour down our throats, which taste good or make us feel good, but which our basic organism is just not prepared to handle. We know today more than ever the importance that diet plays in maintaining good health. The GI tract is the front line that's the first to show the effects of all the dietary decisions we make. A closer look at contemporarily lifestyles makes it clear why our generation is increasingly suffering from a whole panoply of gastrointestinal ailments.

Recipes for an Unhealthy GI Tract

Baby boomers in particular are highly susceptible to GI ailments. Let's look at some of the reasons.

Infancy: Bad Beginnings

We can start at the beginning of a child's life here in America. For many years since the onset of the baby boom, it has been fashionable to birth babies in hospitals. In fact, the opposite used to be true — people had their babies at home, and the only time you went to the hospital was to die!

When a child is born, the gastrointestinal tract is sterile. There are no bacteria. In the first month of life, the baby's gut becomes populated with microorganisms, usually acquired by the newborn from exposure to the mother. By birthing babies in hospitals, we expose them to extremely pathogenic bacteria that are antibiotic resistant, and this can potentially lead to the development of an improper blend of GI flora.

The next culprit is the bottle. In the past, it wasn't fashionable to breast-feed. This was especially true for mothers of baby boomers. Our mothers were encouraged to bottle-feed their infants — only the very poor, who couldn't afford the formulas and accoutrements of bottle-feeding, gave their babies the breast! Fortunately, we now know the numerous benefits of breast-feeding, and it has regained popularity with modern mothers.

The composition of human breast milk is designed to nurture the human infant perfectly. It's a pretty simple concept: human milk for a human child. For a child, it is the most hypoallergenic food available. On the contrary, cow's milk is designed for calves, and the composition differs in some major ways. For instance, human milk is higher in sugar and water content and lower in calcium and fat. Premature administration of cow's milk also produces allergies in many infants. On a microscopic level, it can cause bleeding in the lining of the gut and has been known to cause anemia in infants.

Besides the advantage of human breast milk's composition, another important benefit of breast-feeding is colostrum, which is produced by a nursing mother's breast before her milk "lets down." Colostrum is a yellow-ish runny substance, rich in nutrients and mother's antibodies. It stimulates the lymphatic tissue in the baby's GI tract by providing messages from the mother's immune system.

Finally, after exposing infants to dangerous bacteria and impairing their natural immune defenses, we fluoridate and chlorinate their mouths and their GI tracts with our treated drinking water. The fluoride and chlorine in tap water literally sterilize the flora in the GI tract. This inadvertent chemi-cal poisoning can contribute to GI ills.

Diet: You Are What You Eat

Baby boomers' diets have changed considerably from those of our parents and grandparents. If it were literally true, the old adage "you are what you eat" would strike terror into most of our hearts! My own childhood eating habits can be epitomized by a Hostess Twinkie and a glass of milk — staples of many a baby boomer's diet.

Dietary changes from our parents' days include the introduction of processed foods, the prevalence of nutrient-deficient foods and low-fiber foods, and the introduction of larger amounts of sugar in our foods. The result is a diet devoid of the benefits of whole foods and their assorted nutrients, which has a serious impact on the GI tract. Some of the characteristics of the typical modern diet are these:

LOW FIBER

Besides constipation and hemorrhoids, the low-fiber diet can contribute to the development of diverticulosis, gallbladder disease, colon cancer, and appendicitis. Low fiber can even increase the risk of breast cancer, since sufficient fiber in the diet can act like a sponge, absorbing excess estrogen and harmlessly passing it out with the stool.

HIGH SUGAR

Most packaged foods, from cold cereals to bacon, contain sugar in some form. Although sugar is frequently disguised in labels under another name, whether as fructose, sucrose, corn syrup, dextrose, lactose, or maltodextrose, it's still sugar. High-sugar diets contribute to the development of Syndrome X, yeast infections of all types, obesity, diabetes, hypoglycemia, gallbladder disease, and some types of psychological problems, especially depression and premenstrual syndrome.

PROCESSED FOODS AND JUNK FOOD

These foods are synonymous with "fast food." They are devoid of sound nutrition and high in sugar, fat, salt, and chemical preservatives. Foods in this group are sugary cold cereal (be careful of "health store" brands that are "fruit-juice sweetened" — same thing!), processed meats like sausage, hot dogs, bacon and cold cuts, soda pop, potato chips and French fries, instant desserts, ice cream products, ketchup, and burgers.

HIGH FAT

Fat tastes good, and it satisfies hunger because it is metabolized slowly. But we eat too much of it! Besides being present in animal meats like beef, pork, chicken, and lamb, fat is also present in fast foods, cheese and whole milk products, lard, tropical oils like palm and coconut oil, nondairy creamers, cookies and baked goods, crackers, nuts, and avocados. A high-fat diet can contribute to obesity, colon cancer, pancreatic cancer, gallbladder disease, heart disease, and possibly breast cancer.

Antibiotics: A Mixed Blessing

While the miracle drugs of today have saved many lives, the antibiotic treatment of infections can play havoc with a healthy GI tract. Besides ridding us of harmful bacteria, antibiotics assault the normal communities of "good" bacteria that reside in the GI tract. This can result in fungus infections such as *Candida* or the proliferation of other bacteria like dangerous *Staphylococcus*.

Antibiotics are also inadvertently introduced into our systems by the eating of poultry, meat, or milk products from animals that were treated with antibiotics to keep them healthy under cramped and unhealthy feedlot conditions.

Antacids: Not the "Anti" You Think They Are

Baby boomers use a lot of antacids to deal with many different types of GI problems. The old-fashioned Rolaids commercials with the "drip-drip-drip" and the claim that it "consumes forty times its weight in excess stomach acid" is our model solution for any GI problem. It's a model that has successfully sold billions of dollars of over-the-counter antacids. Now, baby boomers who fear osteoporosis are exhorted to take Tums, giving new life to the old remedy. Now, powerful acid blockers are available over the counter that were formerly obtained only by prescription.

The fact is, however, that most upset stomachs are caused not by too much stomach acid but by the wrong food or too much food. If the culprit is identified or destructive eating patterns are changed, the problem can virtually always be corrected without antacids.

The other problem with using antacids for an upset stomach is that they don't work. "What?!" you say. "I can tell the difference after I take it!" Actually, unless you have an ulcer, this is probably a placebo effect. Antacids were clinically proven ineffective by a Swedish study in 1986. In fact, antacids will sometimes cause your stomach to produce *more* acid — a condition called acid rebound, which worsens your GI problem.[1] Also, antacids change the pH environment of the gut, potentially causing an imbalance of friendly flora and putting you at risk for infection by the unfriendly types. Some believe that antacids may even help set the stage for infection with *Helicobacter pylori*, the bacterium that causes ulcers.

Overeating

We are a nation of overeaters. "All you can eat" dinners and smorgasbords were the dining rage of middle America as we grew up, and they typify the erroneous philosophy that more is better. Even in our supposedly health-conscious age, statistics have shown that our average yearly food intake actually increased during a recent ten-year period. Overeating leads to a host of GI problems: abdominal pain, bloating, gas, diarrhea, constipation, hemorrhoids, and overnutrition. How many of us have *not* suffered from one or more of these consequences at some point when we've overindulged on that special occasion? Many of us should ask ourselves whether we are overindulging regularly and experiencing these symptoms all the time. If you combine chronic overeating with your food allergies, you can imagine why you're miserable!

In the absence of purging or bulimia, obesity is the most obvious complication of overeating. Commercial weight-loss programs are a billion-dollar industry in this country. An estimated thirty-four million Americans aged twenty to seventy-five weigh more than the recommended figures for their age and height — a startling 26 percent![2] Of these, a high percentage are food addicts.[3] According to medical experts, an increase of just 20 percent over ideal body weight is considered a bona fide health hazard.[4]

Chemical Ills: Caffeine, Alcohol, and Smoking

In addition to eating too much, Americans bombard their systems with nonfoods that are nothing but pure mood-changers.

CAFFEINE

Some people pour huge amounts of caffeine into their GI tracts. Caffeine is highly addictive stuff, with distinct physiological withdrawal symptoms, including headaches. Besides coffee and tea, many popular soft drinks have a high caffeine content. Other sources of hidden caffeine are chocolate and cocoa products, pain relievers like Anacin and Excedrin, and many over-the-counter cold remedies. (Make sure you read the ingredients on the labels!)

As a drug, caffeine stimulates gastric secretions, thereby increasing appetite. It also overstimulates the normal rhythmic contractions of the bowels, causes malabsorption of nutrients — especially calcium and magnesium — and blocks prostaglandin production.

In addition to caffeine, the oils contained in coffee — even decaffeinated coffee — can have powerful effects on the digestive tract, acting to increase acid production in the stomach. This can contribute to a host of GI problems, including ulcers and irritable bowel syndrome, also known as spastic colon. People vary widely in their tolerance for caffeine. Some can drink two or three cups a day with no ill effects; others would be advised to swear off it completely.

A word of caution about quitting caffeine: taper it off slowly over several days. Gradually switch from caffeinated to decaffeinated beverages. Cut the caffeine beverages back one-half cup a day, replacing them with decaffeinated. (If you drink three cups of coffee every day, go to two and a half cups the next day, then two cups, then a cup and a half, etc.) If you start to get headaches, taper it even more slowly.

ALCOHOL

Although alcohol can deliver some health benefits in small quantities, in excess it acts as a dangerous toxin in the human body. Excess alcohol can inflame the lining of the esophagus, stomach, and intestine; it can sterilize the gut by killing bacteria and normal intestinal flora, leading to indigestion and diarrhea. Alcohol also impairs digestion by reducing stomach acid and digestive enzymes. Because it contains calories, alcohol consumed at high levels can act as an appetite suppressant, though generally it relaxes you and promotes appetite. Finally, excess alcohol use leads to nutritional deficits as well: it is the number-one cause of malnutrition in otherwise healthy people.

If you have digestive difficulties that may be related to alcohol use, try cutting back and see whether there's improvement. If you're unable to cut back or stop drinking, consult your physician and/or Alcoholics Anonymous.

CIGARETTES

Cigarette smoke contains over 150 poisonous gases, one of which is nicotine—a very powerful stimulant that is highly addictive. Why mention cigarettes here? Because smoking contributes to indigestion or heartburn by increasing the amount of acid produced in the stomach and decreasing the amount of bicarbonate produced by the pancreas. This bicarbonate is essential to neutralize stomach acid. Consequently, smokers are more prone to gastric and duodenal ulcers than are nonsmokers. Smoking also accelerates gastric emptying and intestinal motility. (See chapter 13 for details on how I have helped many people give up smoking.)

An Unsettled Age

The factors outlined above are the major causes of gastrointestinal distress for the healthy individual. It is possible to completely eradicate most GI complaints by avoiding cigarettes and excess coffee or alcohol, improving the diet, reducing the amount of food eaten, and stopping the use of antacids. There are some additional remedies for the common gastrointestinal symptoms, including indigestion, constipation, diarrhea, and flatulence.

Indigestion

Indigestion, or heartburn, affects at least 10 percent of Americans every day. It usually feels like a burning pain in the middle of the chest. Acid reflux, the sour taste of stomach contents momentarily "backing up" in the throat, frequently accompanies indigestion.

Sometimes heartburn can't be avoided, like the normal heartburn that goes with pregnancy and usually passes after the baby is born. But much heartburn is caused by some of our excesses and habits. Here are a few contributors to indigestion:

- Being overweight.
- Smoking.
- Drinking alcohol.
- Overeating.
- Eating certain foods: fried and fatty foods, tomatoes, citrus, chocolate, coffee, foods to which a person is intolerant.
- Age. As you get older, so does your gut. The sphincter at the base of the esophagus that prevents stomach backwash can become looser with age. Hiatal hernia, a benign condition in which part of the stomach can herniate through the diaphragm, affects many older people and is a frequent cause of heartburn. It affects an estimated 50 percent of people aged 50 and older.

Sometimes eliminating the offending food or drink, quitting smoking, cutting back on your eating, and losing weight will take care of the problem. Other things that may help relieve occasional heartburn are

- Aloe vera and bismuth (the active ingredient in Pepto-Bismol). This is helpful for indigestion and reflux.
- Supplemental hydrochloric acid, generally in the form of betaine hydrochloride. Paradoxically, heartburn and reflux are sometimes caused by insufficient production of hydrochloric acid.
- Staying vertical and not lying down for one to one and a half hours after meals.
- DGL, deglycerrhizinated licorice, acts as a natural anti-inflammatory.

Constipation

Constipation is usually defined as the inability to have a bowel movement after more than three days. In our country, it is a very common gastrointestinal complaint. I believe the main causes of constipation are

- Too much fat and sugar
- Not enough fiber
- Not enough exercise

Chronic constipation may also be related to stress, and a long-term program of relaxation techniques, yoga, or meditation can affect this problem. Other possible causes of constipation are inadequate water intake, magnesium deficiency, excess meat in the diet, hormonal imbalance, and certain medications, including some high blood pressure medications and over-the-counter antacids. The following measures are usually effective in treating constipation:

- Reduce fat and sugar intake!
- Increase fiber!
- Exercise!

This is not to be flippant, but those three measures will usually take care of the problem. You can add fiber to your diet in the form of raw, unprocessed wheat bran or ground psyllium seed (the main ingredient in Metamucil without the sugar or additives), or by increasing your intake of fruit and vegetables. Another constipation-buster is to increase your water consumption — doctors and nutritionists have long extolled the benefits of eight glasses of water a day. Not only is it good for your digestive system, but it benefits the entire body by flushing it of toxins, chemicals, and the byproducts of metabolism. The body needs two and a half gallons of water just to process food through the digestive system; if you're not drinking enough water, too much toxic material is reabsorbed by the large intestine. Be sure, though that you're drinking spring or well water. Steady consumption of the highly chlorinated tap water of many cities and communities may increase your cancer risk.

Other remedies for constipation include

- **Herbal treatments.** For occasional relief of constipation, take a tablespoon of goldenseal, buckthorn bark, flaxseed, or linseed in a glass of water. (But be careful — certain herbal laxatives can be habit-forming, too!)

- **Prunes (the old standby) or Rhubarb.** Fresh rhubarb stalks work wonders for constipation.
- **Colonics.** Enemas have been used since ancient times as a cure for constipation. Colonics are thorough enemas that gently cleanse the entire colon.
- **Magnesium** can be helpful in two ways. It restores tone to the muscles of the digestive tract, taking them out of spasm and enhancing peristalsis, which is the natural pulse that moves food through the intestine. It also acts as a natural laxative by pulling water into the intestine, in addition to its physical effect. The standard remedy, Milk of Magnesia, is magnesium hydroxide, but I prefer magnesium citrate. In very heavy doses, magnesium citrate is a physic — a powerful laxative — but in moderate doses can gently aid the digestive process.

RECOMMENDED DOSAGE: 150 mg two or three times daily. (Caution should be exercised by the elderly or those with diminished kidney function as revealed on a standard blood test.)

Diarrhea

Most diarrhea is acute and is usually related to food poisoning, a virus or bacterial infection, or a food intolerance. It is usually self-limiting and passes in a few days, clearing up on its own. Here are some things you can do to help:

- **Rule out infection.** If your diarrhea won't go away after a few days, you should consult a doctor and rule out a parasitic or bacterial infection, or an inflammatory condition like ulcerative colitis or Crohn's disease.
- **Avoid laxative foods.** These include foods like raw salads, most dairy products (except yogurt), raw vegetables and fruits, beans, fruit and vegetable juices, caffeine, and carbonated beverages.
- **Eat the "BRAT diet."** Bananas, rice (white), applesauce, and tea (herbal, especially chamomile) — this food list is often recommended by pediatricians for children with diarrhea.
- **Eat yogurt** with live culture of acidophilus or bifido, or take **acidophilus supplements.** (Flavor yogurt with cinnamon or vanilla rather than eating the highly sweetened fruit flavors.)
- **Eat cooler, lukewarm (not cold) foods.** Heat speeds up the movement of food through the intestine.
- **Use natural medications.** Certain natural clays can help absorb toxins from bacterial overgrowth and also firm up the stool. Bentonite

is one of these, and so is kaolin, which is found in the the over-the-counter remedy Kaopectate (which also contains pectin, a soft fiber.) These are not toxic. If you look at them under a microscope, you'll see particles that look like little golf balls with dimples, which are sites that attract the diarrhea-causing endotoxins produced by bacteria in the intestine.

- **Take a bismuth compound.** Pepto-Bismol is a good over-the-counter remedy that contains both bismuth and pepsin. You can also ask your doctor for a prescription-only pure bismuth citrate. I often prescribe a compound called "B and B": a mixture of bentonite and bismuth.
- **Avoid antimotility drugs.** Drugs like Lomotil, Imodium, and some others work by paralyzing the nerve endings in the bowel to slow intestinal transit time, but they do not remove the diarrhea-causing toxins and can actually cause them to linger.

Make sure to see a doctor if your diarrhea won't go away after a few days. Infants, the very elderly, and the immunosuppressed should be seen right away.

Flatulence

The present vogue for high-fiber, whole-grain vegetarian dishes is generally all to the good, but it can have an annoying side effect. Here are some tips to avoid flatulence:

FOOD COMBINING

Avoid mixing sugar, fruit, or fruit juice with starches. The resulting mix can ferment in your gut, causing flatulence and bloating. Dishes to avoid: sweetened granola with fruit, sweetened oatmeal with raisins, fruit pies, fruit muffins, "low-fat" cookies sweetened with fruit juice.

ACTIVATED CHARCOAL

Tablets of activated charcoal are effective in relieving gas, and the charcoal is not absorbed by your system. (It will also combine with vitamins and medications, so use your judgement.)

DIGESTIVE ENZYMES

Beano is one well-known product that contains a digestive enzyme prepared from *Aspergillus*, a natural vegetarian source. Some people are allergic to *Aspergillus*, a fungus related to *Candida*, and people who have

Candida infections would be advised against using it. But it's generally helpful for people who have difficulty digesting carbohydrates. Another option is to use a product containing pancreatic enzymes from extract of bovine or pork pancreas, although these may be less appealing to strict vegetarians.

CHEW SLOWLY

Chew your food as slowly and as many times as you can.

ELIMINATE SORBITOL

Dietetic candies and gum can contain sorbitol which can't be digested and causes gas.

ELIMINATE MILK PRODUCTS

Except for yogurt and certain cheeses many people are unable to digest milk, a condition called lactose intolerance. Are you one of them? Try eliminating milk and milk products from your diet for a week, and see if your symptoms are alleviated. Try Lactaid milk as an alternative.

Maintaining GI Health

Chapter 16 will help you with an overall approach to a healthy diet, but here are some basic recommendations for optimizing your GI health through your diet.

- **Increase fiber intake**
- **Reduce sugar and fat intake**
- **Avoid processed or fast food**
- **Eat five or more vegetable servings a day**
- **Avoid overeating!**
- **Limit fruits to three a day.** Fruit contains fructose — it's still sugar! Furthermore, some researchers estimate that as many people suffer from fructose intolerance as do from lactose intolerance, or even more.
- **Drink eight or more glasses of water a day.** Water is important for digestion and metabolism — it flushes out the end-products of these processes.
- **Chew thoroughly and slowly.** Digestion starts in the mouth. Chewing

and the action of the enzyme amylase, present in saliva, starts the breakdown of starches.
- **Take supplements as needed.** See below.

On Fiber

In the 1940s, a British gastroenterologist named Dennis Burkitt traveled around the world to study how eating patterns affect gastrointestinal health. He analyzed factors like diet, people's weight, the type of stools they had, and the incidence of different diseases. He was able to conclude from his research that the main problem with the Western diet was that it lacked fiber. He based his entire career on demonstrating that many modern diseases are fiber-deficiency conditions. They run the gamut from coronary artery disease to diverticulosis and colon cancer.

We know that including fiber in our diet is important, but it's important not to overdo it. Fiber has been emphasized to such a degree that it's a wonder some fiber fanatics can keep their feet solidly on the ground — because their intestines are filled with so much gas! While a high-fiber diet works for some problems, it won't work for all. For instance, a *high* fiber diet is not recommended for irritable bowel syndrome, Crohn's disease, or ulcerative colitis.

It's important to include fiber in the diet, but in moderation, according to individual needs. Fiber should be added gradually. Those with heart disease and atherosclerosis will want to add oat bran and psyllium to their diet, as these types of fiber lower cholesterol levels.

On Supplements

Several supplemental nutrients or helpful microbes are beneficial to the gastrointestinal tract. See chapter 16 for recommended supplemental levels on the nutrients listed below, unless otherwise noted.

- **Antioxidants:** vitamin C, vitamin E, the carotenoids, and selenium, to name a few. They have anti-inflammatory and cancer-preventive properties.
- **Calcium and vitamin D** nourish the colon. Milk consumption has been linked to lower rates of colon cancer. Recommended: calcium, 800–1000 milligrams daily; vitamin D, 400 to 1000 International Units daily.
- **Omega-3 oils** like flaxseed oil and fish oil contain "good" prostaglandins with anti-inflammatory properties. Raw flaxseed has a regulatory effect on the gastrointestinal system and prevents constipation. A tablespoon a day sprinkled on cereal or salad is beneficial both for its fiber

and for its oil content. To get the benefits of fish oil, eat fresh cold-water fish — salmon, trout, or mackerel — once or twice a week. If you can't find them easily, take a teaspoon to a tablespoon of cod-liver oil or flaxseed oil daily as a supplement, or three 1000-milligram capsules of flaxseed or cod-liver oil.

- *Lactobacillus acidophilus*: beneficial intestinal flora, found in some yogurt cultures (look on the container) and also available in supplemental capsules. A yogurt a day is advised, but not a frozen yogurt, which has no live cultures. Recommended supplemental dosage: One 500-milligram capsule twice daily, or ¼ to ½ teaspoon two or three times daily.
- **Bifidos bacteria**: beneficial intestinal flora that complement acidophilus, sometimes found in yogurt cultures. Recommended supplemental dosage: One 500-milligram capsule twice daily.
- **Fructoseoligosaccharides.** These organic compounds promote the growth of beneficial intestinal bacteria. They are found in the Jerusalem artichoke and in artichoke flour. Recommended supplemental dosage: Two 500-milligram capsules three times daily or ½ to 1 teaspoon powder three times daily.
- **L-glutamine:** an amino acid that nourishes the enterocytes: cells that line the intestinal wall. High dosages of L-glutamine have been shown to prompt recovery from ulcers and intestinal inflammatory disorders like colitis and Crohn's disease. Preventive supplemental dosage: 500 to 1000-milligram capsules, twice daily. (It's also available in powder form.) In cases of severe GI problems, amounts of up to 40 to 60 grams have been administered with good results.
- *Saccharomyces boulardii*: a fungus that is the Western European version of acidophilus. It is a standard ingredient in over-the-counter antidiarrheal agents taken with antibiotics. It has been shown to reduce the incidence of *Clostridium difficile* infection, a devastating intestinal condition that is sometimes the sequel to antibiotic overuse. As a supplement: 500 milligrams twice daily.
- **Folic acid.** High doses prevent transformation of precancerous cells to cancer and may reduce inflammation in colitis. Recommended therapeutic dosage: 1 milligram (1000 micrograms) daily.
- **Bioflavonoids,** including quercetin and *Ginkgo biloba,* may quench inflammation naturally. Recommended dosages: *Ginkgo biloba,* 60 milligrams of the 24 percent standardized preparation three times daily; quercetin, 100 milligrams three times daily.

By eating healthier diets and taking the appropriate supplements, we can prevent or halt many gastrointestinal illnesses. Although it is difficult to change lifelong eating habits, to give up a cherished food allergen, or to stop eating sugar or fats, it's a small sacrifice to make for the huge improvement you'll notice in your health and sense of well-being—and you'll be around longer to appreciate it.

Fasting

If your health is good, an occasional fast gives your digestive tract a break. The practice of fasting, which dates back to ancient times, was and is used to help a person purify himself or herself spiritually as well as physically.

I believe fasting should last for only a day or so. Drink three to eight glasses of spring water, diluted vegetable broth or juice, miso broth, herbal teas, carrot juice, or watermelon juice throughout the day. If you find you are thirsty, drink more.

Work or light exercise is fine, but don't undertake strenuous activity.

Soak some dried fruit overnight in water or apple juice for your breakfast the next day. This is very easy food for the body to digest, and it contains pectin and vitamins.

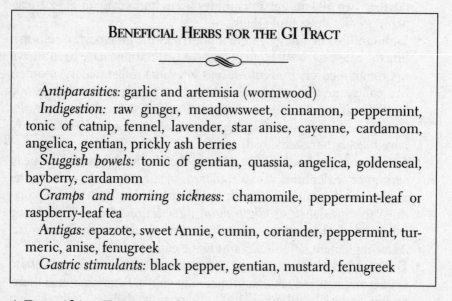

BENEFICIAL HERBS FOR THE GI TRACT

Antiparasitics: garlic and artemisia (wormwood)

Indigestion: raw ginger, meadowsweet, cinnamon, peppermint, tonic of catnip, fennel, lavender, star anise, cayenne, cardamom, angelica, gentian, prickly ash berries

Sluggish bowels: tonic of gentian, quassia, angelica, goldenseal, bayberry, cardamom

Cramps and morning sickness: chamomile, peppermint-leaf or raspberry-leaf tea

Antigas: epazote, sweet Annie, cumin, coriander, peppermint, turmeric, anise, fenugreek

Gastric stimulants: black pepper, gentian, mustard, fenugreek

A Detoxifying Feast

I often suggest that my patients undertake a program of natural cleansing, a diet that promotes the discharge of accumulated toxins and is especially valuable for cleaning out the GI tract. It is not a fast, but rather a *feast*, designed to promote optimal natural vitamins, minerals, and enzymes while restricting proteins, fats, and excessive carbohydrates that burden the system and interfere with natural elimination. Duration: three to seven days, unless you are under a doctor's supervision.

On arising: One glass of spring water with juice of one-half lemon.

Breakfast: Fresh fruits: one bowl of apples, oranges, bananas, grapes, grapefruits, or any available berries and fruits in season. All fruits should be organic, and preferably grown in your own locality and environment.

Midmorning: One glass of green vegetable juice.

Lunch: Vegetable salad. A hearty serving of romaine lettuce, watercress, celery, spinach, carrots, sprouts, or other vegetables available in season. Dressing can be made from lemon juice and cold-pressed olive oil with garlic and herbs to taste.

Midafternoon: Fresh fruit: one apple, pear, or melon in season.

Before dinner: One glass of green vegetable juice.

Dinner: Mixed, sauteed vegetables: carrots, string beans, parsnips, squash, peas, etc. Sauté in cold-pressed oil or ghee.

Bedtime snack: Warm mug of vegetable broth (see recipe).

VEGETABLE BROTH

2 large potatoes, chopped or sliced to approximately half-inch pieces
1 cup carrots, shredded or sliced
1 cup celery, chopped or shredded, leaves and all
1 cup any other available vegetable or green: beet tops, turnip tops, parsley or a little of everything. It's fine to vary this and experiment. However, a valuable broth can be made with only the basic ingredients of potatoes, carrots, and celery.

Optional: Add some garlic, onion, or any of the natural herbal spices. Put all vegetables into a stainless steel cooking pot. Add 1½ quarts of spring water, bring to a boil, then immediately lower heat, cover, and simmer for about half an hour. Strain, toss out the vegetables, cool the broth until just warm, and serve. If not used immediately, keep in refrigerator for up to eight hours and heat before serving.

Allergies and Food Intolerances

So far we've been talking about relatively minor problems, or problems that come and go in most people's lives. By contrast, food allergies and food intolerances are long-term and chronic. They can cause problems that many fail to associate with eating or digestion at all. Besides upset stomach and indigestion, allergies and sensitivities can cause fatigue, anxiety, depression, irritability, skin problems, chronic sinusitis, headaches, and asthma. Over and over again I see patients who suffer from long-term, seemingly intractable problems that we are able to diagnose and "treat" by identifying problem foods and eliminating them from their diets.

Before going any further, though, we should make the distinction between a true food allergy and a food intolerance or sensitivity. Allergies, by definition, are reactions to substances that cause an immune response. A food intolerance, on the other hand, is a genetic glitch or peculiarity in body chemistry or enzyme activity that prevents normal digestion or utilization of some types of foods. The immune system isn't involved; if you could induce the same glitch in another individual, it would cause the same problems.

With a true food allergy, on the other hand, the immune system has somehow become sensitized to respond to a food or food component as if it were a dangerous toxin or invader. The whole array of the immune response — from antibodies to T cells — gets called into play, and the result is a range of symptoms that mimic illness.

True food allergies are fairly rare, though they can cause life-threatening reactions. When it comes to GI problems, the distinction between allergies and intolerances is blurred because the effects are so much alike. I'll generally use the term *allergy* to refer to both allergies and intolerances in this chapter.

Whichever we're dealing with, there is some evidence that food allergies and intolerances are on the rise because of a whole range of factors. One is the increased availability of new foodstuffs, some artificially created, some imported from around the world. People in most cultures around the world used to eat a much more limited diet than we now have available. Many of these new foodstuffs are processed with chemicals, chock-full of preservatives and other additives, refrigerated, or transported or stored for long periods. Some have estimated that the contemporary American diet contains some four hundred different nutrient foodstuffs and twenty-seven hundred chemical additives! As we keep creating new comestibles, the odds are that many of them will trigger allergic reactions in some percentage of the population.

The problem is compounded by underdiagnosis of even the most common food allergies. People are just not accustomed to thinking of materials like milk, eggs, wheat, fish, and nuts as possible causes of illness, ranging from asthma to skin rashes to gas, cramps, or diarrhea. And not enough doctors consider the possibility of allergies as a cause of chronic symptoms.

Wheat is one of the most common causes of food allergy or intolerance. Some individuals experience a profound sensitivity to all wheat products. In their systems, improperly digested wheat fragments appear to mimic powerful neurotransmitters that are similar to opium. This results in symptoms of being tired, feeling "stoned" or "high" because of the opiate-like compound, intestinal bloating, and possibly constipation. These individuals may develop food cravings for the offending substance that can lead to binge eating!

Allergy to wheat is not something that can be diagnosed by standard skin or blood allergy tests. However, if a person who has this allergy or food intolerance eats wheat products, he or she will feel fatigued. Conversely, such an individual who removes wheat products from the diet will notice a rapid improvement in energy level within a few days to a week.

A recent theory by the British researcher J. O. Hunter suggests that the microbe balance in the gut can also affect the allergic response to foods. Certain microbes may literally ferment sugar into alcohol, while others may break it down into toxic aldehydes. Both processes can create profound fatigue, since alcohol and aldehydes stress the whole system, particularly the liver. Some of these microbial byproducts may induce an allergic reaction, while others may act as neurotransmitters in the brain. This process may vary from individual to individual, since everyone carries around a unique balance of gut bacteria. One person may literally get "drunk" from fruit juice, while another can drink it with no such effect. One individual may get a lift from eating meat, while another may feel drowsy as a lion after devouring its prey.

Perhaps the most frustrating aspect of food sensitivities is the fact that many people are intolerant of their favorite foods — the ones they like to eat every day! For them, the thought of giving up those beloved foods is pure anguish. But the good news is that when the offending food is eliminated for several months, in most cases they will be able to tolerate it again, as long as it is limited to once or twice a week. The key to the success of this method is moderation.

Allergy Testing

Your doctor can test for food allergies in several ways, including blood and skin tests. Such tests are helpful, but they do not tell the whole story of food allergy. Food reactions can be very hard to pin down; they may occur instantly or several hours after the ingestion of a particular food, they can trigger a whole range of symptoms, and they can wax and wane. Some food allergies worsen during times of great stress or can be seasonal. For instance, a person with hay fever may find that other allergies surface during the hay-fever season.

The one sure-fire way to find out whether you're allergic, intolerant, or sensitive to a food is to eliminate it from your diet. After four days, reintroduce it. Your symptoms may reappear in a marked and obvious manner, since your body has "de-adapted" to the offending food. There'll then be no doubt about whether you are allergic or not. The elimination diet is highly effective and should be overseen by your doctor. You need to be monitored carefully. In many cases, the food should be reintroduced in small amounts, as little as half a teaspoon, to prevent highly unpleasant reactions.

Food allergies might seem to be the easiest to treat. You just avoid the problem food, right? But that's not always so easy. In this day of highly processed foods, we don't always know what foods or additives have been used in the preparation of a dish. This is especially true of restaurant meals. It is common for many potentially allergy-producing foods to be used in the preparation of an entree or dish: wheat flour, eggs, corn in the form of cornstarch and corn syrup. Casein, a milk protein, is commonly used in breads, sauces, and baked goods. Peanut oil—peanuts are a very common allergy—is used in many commercial baked goods, potato chips, and candies. For many people with food allergies or sensitivities, this inadvertent exposure is simply annoying; they sniffle and sneeze, and eventually it wears off. For other people, the ingestion of the offending substance is life-threatening—they may go into anaphylactic shock, a condition of cardiovascular collapse. The most common life-threatening allergies are those to shellfish, eggs, and peanuts. People with severe food allergies may find that asking the waiter how the food is prepared is not enough protection for them. They may also find it difficult to travel outside the United States, as other countries are not as stringent in the labeling of food products. These individuals may want to have "safe" food sent ahead to their destination. If you don't have this type of allergy problem, simple vigilance should suffice.

Dysbiosis

As part of our fundamental shift in how we look at the gastrointestinal tract, researchers have developed the concept of dysbiosis, a state of bacterial imbalance in the GI tract. It is not a disease but a biological concept. Dysbiosis can affect the small intestine and the large intestine. The microorganisms in the stomach and small bowel are different from those in the large bowel. Overgrowth of certain organisms in either the large or the small bowel can cause different problems and can also predispose an individual to certain disease conditions. Some diseases that are known or thought to be related to small or large bowel dysbiosis are these:

- Atopic eczema. Researchers have established a link between eczema, a skin disease, and small bowel dysbiosis.
- Irritable bowel syndrome. IBS may be caused by the overgrowth of bacterial flora in the large intestine.

- Inflammatory bowel disease. There's a possible connection with exaggerated autoimmune responses to normal intestinal flora.
- Arthritis and ankylosing spondylitis. There's a definite connection between these diseases and abnormal overgrowth of certain bacteria in the small and large intestines.

Some causes of small and large bowel dysbiosis are these:

- **Antacid overuse.** Most cases of small bowel dysbiosis are a complication of antacid overuse, which causes hypochlorhydria, a condition of low gastric acid production.
- **Slow motility.** A slow small intestine may permit food material to rest for longer periods in the intestine, promoting bacterial imbalance.
- **Structural problems.** Surgical "blind loops," fistulas, or strictures can interfere with normal intestinal movement.
- **Immune deficiency.** Chronic disease or drugs like prednisone can induce this condition.
- **Antibiotics.** Long courses of treatment with high-powered antibiotics generally kill off much of the intestinal flora, which can then grow back in unhealthy proportions.
- **Malnutrition** and lack of specific nutrients.

Treatment of large and small bowel dysbiosis, under a physician's care, may involve

- **Changing the diet.** Some patients respond to a low-sugar/low-carbohydrate/high-fiber diet or to the specific carbohydrate diet (see page 193 below).
- **Mineral-based detoxicants.** Bentonite, bismuth, or heilmoor.
- **Carbohydrate supplementation** with specific compounds such as the fructoseoliogosaccharides.
- **Fiber supplements** such as cellulose, psyllium, or pectin.
- **Herbal antimicrobials.** Useful herbal remedies include extracts from *Artemisia annua* and citrus seeds, also goldenseal, and a *Gentiana* or sanguinaria mixture.
- **Replenishing normal intestinal flora** with the appropriate microorganisms like bifidobacteria, *Lactobacillus,* and *Saccharomyces boulardii.*

Leaky Gut Syndrome

Leaky gut syndrome is another condition that can cause problems beyond the immediate digestive organs. It is a problem of nutrient absorption in the small intestine, the true site of digestive absorption. It affects numerous body systems other than the GI tract, producing apparently unrelated symptoms including general malaise, arthritis, headaches, and skin problems. This is because the GI tract interfaces with both the circulatory and the immune systems.

The syndrome is caused by chronic inflammation of the small intestine, which leads to absorption of food particles that are more macromolecular, or larger, than the ideal size for proper metabolism as well as the absorption of immune-reactive materials across the intestinal wall. Although widely known and understood by physicians like myself who are in the vanguard of practicing holistic, nutritional medicine, leaky gut syndrome is not yet an accepted disease syndrome in the conventional medical community. Even so, medical studies have long confirmed the link between intestinal absorption of allergy-producing substances and autoimmune diseases like rheumatoid arthritis and ankylosing spondylitis (a degenerative arthritic condition that affects the spine).

For the baby boomer, several factors may contribute to the development of leaky gut syndrome:

- **Antacids** prevent proper breakdown of nutrients and further inflame the intestinal wall. Food particles are then absorbed indiscriminately.
- **NSAIDs** — nonsteroidal anti-inflammatory drugs such as aspirin and ibuprofren (whose trade names are Advil, Nuprin, Motrin) have been shown to cause gastritis and ulcers. In addition to causing bleeding of the stomach wall, the NSAIDs cause microhemorrhages in the wall of the small intestine.
- **Food allergies** can cause local inflammation of the gut wall.
- **Candidiasis,** an overgrowth of *Candida albicans,* causes inflammation of the intestinal wall.

The test performed for leaky gut syndrome, the intestinal permeability test, evaluates whether a person is passing very large molecules, which normally couldn't be absorbed, through the intestinal wall.

Leaky gut is treated through diet modification, avoidance of antacids and NSAIDs, identification of allergies or food sensitivities, and treatment of candidiasis if present. L-glutamine and quercetin supplements can be helpful. Cromolyn sodium is an effective medication.

A Fungus Among Us

Civilization would be much the poorer without yeast, a fungal microorganism that we use to raise bread and ferment beer. But yeast gets even more intimate with us than that. One variety, *Candida albicans,* is a living microorganism that is part of the beneficial flora that populate our bodies. Like friendly bacteria, it usually coexists peacefully with us on the surfaces of our skin and the mucous membranes of the throat, gastrointestinal tract, and, for women, in the vagina. The overgrowth of yeast, a condition called candidiasis, alters the balance of the normal flora and can affect the body in many ways, resulting in allergic reactions, acne, migraines, premenstrual symptoms, respiratory problems, lethargy, depression, and gastrointestinal complaints.

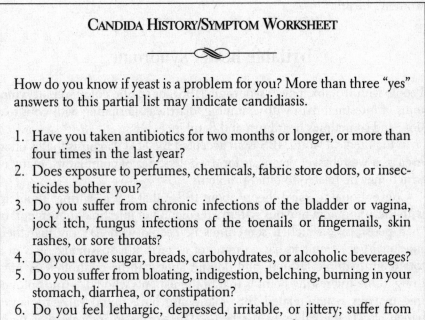

CANDIDA HISTORY/SYMPTOM WORKSHEET

How do you know if yeast is a problem for you? More than three "yes" answers to this partial list may indicate candidiasis.

1. Have you taken antibiotics for two months or longer, or more than four times in the last year?
2. Does exposure to perfumes, chemicals, fabric store odors, or insecticides bother you?
3. Do you suffer from chronic infections of the bladder or vagina, jock itch, fungus infections of the toenails or fingernails, skin rashes, or sore throats?
4. Do you crave sugar, breads, carbohydrates, or alcoholic beverages?
5. Do you suffer from bloating, indigestion, belching, burning in your stomach, diarrhea, or constipation?
6. Do you feel lethargic, depressed, irritable, or jittery; suffer from mood swings; or have dizziness or poor coordination?
7. Do you or have you taken birth control pills or steroids?

Indigestion, bloating, diarrhea, and constipation are frequently related to an overgrowth of yeast in the intestines. You would notice a worsening of symptoms after ingesting a meal high in carbohydrates or sugar, because yeast thrives on these types of foods. Many people with yeast infections subsequently develop an allergy to yeast. Dr. C. Orian Truss was the first allergist to identify the connection between yeast and a wide variety of allergic reactions.

Candidiasis and *Candida* allergy are treatable. Simply eliminating medicine and foods that promote yeast overgrowth are usually enough. Foods that encourage *Candida* are:

- Sugar
- Starchy foods
- Fruits and fruit juices
- Alcohol
- Breads and yeast products
- Antibiotic-laden meat products

With *Candida* infections that are deeply entrenched, prescription anti-fungal agents like Nystatin, Nizoral, Diflucan, or Sporonox may be called for. Women may look in chapter 10 for more on candidiasis in relation to women's health.

Irritable Bowel Syndrome

People with irritable bowel syndrome (IBS), or spastic colon, report symptoms of intestinal pain with cramping, diarrhea alternating with constipation, and sometimes heartburn and flatulence.

In the medical world, IBS is an accepted medical diagnosis that is often used as a wastebasket diagnosis for a whole series of complaints, many of which may be related to other problems.

Conventional medical theory about IBS is that it is a "wiring" problem with the autonomic nervous system's regulation of intestinal movement, or "bad peristalsis," which it sometimes is. People with IBS say that their intestinal tract seems to have a mind of its own: it is spasmodic, acts in a totally unrhythmic fashion, and doesn't appear to be controlled by anything. (One interesting point is that of the patients who have true autonomic nervous system-related IBS, many also have mitral valve prolapse, which affects the valves of the heart. This seems to indicate that these patients really do have "faulty wiring" or an altered autonomic nervous system.)

Doctors are fond of blaming IBS on the patient, labeling it a stress disorder. They think of IBS patients as being neurotic, infantile, and obsessive about their bowel problems. Granted, some patients are a little obsessive, but the unpredictability of their bowel function strikes them where they live. One of the things that heralds the passage from infancy to childhood, and consequently to adulthood, is our ability to control and regulate our elimination habits. Irritable bowel syndrome sometimes seems like an involuntary regression toward childhood helplessness.

For some people, IBS can be incapacitating, interfering with their patterns of daily living; they may be hindered even in their ability to travel or commute because of the need to be constantly within range of a bathroom.

The physician's usual treatment of IBS is to diagnose the problem, recommend Metamucil or a fiber product, tell the patient to watch stress levels, and prescribe an antispasmodic medication. For many patients, this treatment is satisfactory. In my experience with IBS, I have found that what appears to be IBS can actually be symptoms related to food allergy, food intolerance, or dysbiosis. Therefore, I believe it is important to rule out all possible causes of the IBS-type symptoms. Although this approach may be considered unconventional, my colleagues and I have found it to be effective in treating and diagnosing IBS and symptoms that mimic it. In fact, in one recent study, nearly 50 percent of patients thought to have just irritable bowel syndrome turned out to have giardiasis, a parasitic infection that can cause intermittent diarrhea.[5]

Here are some alternate causes for IBS-like symptoms:

- **Dysbiosis.** IBS may be due to an imbalance of bacterial flora with overgrowth of yeast, or to parasites in the intestine.
- **Food allergies and food intolerances.** The intestine may attempt to "purge" itself of the offending substances. Allergies may inflame the intestinal wall, resulting in impaired digestion and spasms.
- **Too much food.** Overeaters often report intestinal difficulties, including spastic colon, flatulence, constipation, and diarrhea.
- **Lack of fiber or excess of fiber.** Too little can result in constipation; too much can cause spasms, bloating, and diarrhea.
- **Carbohydrate intolerance.** Some people can't digest milk products (which contain lactose); others can't eat fructose-laden fruits or juices; still others can't handle grains.
- **Nervous tension.** Some people really do have an imbalance of the autonomic nervous system. They report that their GI system seems to act in concert with their moods and anxieties; if nervous, they "go all the time, like a baby!"

Treatment of IBS

At least 40 percent of cases can be improved by diet changes: the elimination of a specific food, the avoidance of lactose (milk sugar), the removal or addition of fiber, or the adoption of a gluten-free diet. It is also recommended that patients with symptoms of IBS have a comprehensive digestion and stool analysis to rule out dysbiosis or the presence of intestinal parasites.

Once all possible physical causes are ruled out and it is established that the IBS is related to stress reactions and the autonomic nervous system, I prefer a holistic approach in treatment rather than conventional drug therapy. The medications doctors usually prescribe are bowel tranquilizers:

Librax, Donnatal, Levsin, Levsinex, and Imodium. The problem with them is that they are not specific in their focus and they cause side effects. They may quiet the symptoms, but they also cause dry mouth, lethargy, and sometimes urinary retention, especially in men with prostate problems.

These are my recommendations for true IBS caused by a jumpy autonomic nervous system:

- **Relaxation programs.** There are exercises and yoga postures that actually help to train the autonomic nervous system and can relieve symptoms of IBS.
- **Acupuncture.** Acupuncture helps to send regulatory messages to the autonomic nervous system.
- **Herbal therapy.** Peppermint has a soothing effect on the lower GI tract. Look for the enteric-coated variety, which acts selectively on the intestine. Ginger is a settling herb which is also good for nausea.
- **A low-fat, high fiber diet** will put less physical stress on the bowels.
- **Cognitive psychotherapy** and even **hypnosis** have been known to help some patients.

Gastric Ulcers

Ulcer pain is usually sharp and constant and occurs somewhere between the navel and the breastbone. It may be worse between meals and feel better after eating, or the reverse may be true. Some foods may worsen symptoms.

The way modern medicine views the pathology of gastric ulcers has completely and irrevocably changed. For fifty years, doctors believed that gastric and peptic ulcers were a psychosomatic disorder caused by a person's abnormal reactions to the stressors in their life and excessive acid secretion by the stomach. The pharmaceutical and over-the-counter drug industries banked big on the theory that ulcers were caused by this overproduction of gastric acid, and the biggest-selling drugs in the industry were born out of this theory.

We now know that a microorganism is responsible for most gastric and peptic ulcers, and usually *not* excessive gastric acid production. The name of this microbe is *Helicobacter pylori*, sometimes abbreviated to *H. pylori*. Now that we know a microorganism causes most ulcers and that they aren't related to a stressful lifestyle, we can stop blaming patients for coming down with them! Treatment for *H. pylori* infection is now much simpler than lifelong dependency on an antacid. A simple two-week course of antibiotics, combined with a bismuth preparation like Pepto-Bismol, seems to do the trick just fine. The "find a bug, give a drug" theory of medicine is certainly right on target here — and it couldn't have found a more appropriate disease to eradicate!

Gallbladder Disease

Gallbladder disease is a modern illness. An estimated twenty million Americans have gallbladder disease. Why are we including the gallbladder in this chapter? Because its sole function is to store bile, which is produced in the liver and aids in the digestion of fats in the small intestine. The gallbladder has become a prime target for surgical intervention; in fact, this is the most common type of major surgery. Sometimes it's done to reduce pain, sometimes to remove gallstones. It's especially common among women who are receiving estrogen replacement therapy, since estrogen stimulates the production of gallstones. (Accordingly, women with gallstone problems are probably not good candidates for oral estrogen replacement; they might do better with a transdermal estrogen patch.) This is a degenerative disease that's clearly related to diet. A study performed at the University Hospital of Riyadh, Saudi Arabia, found that the incidence of gallbladder surgery went up by 600 percent in that country as the people shifted from a simpler, nomadic existence, eating traditional foods, to a more sedentary lifestyle "enriched" by all the sugary, fat-laden foods of the developed world.

In gallbladder disease, bile in the gallbladder becomes concentrated and thickens. Gallstones are born out of this sludge from cholesterol and bile salts. The end result of the disease process is inflammation (cholecystitis) or stones (cholelithiasis). A gallbladder attack occurs when the gallstone blocks the flow of bile from the gallbladder and is manifested as a pain in the right side (sometimes perceived in the right shoulder because of referred pain) as severe as the excruciating pain of a heart attack.

Some factors that contribute to the development of gallbladder disease are

- **Heredity.** Gallstones occur slightly more frequently in Mexican Americans and Native Americans but are also common in people of northern European stock.
- **Age.** Gallbladder disease often strikes people over sixty years of age.
- **Gender.** In medical school, the "five F's" help doctors to remember the usual patient with gallbladder disease: "fair, fat, forty, fertile, and female." Sexist as it sounds, it describes the group most frequently affected by gallbladder disease: overweight middle-aged white women with a history of several pregnancies. Excess estrogen may be implicated, since hormone replacement after menopause increases the likelihood of stones.
- **Diet.** The propensity of Western diet to predispose one to gallbladder disease was commemorated by journalists during the Persian Gulf War—the prevalence of gallbladder disease among Saudis had gone up 600 percent since the 1940s, when they began "enjoying" more and

more Western foods! Most people know that there is an established link between fat intake and gallbladder disease, but many don't realize that there is also a significant correlation with high sugar intake as well.

- **Obesity.** In comparison with people of normal weight, the bile of obese people is supersaturated with cholesterol, predisposing them to the development of gallbladder illness.
- **Slow intestinal transit.** Medical professionals have long known that constipation is common in patients who have gallbladder disease. Studies confirm that slow intestinal transit contributes to the formation of gallstones in women of normal weight.[6]

Having gallstones doesn't mean that one should rush right out, consult a surgeon, and schedule major surgery. You can live with gallstones and be symptom free. Physicians have noticed that certain foods can initiate a gallbladder attack in patients who have gallstones. When these foods were eliminated from their diet, their gallbladder symptoms disappeared. In explanation, it is thought there might be a food allergy mechanism at work, wherein the gallbladder responds to the allergy-producing food with symptoms of a gallbladder attack.

The most frequently offending foods are eggs, pork, onions, poultry, milk, coffee, oranges, corn, beans, and nuts.

Rose, a sixty-one-year-old woman from Virginia, came into my office for gallbladder complaints. She had been advised to have surgery, but her daughter encouraged her to get a second opinion. I determined that she was not in any immediate danger and gave her a modified version of the "gallbladder disease elimination diet" by Dr. James Breneman. (This is not a "do-it-yourself" diet but should be monitored by a physician.) This diet eliminates the most commonly offending foods outlined above. Besides having Rose increase the fiber in her diet, I also gave her lecithin and certain herbs, like artichoke and dandelion, that help drain bile from the gallbladder. For several weeks, Rose was symptom free, except on one occasion when she slipped from her diet. This was a gradual, gentle diet plan — crash diets can actually precipitate gallstones.

Still on the diet after three months, she had lost twelve pounds, had a 65-point reduction in her cholesterol level, was symptom free, and felt great. Fifteen years later, she still hasn't required surgery, even though surgical methods are simpler now and are prescribed more often.

With the advent of laser laparoscopy surgery in this country, it's much easier to take gallbladders out. As a result, the surgery rates for this disease have almost doubled. Does it make sense to perform so much more surgery merely because its easier? To some extent, yes, because it's not as perilous as before and doesn't require such a long hospital stay. But this new technique has made the gallbladder an easier and more tempting target for surgeons, and has it made people less reluctant to undergo surgery that may not be entirely necessary.

A reaction is setting in, however, as more doctors realize that most painful gallbladders can be left alone once they're mostly quiescent, with just the occasional painful attack. In fact, the pain can generally be reduced by dietary measures: lowering fat and sugar intake or avoiding problem foods like eggs, poultry, or pork. The presence of gallstones in itself doesn't seem to warrant surgery — the new belief is that you can happily take them to your grave. There are some exceptions: people with diabetes in particular may be well advised to have the surgery. Since they sometimes have nerve difficulties and don't get clear-cut pain signals, they run the risk of complications from silent or unperceived gallbladder attacks, and might wind up with a ruptured gallbladder. Surgeons are aware of this, and they operate decisively in these cases.

I've seen many people, however, who suffered from gallbladder pain, had the operation, and then suffered from a postoperative syndrome: the stones were out but they still had pain. And that's pretty aggravating, because their doctor suggested that the stones were the source of the pain. In some cases, the gallbladder is removed only to reveal that it wasn't the source of the pain, that there was some other somatic cause unrelated to whatever stones or sludge might have appeared in the gallbladder.

So if your gallbladder is really shot and if you're having pain all the time, have it out. But most people can pretty well poke along with an asymptomatic gallbladder. Sporadic gallbladder attacks that respond to diet changes, and the presence of gallstones identified by sonogram, are not in themselves an indication for surgery. The pain can be brought under control with dietary modification, and the presence of the stones by itself doesn't mean you need to have them taken out. But this is how it's presented to people. Surgeons will show you a sonogram of a gallbladder laden with stones as a selling point to get you on board for the surgery. It can be hard to resist this kind of pitch from a medical expert, but unfortunately this represents a situation that patients often find themselves in.

If needed, there several surgical methods of treatment available as well as medical treatments for gallbladder disease. They include

• **Laser laparoscopic cholecystectomy.** No longer do patients have to suffer the agony of long incision lines just below the rib cage, making postoperative recovery difficult. Surgeons are removing gallbladders using lasers and a fiberoptic laparoscope (a flexible fiberoptic tube). But if you opt for this surgery, beware! This type of "key-hole surgery" takes considerable skill on the part of the surgeon. A few unfortunate deaths have been related to lack of proper training and experience in this delicate procedure; complication rates have actually increased since its introduction. Make sure you ask the surgeon where he or she received training in the procedure and how many he or she has performed. Some states impose regulations regarding the training and practice of physicians performing this operation.

Though press and publicity for these surgical procedures touts one-day hospital stays, the actual stay is generally three to three and a half days. In some cases there's a need to revert to the older procedure after the laser procedure is attempted.

• **Small-incision cholecystectomy.** This is an alternative to the laser procedure. It's a variation of the traditional gallbladder operation but with a much smaller incision, averaging 2 to 3 inches instead of the much larger standard incision. The operation is shorter than the laser procedure, the hospital release time is the same, and the rate of need for reversion to the older surgery is the same. The more sophisticated procedures may not be an improvement.

• **Medication.** Actigall, or ursodeoxycholic acid, is taken orally to dissolve stones made of cholesterol. It takes one to two years for complete dissolution of stones. Only sufficiently small stones of a certain type are treatable with this drug.

Unfortunately, many people think they can eat fats with impunity after surgery. In reality, gallbladder disease is a warning sign that your dietary excess is hurting you! People who suffer from gallbladder disease often have other concurrent metabolic disorders, like a predisposition to cardiovascular disease and diabetes.

Prevention of gallbladder disease is still the best approach. Here are some things you can do to decrease your risk:

• **Lose excess weight.** But don't crash diet! Rapid weight loss contributes to the formation of gallstones.

• **Eat a healthy diet.** A diet that is low in fat, low in cholesterol, low in sugar, and high in fiber will help prevent gallbladder disease. Fat, cholesterol, and sugar all contribute to gallbladder disease. Slow intestinal transit can be prevented by increasing fiber in the diet. And eat more vegetables! A British study showed that vegetarians have a lower incidence of gallbladder disease.

• **Avoid food triggers.** As mentioned before, there's a correlation between gallbladder attack symptoms and certain foods in people who are sensitive to them. Be on the lookout for food triggers.

• **Take fish oil and nutrients.** Omega-3 oil, found in fish, may block cholesterol formation in bile. People with a tendency toward gallstones can take a higher dose than normal: four to six 1000-milligram capsules of fish oil a day. Lecithin has an emulsifying effect on bile, and taurine, an amino acid, binds to bile salts and accelerates their elimination.

Inflammatory Bowel Disease

Inflammatory bowel disease (IBD) refers to two distinct diseases: ulcerative colitis and Crohn's disease. Between one and two million Americans suffer from inflammatory bowel disease. The two inflammatory bowel diseases, while not identical, form a clinical spectrum. Sometimes it is difficult to precisely differentiate one from the other.

The symptoms of IBD can be mild to severe and include excessive intestinal gas, bloating, cramping, fever, frequent bouts of bloody diarrhea, pus or mucus in the stool, pencil-like or ribbonlike stools, and rectal itching.

Crohn's disease may affect the colon, small intestine, or both. The inflammatory process of Crohn's disease goes deep into the intestinal wall, sometimes perforating it or spreading to other organs like the bladder. Ulcerative colitis differs from Crohn's disease in that it is limited to the colon. The colon's lining becomes inflamed and ulcerated, and it bleeds.

Both ulcerative colitis and Crohn's disease can have serious complications if left untreated. Besides the risk of infections and perforations of the intestinal wall, malnutrition and dehydration are the everyday consequences of IBD. In severe cases, surgery to remove all or part of the small intestine or colon may be necessary.

The usual medical treatment involves steroids, antiinflammatory medications, and antibiotics. Unfortunately, the medical world has long persisted in ignoring the fact that the food that passes through the gastrointestinal tract can have an impact on the lining of this organ. This may seem like a common-sense notion, but it is frequently ignored in the practice of gastroenterology. Many research studies support the notion that elimination diets and food allergy detection can alleviate inflammatory bowel disease, but instead a drug approach is favored, sometimes leading to surgery. As in asthma, powerful immunosuppressive drugs like prednisone are often prescribed. The benefits of supplementary nutrients, acupuncture, and herbal remedies remain unrecognized. New techniques of immunotherapy developed in Great Britain promise alleviation of inflammatory bowel disease when simple diet modification does not suffice.

People with IBD usually have a second inflammatory disorder like arthritis, eczema, or psoriasis. This confirms what many studies have found: that food allergies are a contributing factor in the development of inflammatory bowel disease. In fact, doctors and laypersons alike have discovered that a diet that addresses food allergies is often successful in decreasing or eliminating symptoms of IBD.

One diet that has had great success with IBD patients is the specific carbohydrate diet. Elaine Gottschall, in her book *Breaking the Vicious Cycle*, describes the connection between carbohydrate intolerance and IBD. In 1958, her eight-year-old daughter was diagnosed with incurable, progressive ulcerative colitis. After consulting physicians, she gave her the specific carbohydrate diet. Her daughter was free of ulcerative colitis symptoms within two years! After another two years, she was able to eat a normal diet. Some thirty years later, her daughter continues to have excellent health.

According to the research, people with IBD have difficulty digesting starches and sugars. The entire process leading up to inflammation and malabsorption is fairly complicated, but one factor contributing to IBD is the fermentation syndrome discussed earlier in this chapter. In simple terms, the fermentation of starches by various yeasts and bacteria in the bowel irritates the intestinal wall, causing it to secrete mucus. This mucus layer prevents the absorption of some carbohydrates and other nutrients.

Elaine Gottschall's book outlines the specific carbohydrate diet very clearly and includes many fine recipes. Her dietary recommendations for IBD fly in the face of traditional nutritional medicine. It excludes many forms of starches: all grains, potatoes, and many beans. The diet permits fruits, certain beans and cheeses, and homemade yogurt. It excludes sucrose and all sugars except glucose sweeteners like honey. Beans and nuts provide the carbohydrates.

After one month on the specific carbohydrate diet, many people with IBD notice improvement. This diet has worked wonders for people with ulcerative colitis, Crohn's disease, and other intestinal problems as well.

Diverticulosis

Diverticulosis is a disease of the colon, in which there develop physical outpocketings or herniations, called diverticula, of the intestinal wall. Dysbiosis or an overgrowth of bacteria sometimes infects the diverticula, causing inflammation, the condition known as diverticulitis.

In severe cases of diverticulitis, diverticula can rupture into the abdominal cavity, resulting in peritonitis, a dangerous infection. Surgical intervention is then necessary to repair the bowel and clean out the infection.

What Causes Diverticulosis?

Diverticulosis is a reflection of the modern Western diet. It was unheard of before 1900. Today *more than half* of all Americans have diverticulosis by the time they reach sixty years of age. In countries like Asia and Africa where the diets are high in fiber, diverticulosis is rare.

Symptoms of diverticular disease include nausea, severe cramping pain in the lower abdomen, gas, bloating, constipation, fever, and chills.

Prevention and Treatment

The dietary recommendations to prevent diverticular disease and to treat it are the same: a high-fiber diet that is low in sugar and fat. Once diverticulitis has been diagnosed, it's very important to prevent the complications, which can be serious. After an attack of diverticulitis, try one week on a soft-fiber diet, staying away from whole grains and raw vegetables. I recommend the following foods:

- Steamed root vegetables, soups of cooked tomatoes, squash, or peeled cucumbers
- Cantaloupe, watermelon, peeled pears, soaked prunes, olives, tofu, white rice
- Carrot juice, teas from demulcent herbs like slippery elm, and mullein

After the second week, other soft-fiber foods like beans, oats, miso, and cooked leafy vegetables can be added to the diet.

To relieve constipation:

- Soak 1 teaspoon of psyllium overnight in a cup of water with raisins and prunes. At breakfast, combine with grated and peeled apples and pears.

To help heal the colon:

- Aloe vera gel, chlorophyll capsules, garlic, acidophilus supplements
- The herbs gentian, uva ursi, goldenseal, and grapefruit seed extract, which act as natural antibiotics

You must avoid:

- Whole nuts and seeds, beans, fruits and vegetables that contain small seeds, all of which may be caught in the diverticula

The specific carbohydrate diet recommended in Elaine Gottschall's book is also often effective for people with diverticulitis.

Colon Cancer

Colon cancer is the second most common cancer in America. Each year, 60,000 people die of it. Again, like many other digestive diseases we've mentioned, colon cancer is closely associated with a high-fat, low-fiber diet. Familial history is also a significant factor — people who have had relatives with polyps or cancers of the rectum and colon should be on the alert! Symptoms of colon cancer are blood in the stool, rectal bleeding, or a change in bowel habits.

The prevalence of this disease makes colon-cancer screening of utmost importance. All people over the age of forty should have rectal examinations and a test for occult (hidden) fecal blood. This simple chemical test can be performed at home or in the doctor's office. It will reveal the presence of hidden blood in the stool — blood that may indicate a polyp or colon cancer. The test kit can be purchased at any drugstore. A positive result may indicate the presence of a colon polyp, which is sometimes a precursor to the development of cancer but can usually be removed during a colonoscopy. Self-testing is just one thing you can do to prevent colon cancer.

A positive result on a stool specimen for occult fecal blood, however, doesn't necessarily indicate cancer or polyps. Hemorrhoids, rectal tears or fissures, diet, and medication may all cause bleeding and make for a positive result. (But false positives or not, it is imperative that all positive results be followed up by your doctor!) In a study in Minnesota, 10 percent of the participants had positive test results for blood in their stool, but fewer than three in one hundred of these actually had colon cancer.[7]

The most effective screening devices for colon cancer are the sigmoidoscopy and the colonoscopy. They both involve insertion of a flexible fiberoptic tube into the anus in order to facilitate visualizing the interior of the colon. The sigmoidoscopy is a simpler procedure; the colonoscopy covers more territory and requires some advance preparation. Doctors recommend that sigmoidoscopy be performed every three to five years for those over the age of fifty, or earlier for those who have a family history of colon cancer. Although the colonoscopy is a fairly unpleasant procedure, when a doctor recommends it, it may save your life.

Although colon cancer screening is important, prevention is even more important. Diet plays the largest part in the prevention of colon cancer. Here are the recommendations:

• **Fiber.** Fiber decreases the intestinal transit time: the amount of time that feces stays in the colon. This seems to counteract the effects of fats and carcinogens on the intestine. Fiber in your diet can also prevent the development of colon polyps, some of which are precancerous.

- **Low-fat.** Excess fat in the diet is a known risk factor not only in colon cancer but in many types of cancer.
- **Add vegetables.** Five or more servings of vegetables a day provide good cancer prevention, according to The National Cancer Institute. Vegetables contain many cancer-preventive chemicals, especially the cruciferous vegetables: cabbage, broccoli, Brussels sprouts, collard greens, turnips, and cauliflower. Mixed carotenoids from vegetables like carrots are also important for health.
- **Add calcium.** Calcium has an important role in colon-cancer prevention. Many fruits and vegetables are high in calcium. Calcium combines with bile and harmful fatty acids, inactivating them until they are excreted.
- **Add nutrients.** Adding nutrients like omega-3 oils, found in flaxseed oil and fish; butyrate, found in goat cheese; and fructose oligosacchardies (FOS) derived from Jerusalem artichoke gives you further protection. These nutrients have tumor-inhibiting properties and exert anti-inflammatory action. Vitamins A, E, and C, as well as selenium, help to counter the effects of free radicals and antioxidants in your system, reducing the risk of cancer. Vitamin D, too, has been indicated in cancer prevention. So has folic acid, in doses higher than those commonly available over the counter: 2 to 5 milligrams a day has been shown to be preventive.
- **Consider an aspirin a day.** While potential side effects like bleeding don't warrant its use in everyone, those especially prone to colon cancer (such as near relatives of colon-cancer patients, or individuals with a history of precancerous polyps) might want to opt for it.

By adopting dietary modifications and proper colon-cancer screening measures, we should be able to greatly improve the somewhat scary statistics.

A Look to the Future

Most, if not all, of the gastrointestinal problems encountered today are a result of our dietary habits and the American way of life. Diets high in sugar, high in fat, and low in fiber contribute to the development of colon cancer, diverticulosis, gallbladder disease, leaky gut syndrome, dysbiosis, and candidiasis. High-sugar diets contribute to the development of Crohn's disease: in seventeen studies on Crohn's disease, all reported that those patients consumed more sucrose than people without the disease — from 20 to 220 percent more![8]

We need to revise our thinking about the foods we eat, the way we eat them, and their effect on our health. We need to continue to look for the causes of gastrointestinal ills and be willing to change old concepts that are no longer useful. Many of the prevailing concepts held by gastroenterologists leave a lot of patients high and dry. Their GI problems are poorly treated or untreated, or they're offered temporary symptomatic relief without resolution of the underlying problems.

We need to pay better attention to what the research is telling us and to incorporate this new information into the medical treatment of gastrointestinal problems. We also need to apply some basic common sense.

CHAPTER TEN

Mostly for Women

I frequently see women in my office who have been plagued with a host of gynecological troubles in their forties. They're angry, they're hurt, and they want and deserve answers. They are no longer satisfied with the standard answers and treatment options they've been getting from the medical community. They've lost their faith in the medical establishment.

There are two reasons for this dissatisfaction. First, the medical attitude toward women is in general a macho one — invasive and heroic. Also, the shift away from extended family systems to the isolated nuclear system has meant the loss of elder female mentors, such as the midwife. Macho attitudes in medicine extend to the specialty of gynecology, which even today is still affected by erroneous myths regarding female anatomy, physiology, and psychology — beliefs that date back several hundred years.[1]

The Hysteria Myth

From ancient Greece down through the ages, the womb was thought to be the cause of nearly all diseases in women. The words *hysteria* and *hysterectomy* are derived from the Greek word *hystera*, or "womb." Many types of female problems — "hysteria," "excessive emotions," headaches, dizzy spells, and diseases of the stomach, heart, and other organs — were attributed to the influences of a woman's womb.[2] Only a hundred years ago, hysterectomies were commonly performed as a way of preventing female orgasm and sexual desire, which were thought to be abnormal in women! Not until this century, through the work of Dr. Robert Greenblatt, a pioneer in female endocrinology, was it slowly accepted by the medical establishment that women indeed had sexual desires and produced many types of female hormones.[3]

Today, hysterectomies are still performed to treat anemia, bleeding, benign ovarian cysts and uterine fibroids, pain, endometriosis, uterine prolapse, and the "prevention" of uterine and ovarian cancer. Most hysterectomies are performed on women of childbearing age: a startling 60.2 percent in 1984.[4] Between 1965 and 1984, an estimated 12.6 million hysterectomies were performed in the United States; an estimated 670,000 hysterectomies are performed annually. According to speakers at the annual meeting of the North American Menopause Society in 1995, too many women are still getting hysterectomies for benign conditions. Even though the rates have dropped over the last decade, at least half of women are still prescribed a hysterectomy at some time during their lives. One study at San Diego Naval Hospital showed that 15 percent of 584 hysterectomies were performed for cancer or malignant diseases.[5] Extremely high numbers of hysterectomies have been performed in some individual hospitals and in some states, unjustified by any special health patterns in the population.

In the past, it was believed that the uterus served no real function after childbearing days had passed. Simply removing the uterus and leaving the hormones intact would "take care of the hormone problem" while alleviating a host of "pesky" gynecological problems like "messy periods" or "possible cancer." We know now that the uterus is an important source of prostaglandins and other hormones that help keep a woman in balance. In addition, the removal of the uterus impedes the blood circulation to the remaining ovaries, creating an estrogen dominance situation, and, in many cases, resulting in premature menopause.[6]

Women are becoming increasingly aware that hysterectomy is being called into question as a standard remedy for various female ailments. Just as one example, I treated a woman who was told she needed a hysterectomy because of large fibroids in her uterus that were pressing on her bladder. Now, fibroids naturally shrink during menopause because of reduced estrogen levels. Clara was in her early forties, and the surgeon told her that there was no point in waiting for menopause, since it was at least five or six years away. But she was very adamant about seeking alternatives, and she held off. The result was gratifying. She came to see me one day when she was forty-five and told me she'd missed her period. I did a blood test, to see if this was related to the fibroids, and it confirmed that she was going through menopause. She was quite relieved; her delaying tactics had paid off, and she'd avoided an unnecessary surgery. We were then able to relieve her menopausal symptoms by using topical progesterone cream, which unlike estrogen doesn't stimulate the fibroids.

Today, greater awareness about the role of the female reproductive system in maintaining wellness in women is changing attitudes in the medical community. The use of advanced diagnostic techniques and procedures like laparascopy, vaginal ultrasound, colposcopy, laser surgery, and improved medical management with hormonal, innovative surgical, and nutritional therapy will hopefully prompt a steady decline in the number of hysterectomies performed.

Some may say the change in medicine is due to the increased number of women in medicine. But being a female doctor doesn't necessarily engender a higher consciousness toward women and their problems, as my colleague Dr. Vicki Hufnagel, author of *No More Hysterectomies*, will attest. Women physicians are educated in the same way as their male counterparts, handed down the same protocols and treatment options for a range of gynecological problems. Unless there's a continued evolution in gynecological treatment, many female doctors will be conditioned to treat problems in the same search-and-destroy fashion.

Medicine and the Baby-Boomer Woman

For a baby-boomer woman in her forties, "when you're ready, we'll put you on estrogen" is the response she'll commonly hear from the medical community. Beyond this cursory comment, women haven't been prepared culturally and medically for menopause. Suddenly, a woman in her forties can find that all the bad influences of her twenties and thirties — stress, poor nutrition, drugs or alcohol, exposure to sexually transmitted diseases, too much work and too little sleep, being "super-mom" or "super-woman" — meet the biological changes of her forties. She can then experience a dramatic biological shift that stops her in her tracks. This shift can take her out of her career or very involved parental responsibilities and encourage her to take stock of some very real physical problems brought on by premenopause or menopause. These can include Syndrome X, exacerbation of asthma and allergies, migraines, immune symptom problems, fibromyalgia symptoms, arthritis, and more. Many problems that women may have had in their twenties or thirties quickly become unmanageable in their forties. Suddenly, they are forced to start taking their health seriously and make changes in their lifestyles.

Menopause: A Natural Stage of Life

A dubious term for menopause is now making the rounds — "ovarian failure." The implication is that menopause is a pathological situation requiring a medical solution — all that needs to be done is replace hormones, and women can go on with their lives. This medicalization of a natural stage of life is preposterous. It's matched only by the medicalization of other important moments, with the result that we now feel that birth and death must take place in a hospital, never in the home.

Still, the forties for many women catch them completely off guard. Significant hormonal stages render them a little less stable, a little less resilient. These changes begin very early in the forties and sometimes even in the thirties. It's a gradual progression, a broad period of transition. This is ideally a time for women to consolidate their health strategies — a time of real challenge and self-mastery. It presents women with a biological challenge that can be a tremendously empowering project as they make the appropriate psychological, physical, and dietary adjustments.

Here's one example of the difficult transition a colleague of mine went through. Ilana (we'll call her), a well-known and effective sex therapist, who is considered a world authority on female sexuality, began to feel quite sick about the age of thirty-nine. She thought she had chronic fatigue syndrome or was suffering from depression. She had no typical signals of menopause, no change in her cycles, and no hot flashes or vaginal dryness, but she felt sick in an indefinable way. After some years of trying to cope, she went to a gynecologist, who correctly told her, "You're beginning to have premenopausal symptoms." Testing showed borderline hormone levels — classic indicators of menopause. (Testing is, in fact, not always effective in indicating menopause and sometimes reveals no change when there is actually a premenopausal drift.)

Ilana was given hormone replacement therapy and got a psychological lift but developed side effects: increased appetite and breast tenderness. It didn't feel natural to her, and she didn't like the experience. So she embarked on a journey toward natural strategies to deal with her menopausal symptoms. She began a herbal program, taking certain vitamins and a natural estrogen, and using a natural progesterone cream called Pro-Gest. (Details on all these later in this chapter.) She mastered the challenge. Since her experience, she has taken to lecturing on postmenopausal sexuality.

Premenopause

In Chinese medicine, there is an understanding that women undergo a distinct, prolonged premenopausal stage. Chinese doctors understand this as a change in what they call the kidney energy, which is the reproductive, hormonal energy of the body. They theorize that this change in energy allows certain symptoms to appear, such as intensified allergies or respiratory problems, achy body, hot flashes, anxiety, or depression. We too are beginning to identify premenopausal symptoms that relate to excess estrogen or lowered estrogen during this time.

The premenopausal phase, which can occur anytime between the ages of thirty-eight and fifty, is a critical time. Although estrogen levels eventually fall by the end of menopause, it's common during this early phase for some women to experience increased estrogen levels, or estrogen dominance. This can lead to weight gain, hypoglycemia, menstrual disturbances, and other problems. Fortunately, we can take preventive action by adjusting the diet to forestall some of these problems. (See the section on estrogen dominance syndrome later in this chapter.)

Within the premenopausal phase, women may experience changes in body weight, along with a greater susceptibility to carbohydrate craving, which can lead to insulin fluctuations and Syndrome X (see chapter 6). Some women have no changes, while others have exaggerated changes in their capacity for handling carbohydrates. If they don't recognize this early, they could end up far down a slope of decline, with a seemingly irretrievable weight gain, body change, and loss of their youthful slender figures. Worse, insulin imbalance and Syndrome X are significant risk factors for diabetes and heart disease. The key to prevention is a healthy diet that avoids the kinds of pasta dishes and low-fat desserts, usually laden with sugar or starch, that release floods of sugar into the bloodstream, raising insulin levels, and thus cause the body to crave still more carbohydrates. See the section called Putting on Pounds, on page 204.

Menopause: A Hormonal Roller-Coaster

Menopause is not so much a period of hormone deficiency as of hormonal turbulence. Throughout menopause, a woman can expect to have crescendos and decrescendos of estrogen levels. And it's quite a mix of hormones that's fluctuating. The ovaries produce three types of estrogen — estrone, estradiol, estriol — and levels of each can change independently. (All estrogen is synthesized from cholesterol.) Higher levels of estrone and estradiol have tumor-producing effects, and higher levels of estriol will counter these effects.[7] The female body also produces progesterone, the "counterhormone" to the estrogens, which may decrease before estrogen does. There may be surges of pituitary hormones as well.

Progesterone is a multifaceted hormone in the female body, acting in part to slough off the endometrium, the lining of the uterus, resulting in a menstrual period. Progesterone also helps to regulate blood sugar levels.

It's these shifting levels of hormones that cause some of the typical indicators of menopause, including mood swings, insomnia, hot flashes, night sweats, palpitations, carbohydrate cravings, and weight gain. Let's take a look at some of the more common symptoms, and what may be done to alleviate them.

HOT FLASHES

During a hot flash, women report having a sudden rise in body temperature and feeling flushed. They may then start perspiring and sometimes have heart palpitations. This may be followed by chills.

It is not really clear what causes hot flashes. Sometimes they can be related to a surge in estrogen, or they may be due to an imbalance of other female hormones: progesterone deficiency or surges of pituitary hormones. The excess or deficiency of any of these hormones can lead to excesses or deficiencies of others. It is almost as if some women are "allergic" to overproduction of these hormones at the time of menopause. Sometimes, neutralization techniques in an allergy laboratory can provide substantial relief for women who suffer from severe menopausal migraine headaches, hot flashes, and mood changes.

There is also a prostaglandin element to hot flashes. By modifying the production of prostaglandins in the body, favoring the production of "good" prostaglandins over "bad" ones through the use of supplemental nutrients, these symptoms can be wonderfully alleviated. Some of the more effective nutrients include

- Vitamin E. Recommended: 800 International Units daily.
- Gamma linolenic acid (GLA). This is an omega-6 oil found in primrose oil, borage oil and black currant seed oil.

RECOMMENDED DOSAGE: Two to four 240 to 300-milligram capsules daily.

It may also be possible that the hot flashes experienced by some women are actually symptoms of hypoglycemia, which can cause mood changes, food cravings, weight gain, and fatigue. See the section Putting on Pounds below. Adjusting the diet may have multiple benefits, reducing symptoms like hot flashes and assisting with weight control as well. Progesterone therapy through an externally applied cream such as Pro-Gest can also have a mitigating effect. See the section on Estrogen Dominance Syndrome later in this chapter (page 213) for details.

Some practical tips in dealing with hot flashes include wearing layered clothing so that sweaters or outer garments can be removed or put back on, and wearing a cotton shell or t-shirt as a cool inner garment.

Putting on Pounds

There is a natural tendency toward weight gain with menopause, caused partly by the body's changing nutritional needs. Nutritionally, the reproductive cycle requires a certain input in terms of iron, protein, and calories. The higher calorie requirements of menstruation and child bearing evaporate at menopause, but lifetime habits of eating don't change immediately. Women tend to keep eating the same kinds and quantities of food they always have, even though their caloric and nutritional needs are lower. It's important to be conscious of this, but there's no need to try to effect a sudden drastic change of lifetime habits. Allow your eating habits to change gradually, over several years, but do be aware they should change.

Even before menopause, women who have had children will probably have experienced a weight gain because of hormonal and physical changes. In fact, the physical action of carrying a child, during and after pregnancy, as one goes about various activities of daily living, is a form of "squat exercise." These are exercises specifically used by weight trainers to increase physical mass in the hips and legs.

Studies on women and exercise have shown that exercise may be performed at too low an intensity to result in weight loss, and that exercise alone without dietary changes is not effective in producing weight loss.[8] If a woman has the time and means, she should explore a more strenuous, highly aerobic type of workout in order to achieve the weight loss and establish the emotional balance she desires to have during the turbulent menopausal period.

"Squat exercises" aside, estrogen dominance, which is common during menopause, will also contribute to fatty tissue buildup in the hip and thigh area, promoting an "Earth Mother" physique. As mentioned earlier, estrogen dominance coupled with progesterone deficiency can produce symptoms of hypoglycemia and uncontrollable appetite. Many women experience a deterioration in blood sugar metabolism because of estrogen dominance and progesterone deficiency. Because progesterone tends to regulate blood sugar metabolism, these progesterone-deficient women develop carbohydrate cravings, and satisfying these cravings produces an even more pronounced blood sugar fluctuation. This is the pattern that can eventually lead to insulin imbalance and Syndrome X. To avoid hot flashes or other symptoms due to hypoglycemia, I recommend the following guidelines:

- Eliminate or decrease sugar in diet — and that includes low-fat cookies and desserts, which can contain huge amounts of sugar and starch despite their low-fat content.
- Avoid pasta, white bread, and other refined carbohydrates, which release sugars rapidly into the bloodstream.
- Add more protein to buffer carbohydrate release.
- Eat more foods like beans and tofu that release sugar into the blood very slowly. (These also contain natural estrogen mimics called isoflavones.)
- Schedule regular meals and small snacks to avoid severe drops in blood sugar.

See the section on Estrogen Dominance in this chapter, chapter 6 on The Endocrine System, and chapter 16 on Diet and Nutrition for more on managing hypoglycemic reactions.

Libido

Sexual drive may or may not change during menopause. If changes occur, they may be due to psychological factors or possibly to adrenal changes.

The adrenals are the source of a woman's androgenic hormones and the hormone testosterone. The androgenic hormones contribute to libido and enhance energy, drive, and mood. Women normally produce a small amount of testosterone, which also contributes to libido. The steady production of hormones by the adrenals decreases with age — we call this adrenopause — and this can affect sexual drive. A decrease of one of the adrenal hormones, DHEA, or a decrease of testosterone could cause some weakening of sexual libido. For some women who are naturally very low testosterone producers, adrenopause combined with menopause may upset that balance even more, resulting in diminished sexual desire. Women with low testosterone levels may benefit from a drug called Estratest, which is estrogen with a little testosterone in it. The testosterone may provide an impetus toward sexual activity for a woman who has experienced declining libido.

Other women may go through menopause but not go through adrenopause. For these women, the suppression of female hormones allows the androgenic hormones to come to fuller expression. One manifestation of this is the development of facial hair. Women also report feeling stronger, more in control, and empowered by the newly dominant androgenic hormones. Some may even experience an increase in sexual interest and become more sexually active.

Vaginal Dryness

Another side effect of menopause can be vaginal dryness. This is an easily remedied problem, because there is such a range of options to deal with it. Besides the obvious remedy of using a water-soluble vaginal lubricant during sexual intercourse, there are hormonal and vitamin treatments. Several of the following may help:

- Vitamin E suppositories
- Topical progesterone cream inserted vaginally to replenish the tissues.
- Estriol — an estrogen cream

Estriol cream has a more local effect than other estrogen creams. This means less of it is absorbed by the body and it is therefore less potentially carcinogenic. (There is some increase in cancer risk with estrogen therapies.) It can be used as needed or cyclically.

For some women, systemic estrogen/progesterone therapy is indicated for more pronounced symptoms. See the section on Estrogen Dominance later in this chapter.

One specialized menopausal condition of vaginal dryness, called lichen planus, is effectively treated with testosterone cream.

Heart Disease

In their late forties and early fifties, women catch up with men in terms of risk for heart disease. Whatever protective effect their natural estrogen levels may have provided falls away, and women join the risk pool. Women of this age will have to work a little harder to maintain good levels of cholesterol and HDL and to guard against sugar imbalances and Syndrome X.

Many women at this time of life decide to take hormone supplements — estrogen and progesterone — not only to avoid menopausal symptoms but often because they've heard that hormone replacement can lower the risk of heart disease. Statistics do show that across the great spectrum of the population, those who are receiving hormone therapy do have a lower incidence of heart disease and about half the rate of heart attacks. But there is yet no clear explanation of this phenomenon. Hormone therapy may alter blood clotting factors, glucose metabolism, insulin response, blood pressure, and the balance of lipoproteins. It may somehow slow the natural stiffening of the arteries with age. Some researchers, proposing that the benefit may come from the slight blood loss that is a side effect of hormone therapy, have investigated the relationship of iron in the blood to heart disease and have suggested that the blood loss from menstruation has a protective effect by reducing blood levels of iron and that the small amount of blood loss associated with estrogen replacement therapy is enough to account for the statistical benefits.

All in all, it's a hard to know what to make of such statistics, especially when you consider that many of the people in the studies are not exercising, not eating well, and not otherwise reducing their risk factors. It may be that women who choose hormone replacement may also be more conscious of health issues and take better care of themselves. But if you *are* conscientious about exercise, nutrition, and so on, there's not really any evidence that hormones are going to extend your life. And other statistics are of concern: those that show an increased incidence of breast cancer when the hormones are taken. All in all, hormone replacement has to be carefully tailored to the individual. Moreover, new evidence suggests that the cardio-protective effects of estrogen may be reversed by standard synthetic progesterone, which is routinely prescribed. Use of natural micronized progesterone is preferable.

But hormone replacement is not the only special concern for mature women. There is a new awareness of heart disease that is linked to Syndrome

X and involves anginalike chest pains without significant arteriosclerosis, possibly due to a breakdown of the functioning of the microvascular capillaries and arterioles in the heart. This points out a long-standing issue in the management of heart disease. Since two-thirds of patients with the Syndrome X version of heart disease are women, it may be that this is really a "normal" form of heart disease that has simply been overlooked because of a long-standing focus in research and treatment on male patients, who are more at risk from heart attacks at an earlier age. As Kathleen B. King, a professor of nursing at the University of Rochester, has pointed out, "Men often experience what are considered 'textbook' cases of angina and other heart-disease symptoms, because the textbooks were written to describe men's symptoms." It's true that premenopausal women experience fewer heart attacks. But it's also true that women (and African Americans) who have heart disease are given fewer high-tech treatments like balloon angioplasties and bypass operations, fewer medications, and less frequent transfer to top university hospitals. There is clear evidence that chest pains in women tend to be treated as a psychiatric rather than a cardiac ailment. Yet, women are as likely as men to suffer from heart disease as men, though at a later age, and are just as likely to die of it.[9]

What does this mean for women who are moving into the higher-risk ages? Simply that they should take their cardiovascular health just as seriously as men, and should pursue an exercise and nutrition program that will reduce the risk. While women tend to suffer from heart problems later in life than men, the basic groundwork of health or disease is laid at the same time. Also, given the special risks for Syndrome X, or microvascular angina, women should investigate recurring chest pain or anginalike symptoms and not let them be dismissed too easily. We now know that even a negative angiogram doesn't mean there can't be cardiovascular problems. Stress tests that show abnormal EKG patterns or coronary blood flow, and insulin resistance tests, may offer better clues to the Syndrome X type. And the conventional low-fat, high-carbohydrate diet may actually contribute to the problem, especially if there is a high sugar intake. The best bet for prevention or reversal is a diet that is low in simple sugars and processed carbohydrates and includes enough omega-3 and essential oils. Such a diet could be the Mediterranean diet or the Salad and Salmon Diet outlined in chapter 16.

Osteoporosis — Not Just for the Elderly

Many women are concerned with the threat of osteoporosis, and rightly so. Hormone replacement therapy is touted as the solution to this problem, too. While it is true that estrogen is an important promoter of bone retention, recent studies have cast doubt on its long-range benefits. Specifically, it's beginning to seem less useful in helping to prevent fractures in women in their eighties — the age when women are most prone to fractures of the hip and spine. By then, according to studies, there is very little difference in bone strength between women receiving long-term hormone replacement therapy and those who are not. While estrogen can be an important means of forestalling osteoporosis, generally only a minority of women really require it. Instead, most women can use natural bone-builders like calcium and other cofactors for bone mineralization to support bone strength. The following can be useful:

- Calcium, 1000 to 1500 milligrams per day
- Vitamin D, 800 International Units per day
- Magnesium, 500 to 600 milligrams per day
- Manganese, 50 milligrams per day
- Zinc, 45 milligrams per day
- Boron, 6 milligrams per day
- L-lysine, an amino acid, 500 milligrams per day
- Vitamin C, 1000 milligrams per day

As another alternative to estrogen replacement, natural progesterone, applied through a topical cream, has significant bone-enhancing effects, as is pointed out by Dr. John Lee in his research. See also the section on Natural Hormone Replacement Therapy, on page 211, for other ways of promoting bone retention.

Building a few healthy habits can equal or surpass the effects of hormone replacement therapy alone in supporting bone strength. A best bet: Engage in a regular exercise program that involves lifting or resisting weight. This kind of weight-bearing exercise most increases bone mass. But even regular walking can help. A recent study by Elizabeth Krall of the Agricultural Research Service has shown that women who walk about a mile a day, starting during or after menopause, can reduce the risk of serious bone density loss. The study found that women who start a walking program have up to seven years' worth more bone in reserve than nonwalkers.

Finally, it's important to avoid the following: excess coffee consumption, since caffeine leaches calcium from bones; excess protein consumption, which may cause the kidneys to excrete too much calcium; and certainly smoking, which hastens menopause and tends to lower estrogen levels.

Estrogen Replacement Therapy — Less Than a Panacea

Hormone replacement therapy (HRT) is the practice of supplying estrogen and progesterone to substitute for the naturally declining levels after menopause. It is also recommended to women on the basis of its cardioprotective effects.

But, far from being the "be-all and end-all" treatment for menopausal women, hormone replacement therapy can result in the following side effects:

- Hormonal headaches
- Breast swelling and tenderness
- Water retention
- Yeast infections
- Increased appetite
- Sugar cravings and weight gain

Breakthrough bleeding can also be a problem side effect. Estrogen replacement therapy can be managed so that you bleed regularly, or not at all. But bleeding can occur when it's not supposed to.

Certain studies have shown that there is a 30 percent increased risk of breast cancer among women who have undergone estrogen replacement therapy for fifteen years and a 50 percent increased risk of breast cancer for women who undergo estrogen replacement therapy for as long as twenty-five years.[10] It can also double the incidence of gallstones and gallbladder disease among women. The incidence of asthma and blood clots may also increase. Small wonder, then, that many women are not reassured by their doctors' insistence that hormone replacement therapy is innocuous and provides numerous benefits.

So when is hormone replacement therapy necessary — or is it ever? Individual circumstances need to be considered. I find estrogen replacement mostly unnecessary for the relief of hot flashes, depression, and vaginal dryness. These side effects can be significantly relieved with natural agents.

On the other hand, in the few instances where natural therapy fails, estrogen replacement therapy should be considered when there is no history of cancer, a family history of breast cancer, or uterine fibroids, which can be worsened by continued estrogen exposure.

Other reasons to consider hormone replacement are

- **Early onset of menopause,** either because of true premature ovarian failure or because of surgical menopause (hysterectomy or removal of ovaries).
- **Women at risk for osteoporosis:** thin women of northern European extraction, ex-smokers, women with a history of hyperthyroidism, or women whose mothers had severe osteoporosis, and have documented evidence of accelerated bone loss.

Tri-est is a balanced natural estrogen combination used in replacement therapy for the treatment of early menopause, osteoporosis, and severe physical or psychological reactions to menopause. Premarin, a synthetic hormone, is a conjugated or "bound" estrogen (estradiol), which is a copycat of human estrogen.

The estrogen patch Estraderm (estradiol transdermal system) is indicated for women who have reasons to avoid oral estrogen, such as liver or gallbladder disease or susceptibility to blood clots. It is a good alternative for women who tolerate oral estrogen poorly, and it relieves hot flashes, night sweats, and urogenital atrophy. Although it isn't recommended by the manufacturer for the treatment or prevention of postmenopausal osteoporosis, studies have shown that the estradiol transdermal system has effects similar to those of oral estrogen replacement therapy in reducing urinary calcium excretion.[11]

Natural Hormone Replacement Therapy

My preferred alternative to synthetic hormone replacement therapy with drugs like Provera and Premarin is to use natural alternative hormone replacement therapy. This therapy, which uses estrogen and progesterone, more precisely mimics the body's own profile of these hormones during a woman's earlier years. In this way, the estrogen profile can be tailored to favor specific forms of estrogen that have less carcinogenic potential.

One theory is that one reason for an increase in breast cancer is that women may have an imbalance in the types of estrogen they are producing. Favoring less carcinogenic estrogens would be one way of using estrogen to an advantage while mitigating the cancer risks.

NATURAL ESTROGEN SOURCES

Herbal and natural medicines contain an abundance of natural estrogens. Phytoestrogens — including isoflavones, phytosterols, saponins, and lignans — are compounds in plants that are capable of exerting mild estrogenic effects. In high levels, they can have significant effects, which may explain the rarity of hot flashes and other menopausal symptoms in cultures consuming a plant-based diet. Phytoestrogens are found in soy, fennel, celery, parsley, clovers, sprouts, flaxseed, nuts, and seeds. There is an over-the-counter phytoestrogen called genistein, which is an isoflavone derived from soy. Phytoestrogens from the soy plant are also used in estrogen creams. They tend to be unstable when taken orally, but work well topically.

Some women report having relief from hot flashes and other menopausal symptoms when using black cohosh, a medicinal plant known to Native Americans for years and containing large amounts of phytoestrogens, in conjunction with estrogen cream.[12] A herb called *Vitex agnus castii*, or chasteberry, is sometimes helpful for the same symptoms. These can both be found in health food stores in various forms, sometimes as teas or capsules or tinctures.

A study by the U.S. Department of Agriculture showed that natural estrogen levels increased in women taking only 3 milligrams of boron a day in capsule form.

Women who are trying natural hormone therapy should still be monitored through annual mammograms and gynecological examinations, to catch any possible cancerous precursors.

NATURAL PROGESTERONE — AN ADJUNCT THERAPY

Only in the last five years have we recognized the possibility of using a transdermal system for getting progesterone into the body. For years, creams made from wild yam were used as beauty creams by women. It was long recognized that these creams not only were beneficial from a cosmetic standpoint but seemed to have a rejuvenating effect on the women who used them. Research has now shown that wild yam is a potent source of natural progesterone, which is identical to human progesterone. These women had been absorbing natural progesterone, which not only enhanced their well-being but relieved PMS or menopausal symptoms in some instances.

Although not really sanctioned by the medical establishment, these wild yam products are made available by the cosmetic market, and at this point, the FDA hasn't moved to stop the production.

Products like Pro-Gest cream have been successfully used for years by my patients as a source of natural progesterone. These products help relieve some of the symptoms of estrogen excess, which we will outline later, including fibrocystic breast disease, fibroids, PMS, ovarian cysts, endometriosis, and even hot flashes. Also, as a hormone, progesterone has some anticancer effects.

A New Paradigm for Menopause

By making adjustments by use of natural means, women often experience a surge in energy and vitality as they go into their fifties. Taking a proactive stance about menopause can result in a profoundly positive change. Often, women become healthier during and after menopause than they were before menopause.

It's my hope and expectation that in the future women will increasingly find it more easy to adjust to menopause. We need a cultural change in how we view menopause, more and better information made readily available to women, and new and better treatments to help them deal with the many changes it brings.

Estrogen Dominance Syndrome

Though we think of declining estrogen as the hallmark of menopause, it's actually common for women to experience surges of abnormally high estrogen levels during the menopausal and premenopausal periods, and even earlier in life. Dr. John R. Lee has done extensive research into this phenomenon. It is his belief and mine that an excess of estrogen, coupled with a deficiency of progesterone (the counter hormone to estrogen), is the common denominator for a lot of female troubles. Dr. Lee has pioneered the use of natural progesterone as an aid to dealing with this syndrome.

Estrogen dominance can start early on in a women's menstrual cycle. Young women who suffer from this enter menarche with tremendously difficult periods, and doctors sometimes give these teenage girls birth control pills to help regulate the frequency and severity of their periods.

Some women will develop the estrogen dominance syndrome much later in life, sometimes as a result of diet, liver impairment, or environmental factors or also as a result of anovulatory cycles before menopause — that is, menstrual cycles in which no ovulation has occurred.*

Diseases or problems that are thought to be related to or affected by excess estrogen and deficient progesterone in women are

- Weight gain
- Fibrocystic breast disease
- Certain types of PMS
- Migraines
- Menstrual disturbances — irregular and heavy bleeding.
- Endometriosis, the uterine tissue disorder, which is helped by the use of estrogen blockers (see Resetting the Balance on page 215).
- Fibroids, a sign of excess proliferative capacity of the uterus, which may not be balanced with sufficient progesterone.
- Ovarian cysts

Causes of Estrogen Dominance Syndrome

Besides the natural hormonal fluctuations of menopause, certain lifestyle choices and conditions can also contribute to estrogen dominance syndrome, especially a low-fiber diet, overloading the liver with internal toxins, and absorbing toxins from the environment.

---

* Ovulation is necessary in order to produce the *corpus luteum*, (which means "yellow body") that is found on the surface of the ovary after ovulation. Surrounding the ripening egg, the *corpus luteum* remains after ovulation to produce progesterone for the last half of the menstrual cycle. Without ovulation, less progesterone is produced, which can cause estrogen imbalance in some women.

LOW-FIBER DIET

A low-fiber diet causes estrogen levels to be higher, while a diet high in fiber results in decreased estrogen levels in the bloodstream. Why? Excess estrogen is excreted in the bowel. When stool remains in the bowel for a longer time, the estrogen is reabsorbed. Studies have shown that women on a vegetarian/high-fiber diet have lower levels of circulating estrogen.[13] Lower levels of estrogen mean less estrogen stimulation of breast tissue, for example, which reduces the risk of breast cancer.

OVERLOADING THE LIVER

The liver is a filter of sorts. It detoxifies our body, protecting us from the harmful effects of chemicals, elements in food, environmental toxins, and even natural products of our metabolism, including excess estrogen. Anything that impairs liver function or ties up the detoxifying function will result in excess estrogen levels, whether it has a physical basis, as in liver disease, or an external cause, as with exposure to environmental toxins, drugs, or dietary substances.

Estrogen is produced not only internally but also produced in reaction to chemicals and other substances in our food. When it is not broken down adequately, higher levels of estrogen build up. This is true for both men and women, although the effects are more easily recognized in men. Alcoholic men with impaired liver function develop a condition called gynecomastia, with estrogenic characteristics including enlarged breasts, loss of male pubic hair, and eunuch-like features.

In like manner, the estrogen dominance syndrome can be evoked in women by too much alcohol, drugs, or environmental toxins, all of which limit the liver's capacity to cleanse the blood of estrogen. It has been found that circulating estrogen levels increase significantly in women who drink. In one study, blood and urine estrogen levels increased up to 31.9 percent in women who drank just two drinks a day.[14] Consequently, breast cancer risks are higher for women drinkers. Not surprisingly, osteoporosis rates are lower.

ENVIRONMENT

We live in an estrogenic or feminizing environment. Certain chemicals in the environment and our foods, one of which is DDT, cause estrogenic effects. Although banned in 1972, DDT, like its breakdown product DDE, is an estrogenlike substance and is still present in the environment.[15] Chlorine and hormone residues in meats and dairy products can also have estrogenic effects. In men, the estrogenic environment may result in declining quality of sperm or fertility rates. In women, it may lead to an epidemic of female diseases, all traceable to excess estrogen/deficient progesterone.

Resetting the Balance

If you suffer from some of the problems mentioned earlier, and think your diet or toxins may be causing estrogen dominance in your system, you may want to consult with an innovative physician who recognizes the syndrome of estrogen dominance. Such a doctor can measure the levels of hormones in your blood or, in the case of progesterone, in your saliva. Estrogen dominance is not a standard medical diagnosis but is entering the lexicon of alternative-minded physicians. Such a doctor would be likely to recommend the following means of resetting your estrogen balance:

- **Increase dietary fiber.**
- **Use dietary supplements.** Lecithin (a phospholipid) and the sulfur-containing L-taurine and L-methionine amino acids are compounds that will promote bile circulation, which enhances estrogen's excretion out of the body. These lipotropic formulas support the liver metabolism of estrogen. A typical formula might provide the following, sometimes in a base of liver-stimulating herbs like milk thistle, black radish, beet, or dandelion, for twice-daily consumption: choline (a concentrated form of lecithin), 500 milligrams; inositol, 250 milligrams; taurine, 250 milligrams; methionine, 250 milligrams.
- **Use natural progesterone** to balance the excess estrogen, in the form of a cream like Pro-Gest that is absorbed through the skin.
- **Eat soy foods** like bean curd or tofu. They contain the phytoestrogens we've discussed earlier, including diadzin and genistein. They act as estrogen blockers at the tissue level, blocking receptors that could promote cancer.

Breast Cancer: The Great Dilemma

We know quite a bit about breast cancer, but there are great limitations to our knowledge. This paradox presents us constantly with dilemmas of prevention, diagnosis, and treatment that are often difficult to resolve. To cite one example: a young woman named Angela came to see me, with a history of fibrocystic breasts and additionally with heavy menstrual periods and PMS. On top of this, she had uterine fibroids and felt fatigued most of the time as she approached menopause.

Since Angela's mother, sister, and aunt had all had breast cancer, she had been going through the nerve-wracking process of undergoing repeated breast biopsies. Finally, she had opted for bilateral prophylactic mastectomy, or the removal of both her breasts, and the insertion of artificial breast implants. Given her situation, I could almost understand her choice. But it is not the recommendation I would have made to her had she come to me originally before making such an irrevocable and harsh decision.

For one thing, the benefits of prophylactic mastectomies have yet to be proved. A drastic preventive measure, a prophylactic mastectomy removes the entire breast, nipple, and areola. Just as the removal of cancerous tumors is not always 100 percent accurate, one missed breast tissue cell that is potentially cancerous can still set off a cascade of cancer growth.[16]

I believed that her fibrocystic breast disease was a manifestation of an estrogen/progesterone imbalance that could have been treated. Had it been treated, the majority of her symptoms would have been relieved, including the fibrocystic breast disease, and she would have had few or no uterine fibroids. With proper medical monitoring through mammograms, the surgery could have perhaps been avoided.

The Noncancer: Fibrocystic Breast Disease

Fibrocystic breast disease is a common and benign syndrome in premenopausal women. Women with fibrocystic breast disease complain of painful, lumpy breasts that are affected by the menstrual cycle. Although there's no clear link between fibrocystic breast disease and breast cancer, there is a slightly higher rate of breast cancer in women who have fibrocystic breast disease. This may be purely a statistical artifact caused by the fact that these women get more scrutiny and therefore more breast cancer is found.

If the truth be known, the composition of normal breast tissue is not uniform. Fibrocystic breast disease is actually a normal variation in breast tissue, albeit, a painful variation. Without treatment, fibrocystic breast disease generally resolves in menopause. This is not to say to the millions of women who suffer from it that they need to tough it out until menopause. There is a solution.

Treating Fibrocystic Breast Disease

Fibrocystic breast disease, which is also related to progesterone deficiency syndrome, can be largely ameliorated nutritionally. Women will notice an appreciable decrease in their symptoms if they make the following dietary modifications:

- **Give up** coffee, tea, chocolate and caffeinated soft drinks, which contain caffeine or other alkaloids belonging to the methylxanthine family. Theophylline, used in asthma treatment, also has methylxanthine properties. Studies have shown a link between fibrocystic breast disease and these compounds.

- **Add natural progesterone** by eating yams and sweet potatoes or by using topical progesterone cream.
- **Add foods or supplements that are rich in prostaglandin precursors,** the "good" counterinflammatory prostaglandin precursors. These are nutrients like fish oil, flaxseed oil, borage oil, primrose oil, and black currant seed oil. An effective daily dosage: borage oil, three 500-milligram capsules; or primrose oil, six to eight 500-milligram capsules.
- **Add a Vitamin E supplement,** proven effective against fibrocystic breast disease. Dosage: 400 to 800 International Units daily.
- **Add magnesium and iodine to the diet.** They are sometimes helpful. If supplementing with iodine, ask your doctor for a prescription of elemental iodine, now generally available through compounding pharmacies. Usual dosage: magnesium, 200 milligrams twice daily; iodine, 3 milligrams per day.
- **Decrease circulating estrogen** by eating a high-fiber diet.

Also consider getting an evaluation to rule out hidden hypothyroidism, which is often associated with severe PMS and fibrocystic breasts (see chapter 6, The Endocrine System).

Causes of Breast Cancer

Breast cancer embodies the potential precariousness of midlife. There are very few other ways in which you can have your entire health, vitality, and life so suddenly snatched from you. Most life-threatening illnesses are slow, degenerative pathways. In the case of breast cancer, the hormonal vigor of midlife actually contributes to the spread of the disease because of the relationship between estrogen and cancer.

Causes of Breast Cancer

Theories about why there is an overall increased incidence of breast cancer are many. Let's consider some of the likely culprits.

PROLONGED ESTROGEN EXPOSURE

It may be that modern women are exposed to estrogen for longer periods than their ancestors. Today's young women enjoy better nutrition, which results in a lowering of the age of menarche. It's believed that the critical formative time for precancerous breast lesions may be during puberty. Some even speculate that hormonal "priming" for breast cancer may occur in utero.

This lowered age of menarche means that women today go through more menstrual cycles — an estimated two or three times more — than women in colonial America. Women at that time went through menarche at the age of seventeen or eighteen; had many childbirths, with breast-feeding interrupting the cycle of menstruation and estrogen stimulation on the breast tissue; and then went through menopause in their midforties.

GENETIC PREDISPOSITION

Researchers have recently identified a gene marker called the BRCA-1 gene. A genetic mutation, it puts women at risk for developing breast cancer and ovarian cancer.[17] An estimated 600,000 women in the United States may carry the genetic trait.[18]

Commercial tests are now available for the BRCA-1 gene, although, as it with screening for the Alzheimer's disease gene, the desirability of its application is hotly debated.

DIETARY FACTORS

Women with midabdominal girth expansion and obesity produce more estrogen and place themselves at risk for developing breast cancer. Alcohol consumption increases estrogen levels and the incidence of breast cancer in women. Other dietary influences are the eating of grilled and fried meat. Grilling and frying produce some of the same cancer-causing substances that are found in cigarette smoke.[19]

ENVIRONMENTAL HAZARDS

Studies are being done on the effects of environmental hazards like pesticides, power lines and the resulting electromagnetic fields, and PCBs (polycholorinated biphenyls). There are certain pockets of breast cancer, for instance, in Nassau County in Long Island, New York. Women in Nassau County have a 13 percent increased incidence of breast cancer over all other areas of New York State.[20] There's an absolute correlation of breast cancer to industrial sites in that area.

HORMONAL INFLUENCES

Breast cancer is particularly virulent when it develops immediately after childbirth. A recent study confirms a higher incidence of breast cancer in the first postpartum month. This is due to the acceleration of growth in breast cancer tumors that are either estrogen-receptor positive or progesterone-receptor positive; essentially, the hormones speed the tumor activity. Even so, survival from this particularly virulent cancer is possible, and no woman should give up hope.

A patient of mine was thirty-five when she gave birth to her first child. She was found to have breast cancer, and ten lymph nodes were involved. She survived through a combination of chemotherapy and an autologous bone marrow transplant. This involved having some of her bone marrow removed and reserved, since the chemotherapy would kill the bone marrow cells that maintain immune defense. She then received massive doses of chemotherapy to kill tumor cells, after which she was given back her bone marrow. Generous supplements of vitamins, particularly the antioxidants, helped salvage her immune system from the ravages of chemotherapy.

Preventive Measures

STOP SMOKING

Cigarette smoke contains over five hundred toxic, cancer-producing chemicals.

PERFORM BREAST SELF-EXAMINATIONS

All women should perform monthly breast self-examinations. After her menstrual cycle, a woman should examine each breast while in the shower and again while lying flat on her back. Starting at the nipple, run the fingers around each breast in a circular motion, moving outward, taking care also to examine the tissue under the armpit. Any small lumps or hard granules should be noted.

MAMMOGRAPHY

If there is a strong family history of breast cancer, an initial mammography should be performed when a woman is between the ages of thirty-five and forty, and every one to two years thereafter, depending on other risk factors. Some claim efficacy for routine mammograms before the age of fifty, when all agree mammograms should become annual, although a recent National Institutes of Health Consensus Panel deadlocked on the issue, preferring to leave it a matter of "a woman's choice."

NUTRITIONAL RECOMMENDATIONS FOR CANCER PREVENTION:

- **Try a pesco-vegetarian diet** with no milk products, saturated fat, or eggs. Add fish to gain the benefits of fish oil.
- **Use omega-3 oil** from cold water fish or flaxseed, which has preventive effects.
- **Olive oil helps.** Greek women, who derive 40 percent of their calories from fat, mostly olive oil, have reduced rates of breast cancer.
- **A high-fiber, low fat diet** results in decreased circulating estrogen levels.[21]
- **Include soy foods,** which contain the phytoestrogens that act as estrogen blockers at the breast tissue level. Soy in the diet is correlated with reduced breast and prostate cancer.
- **Include cabbage family foods.** In addition to phytosterols, cabbage family foods (cruciferous foods) are major sources of indole-3-carbinol, a proven cancer preventive agent. They include cabbage, Brussels sprouts, cauliflower, kale, broccoli, turnip greens, and radishes.[22]
- **Add prostaglandin precursors** — the counterinflammatory prostaglandins: fish oil, flaxseed oil, and GLA (borage oil).
- **Use vitamin supplements,** especially relatively high doses of vitamin E, up to 800 International Units daily. Vitamin C, mixed carotenoids, zinc, and selenium may be helpful.
- **Eat "five a day"** — simply having five servings of fruits and vegetables every day helps prevent cancer.
- **Eat foods high in carotenoids** — plant substances, some of which are easily converted into vitamin A by our bodies, that have been found to have cancer-preventive qualities. Foods high in carotenoids include spinach, carrots, pumpkin, mango, papaya, apricots, and sweet potato.
- **Be environmentally aware,** especially if you have genetic risk factors. Be aware of pollution: safeguard your water sources or drink bottled water, eat organic produce and meats to avoid risks of insecticides and herbicides, avoid living near industrial plants or EPA "superfund" sites.

DRUG THERAPY

While currently being touted for prevention, the drug Tamoxifen should be used only by women who have a history of breast cancer as a preventive against breast cancer recurrence. It is not a benign drug, having a risk of uterine cancer, liver disease, and other adverse reactions.

Treatment of Breast Cancer

Medical treatment of breast cancer usually involves lumpectomy, radiation, and/or chemotherapy.

The nutritional treatment of breast cancer includes the cancer preventive recommendations, especially the inclusion of the cabbage family vegetables with the indole-3-carbinol phytochemicals. These plants have proven anticancer activity.

Small, frequent, appetizing high-caloric meals are necessary for patients undergoing chemotherapy and radiation. For the woman experiencing anorexia or lack of appetite, food should literally be thought of as medicine: something she has to take! The body has significantly higher caloric needs than normal when fighting and destroying cancer cells. It needs all the fuel it can get to help it in this real-life struggle.

Other Cancer Risks

Of course, breast cancer is not the only form of cancer that specifically attacks women, though it is by far the most common. It's worthwhile being aware of the others, since early detection can often lead to cure. The recommendations for preventive nutrients apply to cervical cancer, ovarian cancer, and uterine cancer just as they do to breast cancer. Nutrient treatment and prevention is especially effective with cervical cancer.

Cervical Cancer

Cervical cancer kills approximately forty-four hundred women a year, but it is absolutely preventable and treatable. No longer should any woman die from this disease.

CAUSES OF CERVICAL CANCER

Studies have shown that the human papilloma virus (HPV), which causes genital warts, is a virus significantly linked to cervical cancer in women. There are many strains of HPV, some of which lead to aggressive cervical cancer. Protection against HPV infection involves safe sex practices: using condoms with spermicide and limiting the number of sexual partners.

Other risk factors for cervical cancer include

- Vitamin deficiencies
- Early sexual activity
- Use of contraceptive pills

- Multiple sexual partners
- Genital herpes virus
- Smoking

PREVENTION AND DETECTION OF CERVICAL CANCER

Besides quitting smoking, limiting the number of sexual partners, and using condoms, prevention of cervical cancer includes having regular pelvic examinations with PAP smears. Women with a history of HPV, genital herpes, or abnormal PAP smears will need to have followup exams every 6 months and, in some cases, every 3 months.

In addition to the PAP smear, a colposcopy examination is highly recommended for women in the high-risk group. A colposcopy examination consists of painting the external area and interior of the vagina and the cervix with a strong solution of vinegar (acetic acid) to highlight any areas of cell changes. After a few minutes to give the acetic acid time to soak in, a colposcope is inserted. A colposcope is a lighted, high-magnification instrument used to visualize the vulva and external genital skin surfaces and the interior of the vagina and cervix.

Cell changes, called dysplasia, appear white because of the effects of the acetic acid. Biopsy specimens are taken from any questionable areas.

SURGICAL TREATMENT OF DYSPLASIA OR CERVICAL CANCER

Surgical treatment of dysplasia and very early cervical cancer involves burning or vaporizing the offending areas. Cryosurgery is the "burning" of tissue by freezing it with liquid nitrogen. Laser therapy is used to vaporize cervical cancer or dysplasia. For cancer that is invasive or involves larger areas of the cervix, more extensive or radical surgical measures may be taken.

NUTRITIONAL PREVENTION

Nutritional therapy is extremely promising for cervical cancer prevention and involves the use of folic acid, mixed carotenoids, vitamin C, and the essential fatty acids. It's been shown that high doses of these vitamins can have a preventive effect against cervical cancer once it has been initially diagnosed to be in the precancerous stage. Proper nutritional therapy can actually halt progression of the disease. (The same nutritional prescription can help with other cancers of similar epithelial tissue, including those of the mouth, throat, lungs, and skin.)

To promote healthy cervical tissue, the following supplements are recommended:

- Vitamin C: 1000 milligrams per day
- Vitamin E: 800 International Units per day
- Vitamin A retinol: 25000 International Units per day (but no more than 5000 International Units daily in case of pregnancy; higher doses of Vitamin A—but not beta-carotene—above around 8000 International Units per day, have been associated with a higher incidence of birth defects)
- Mixed carotenoids: 25,000 International Units per day (no pregnancy limits)
- Selenium: 100 micrograms twice daily
- Zinc: 30 milligrams twice daily
- Folic acid: 10 milligrams twice daily (via a doctor's prescription)
- Flaxseed oil: 1 tablespoon twice daily

Uterine Cancer

Uterine cancer is often associated with obesity and estrogen dominance. Cancers of the uterus generally occur in women in their fifties and sixties. The most common symptom is postmenopausal bleeding. In premenopausal women, severe, irregular, and heavy bleeding could be symptoms of uterine cancer, and women with these symptoms should see a gynecologist.

To diagnose uterine cancer, a dilatation and curettage (D & C, or dilating the cervix and scraping the uterine lining) is commonly done. Endometrial tissue is then sent to the pathology lab for evaluation. Sometimes, a uterine tissue aspiration, simply and easily performed in the office, can quickly indicate the potential for uterine cancer.

Hysteroscopy, the insertion of a fiberoptic tube to visualize the interior of uterus, along with a biopsy of endometrial tissue, may be done instead of the traditional D & C.

The detection of uterine cancer involves regular PAP smears and gynecological examinations. Just being postmenopausal doesn't mean you don't need to be checked! Since obesity and estrogen dominance are risk factors, it's important to keep close watch on them.

Ovarian Cancer

Ovarian cancer is fairly uncommon. It is usually discovered late in the course of the illness, and occurs most frequently in women in their thirties and forties, but sometimes in women in their twenties. New evidence points toward a gene that predisposes certain women to ovarian cancer.

Women who have a familial history of ovarian cancer might opt for routine annual sonograms and a blood test called CA125. The blood test should not be used as an absolute screening test, because false positives and negatives are fairly common.

DETECTION OF OVARIAN CANCER

It's important to be aware of changes in your menstrual cycles and of any unusual pain or pressure. If you are experiencing these symptoms or any changes in bladder or bowel patterns, do see your gynecologist. At the least, an annual pelvic examinations will screen for this rare possibility. Women with a family history of ovarian cancer may want to have more frequent examinations.

Overcoming Vaginal Pain

The baby-boomer woman is experiencing an unprecedented level of environmental stresses that target the vagina. Exposure to vaginal douches and sprays, fragrances and chemicals, birth control pills, diethylstilbestrol (DES), antibiotics, antifungals, bleaches in toilet paper and feminine hygiene products, environmental toxins, genital herpes, and HPV — it's no wonder normal vaginal health is at risk! Too many women suffer from the symptoms of vaginitis: itchy, burning sensations, uncomfortable and malodorous discharge, pain on intercourse.

Causes of Vaginitis

Why is vaginitis such a pervasive a baby-boomer phenomenon? There are several contributing reasons:

- The baby-boomer woman reached her menstrual age after the advent of antibiotics, the main side effect of which is to kill off the "good" vaginal flora and thereby promoting yeast infections, or candidiasis.
- She or her mother may have been exposed to diethystilbestrol (DES), which was used by women of her mother's generation to prevent miscarriage. This exposure may set up an inflammatory condition in the vaginal wall. A mother's DES exposure can result in vaginal malformation in her daughters.
- She is the recipient of the fruits of the sexual revolution, which include a higher incidence of herpes infections and human papillomavirus.
- She may have been taking birth control pills.
- She may consciously defer pregnancy to a later age, with hormonal consequences.
- Chemical sensitivity is another problem: she's been exposed to more chemicals than were previous generations of women. We tend to think of

chemical exposure and sensitivity as affecting primarily the nasal passages, the superficial skin, and the lungs, but vaginal tissue is an ideal target organ for chemical sensitivity. Inadvertent application of chemicals present in water, deliberate applications of chemicals in vaginal deodorants, inadvertent applications of bleaches or dyes present in clothing or in toilet paper and feminine hygiene products — these can all increase the incidence of vaginitis.

Many women haven't been given satisfactory answers about their vaginitis. I'm aware of this because I am very often consulted by women for just this problem.

One problem in the treatment of vaginitis is that in medicine it is treated as an infection with a "find the bug and use a drug" mentality. But there isn't always a bug. Vaginitis may be caused by allergies, a yeast (or *Candida*) infection, a mixed infection, chemical irritation, physical irritation, or a nutritional problem with deficits of essential fatty acids.

To complicate matters, the medications commonly prescribed to treat vaginitis threaten to destroy all the normal vaginal flora. They may cause an allergic reaction, with thinning of the skin and impairment of the local immune system, thus setting the stage for subsequent infection.

Treatment of Vaginitis

The treatment of vaginitis involves identifying the cause, whether it be allergy, chemical or physical irritation, nutritional deficits, mixed infection, or yeast (*Candida*) infection. If possible, the offending agents should be eliminated. In addition, effective treatment may require the incorporation of lifestyle changes that address deep-seated attitudes and habits.

Some general rules for vaginal health are these:

1. *Change your bathing practices.* In this culture, we have an obsession with cleanliness. The vagina is designed to accommodate beneficial bacteria in a synergistic fashion. The bacteria act to repel harmful bacteria just as the colon does. Whenever we use soap, we float the flora away, along with the natural secretions and oils. Long immersions in a bath can have a similar effect on vaginal flora. Remember that soaps, oils, perfumes, and chemicals dissolved in your bath will also affect vaginal tissue. For some women, showers may be a better choice. Also, keep in mind that whatever you shampoo your hair with also trickles down to the vaginal area — and sometimes shampoos can be very caustic to vaginal tissues or the genitals.

2. *Change your style.* Tight, confining clothes and pantyhose are notorious for reducing air flow to the genitals. Wearing pantyhose can bring confining fabric directly into contact with the area. If nylons must be worn, consider using a garter belt and stockings. This, along with the use of loose

cotton underwear instead of nylon or synthetic underwear, will insure proper air flow to the genitals.

3. *Don't douche or deodorize.* Douches and deodorants are unnecessary and change the pH balance of the vagina. It is for culturally misguided reasons that vaginal douches and deodorants are popular, their purpose being to mask natural odors. These odors are caused by pheromones and other sex hormones in combination with normal vaginal bacteria and secretions. The use of sprays and antifungal medications may result in bacterial overgrowth, which can cause odor, irritation, discharge, and pain. Therapeutic douches can be good when they are used for specific problems — *Acidophilus* douches reestablish vaginal flora, and tea tree oil douches have antiseptic effects against bacterial or fungal infections — but douches should not be used routinely. Chemicals and fragrances in these products may cause allergies and result in vaginitis.

4. *Look for and identify allergies.* Food allergies or inhaled allergies can also alter the vaginal balance. Allergies affect all mucous membranes and do not limit themselves to causing runny noses, wheezing, or watery eyes. They can also cause vaginal irritation.

5. *Change your diet.* Vaginitis is more common in people who have diabetes and chronically high blood sugar. Candidiasis, the most common type of vaginitis, is diet related. Women with chronic vaginitis report a vast improvement with diets that are low in sugars, including fruit sugars.

6. *Eliminate environmental chemicals.* Determine whether you have allergies to any inhalants or chemicals in your environment at large. The soaps, chemicals, bleaches, and fragrances in laundry products used to launder underwear can also have an irritant effect on vaginal or genital tissue. Other immediate sources of potentially allergy-producing chemicals are sanitary products, which are chemically treated with bleach in order to make them white and therefore appear sanitary. Many health-food stores stock chemically untreated sanitary products.

After eradication of the culprit or culprits responsible for the vaginitis, it is helpful to restore vaginal pH with vinegar and water douches or an *Acidophilus* douche, which acts to restore normal vaginal flora. Dryness of the skin of the genitals and the vulva can be alleviated nutritionally with supplements of vitamins E and A, as well as zinc.

Restorative douche: 1 to 2 teaspoons of distilled white vinegar to 1 pint distilled water; ½ to 1 teaspoon of acidophilus powder may be added.

Treatment of Candida-induced Vaginitis

Candida is a specific type of yeast that colonizes in humans. It can cause systemic problems such as fatigue, joint pain, memory deficits, and malaise, in addition to the common form of vaginitis. Especially after antibiotic therapy, *Candida* converts from its regular yeast form to an invasive fungal form, which can leave spores of fungi deep in the vaginal tissue. Some women with recurring vaginitis caused by "yeast infections" may undertake an ongoing series of futile applications that temporarily alleviate the problem, never truly eradicating it.

Although the use of antifungal medications or herbs is important in treating *Candida*, complete treatment involves identifying the reason that permitted it to proliferate in the first place.

There are three common sources of recurring *Candida* or yeast infection:

- The GI tract. Many of the fungi that cause vaginitis can be dispersed from the GI tract to the vagina. Diet changes, especially reducing sugars and fermented products, can help. It may be necessary to restore the beneficial flora of the GI tract with *Acidophilus* or live yogurt cultures.
- The vagina itself. Spores of fungi may lie in a dormant form several cells deep in the vaginal tissue, requiring a systemic rather than topical approach to vaginitis, and the use of antifungal drugs such as Nizoral, Diflucan, or Sporonox.
- The sexual partner. For a while it was the vogue to blame the partner for "ping-pong" vaginitis: infection and reinfection. However, new studies indicate that it is rare for any circumcised man to harbor and transmit yeast infections. As a precaution, however, couples who face recurring vaginitis may opt for treating the male preventively for a week or two with topical antifungal medication.

Women with chronic yeast infections should ask themselves these questions:

- Do I eat a high-sugar diet, including sugar from natural sources like fruit or honey?
- Am I consuming many yeast-containing foods, foods like breads, cakes, pretzels, and muffins?
- Do I use antacids? Steroids? Hormones like birth control pills?
- Am I immunosuppressed because of stress? Because of chronic infections like sinusitis? Because of drug or alcohol use?

Bolstering the immune system is crucial in treating yeast infections. Nutrients like vitamins A, C, and E; beta-carotene; zinc; selenium; and primrose oil will help reestablish normal immune defenses.

In a patient with a mild *Candida* infection, herbal medicines usually cure it. These include:

- Grapefruit seed extract. Recommended dosage: 125 to 250 milligrams three times daily
- Pau d'arco. Recommended dosage: Three glasses of freshly brewed tea from tea bags three times daily
- Garlic. Recommended dosage: concentrated garlic capsules, 400 milligrams three times daily
- Caprylic acid. Recommended dosage: 500 to 750 milligrams three times daily

These treatments can be combined and sometimes work synergistically.

The treatment of long-standing *Candida* infections requires use of antifungal medications as well. Some patients may require desensitization to *Candida* through a treatment called provocation-neutralization, a type of immune therapy. This involves injecting tiny amounts of nonliving *Candida* extract under the skin to trigger an immune response. In this way, the body can reconstitute its normal defense mechanism against *Candida* and prevent further infections from developing when herbs or medication are withdrawn in the future.

Overcoming PMS, Cramps, and Heavy Bleeding

While menstruation is a biological fact of life, we're enlightened enough nowadays not to call it "the curse." Yet, for too many women, it still feels like one. They may experience extreme fatigue, moods that swing from anxiety to depression, severe cramps, heavy bleeding, and other unpleasant symptoms. It's not commonly known that many of these symptoms are not inevitable companions of menstruation but are actually induced by dietary and nutritional imbalance.

Premenstrual Syndrome — It's Official

You may have been aware of the recent controversial decision by the American Psychiatric Association to include premenstrual syndrome, or PMS, as an official malady in its diagnostic bible, the DMS-IV listing of psychiatric complaints. Many women's groups argued against this, complaining that it is wrong to turn a common physiological complaint into a psychiatric problem. The psychiatrists, on the other hand, insisted that "their" PMS was a special case of the common syndrome, one affecting only a small percentage of women and involving deep and debilitating depression. The idea was that these women could then get insurance-covered medical treatment. Whatever the merits of the issue, it actually points to a trend in the medical establishment toward taking PMS seriously as a treatable complaint.

Women with premenstrual syndrome complain of symptoms for a week to as long as three weeks prior to their periods. Common symptoms of PMS include

- Mood changes: anxiety, depression, crying spells
- Fatigue and increased need for sleep
- Constipation, intestinal bloating, distention
- Water weight gain
- Breast tenderness

Although there are ideas about the cause of PMS, including the estrogen excess syndrome, there are no definitive answers. There are probably many hormonal influences yet to be discovered and understood. It seems clear, however, that a hormonal imbalance of some type contributes to PMS.

Many women with PMS have low magnesium levels. Interestingly, women often report chocolate cravings immediately before their periods, and cocoa turns out to be rich in magnesium. But unfortunately, chocolate products are high in sugar and contain a stimulating chemical, theobromine. Therefore, we can't really recommend dipping into a box of chocolates as a source of magnesium to combat PMS, since this will more likely contribute to rebound moodiness and irritability.

OVERCOMING PMS

Regular exercise and maintaining an ideal weight helps to alleviate the symptoms.

It is also well known that premenstrual syndrome and the emotional aspects of it are uniquely treatable through a nutritional approach. Women who institute the following measures report having relief from many of the symptoms of PMS:

DIETARY RECOMMENDATIONS:

- Eliminate sugary foods. Hypoglycemia is a major component of PMS — it intensifies the carbohydrate craving, anxiety, and fatigue associated with PMS.
- Reduce saturated fats and increase fiber in the diet. This will reduce high levels of estrogen that may be associated with emotional and physical symptoms.
- Eat foods high in the amino acid tryptophan: milk, chicken, a little turkey. Tryptophan has a calming effect.
- Reduce or eliminate caffeine, which causes breast swelling and tenderness.
- Reduce sodium intake, which can cause excess water retention.

RECOMMENDED NUTRITIONAL SUPPLEMENTS

- (GLA): four to six 240-milligram capsules per day
- Vitamin E: 400 International Units per day
- Vitamin B_6 (regulates ratio of estrogen to progesterone): 50 to 100 milligrams twice daily
- Chromium: 100 micrograms three times a day between meals. This is good for hypoglycemia
- Magnesium: 150 to 200 milligrams twice daily

The above supplements should be taken every day, not just when PMS symptoms occur.

Extreme Cramps and Heavy Bleeding

Severe cramps and heavy menstrual flow can indicate estrogen/progesterone imbalance. Adequate progesterone allows the proliferating endometrium to shrink.

TREATING CRAMPS AND HEAVY BLEEDING

In addition to addressing the possibility of progesterone deficiency, women with extreme cramps and heavy bleeding should stop drinking coffee and alcohol. As noted before, coffee promotes muscle-cramping and alcohol is a culprit in estrogen-dominance/progesterone deficiency.

For relief of menstrual cramps, nutritional recommendations include

- Flaxseed, 1 tablespoon per day
- Borage oil, one 240-milligram capsule four times daily
- Vitamin E, 800 International Units daily
- Magnesium, 600 to 800 milligrams daily

For abnormal or heavy bleeding, women should

- Follow recommendations for progesterone deficiency/estrogen excess syndrome (see page 213).
- Increase dietary intake of foods high in the carotenoids, iron, vitamin A, vitamin C, vitamin E (see chapter 16).
- Increase foods high in bioflavonoids, present in most fruits and vegetables. These reduce capillary leakage.
- Decrease intake of red meat, eggs, dairy products, fatty foods.

Supplements to control heavy bleeding:

- Vitamin E, 400 International Units daily
- Borage oil, 300-milligram capsules two or three times daily
- Ferrous fumarate (iron), 80 milligrams three times daily
- Rutin (a bioflavonoid), 500 milligrams twice daily

A Growing Problem: Amenorrhea

Amenorrhea is a loss of menstrual periods in premenopausal women. The baby-boomer woman is especially prone to amenorrhea because she is likely to be a striver and perfectionist who is newly conscious of the benefits of exercise and the importance of maintaining proper body weight.

One of the most common causes of amenorrhea is intensive exercise. That's why this condition is more common among professional athletes. Intensive aerobic exercise can affect the hypothalamic-pituitary-ovarian balance, reducing hormone production by the ovaries and leading to the condition of athletic amenorrhea.[23]

This happens because the body perceives intense physical exertion and a low caloric intake as an indication of stress and famine. In its evolutionary wisdom, the body decides that this is not a good time to bring a new member of the tribe into existence, because the likelihood of its survival will be poor.

Amenorrhea can also be caused by famine or malnutrition, since it's one of the female body's natural means of energy conservation. Nutritionally, the reproductive cycle requires a certain input of iron, protein, and calories. This is why women at menopause have a tendency to gain weight — the higher calorie requirements of menstruation and child-bearing are gone. A women who is pursuing a very low-calorie diet may send her body into energy-conservation mode, inducing amenorrhea.

What are the hazards of amenorrhea? Well, the number one concern is osteoporosis. Amenorrhea can be perilous in terms of reducing future bone mass. It's a kind of premature menopause accompanied by estrogen deficiency, which puts one at risk for osteoporosis.

Treatment for Amenorrhea

- **Identify and treat stress** — try to cope with stress more effectively through stress management programs, exercise, relaxation therapy, and massage therapy.
- **Exercise moderately** — develop an active exercise style that is not

destructive or punitive. You can be a world-class athlete without punishing training.

- **Eat adequately** — eat to support physical and mental needs.
- **Treat nutritional deficiencies** of essential fatty acids, vitamin E, and
  zinc, which may also cause disturbances in the reproductive cycle.

The medical treatment for amenorrhea may involve the prescription of
Provera, a synthetic progesterone. It was designed to mimic the function of
natural progesterone: to bring on menstrual bleeding. Estrogen causes the
proliferation of the endometrium, the lining of the uterus, while the
counter-hormone progesterone causes it to periodically slough off.

However, there are some problems. As you can see in the table, synthetic
progesterones like Provera actually have some of the opposite effects of
natural progesterone. Consequently, some women taking high doses of
synthetic progesterone report having intense cravings for sweets. What they
need are lower levels of synthetic progesterone and higher levels of natural
progesterone to help control their blood sugar.

Differences in Types of Progesterone

Synthetic	Natural
High doses act as a depressant	Has antidepressant qualities
Can increase appetite, cause cravings	Helps to control blood sugar
May increase edema and swelling	Helps to reduce edema and swelling
Reverses cardioprotective benefits of estrogen	Enhances cardioprotective benefits of estrogen

Endometriosis: The Disease of Liberation (and Civilization)

Endometriosis is a puzzling entity and a baby-boomer phenomenon, affecting an estimated 15 percent of all women during their reproductive years.[24]
It is an overgrowth of the lining of the uterus and a migration of endometrial
tissue to other sites within the body. During a woman's monthly cycle, these
bits of displaced tissue grow and then bleed just as they do in the uterus,
sometimes causing pelvic and abdominal lesions or scarring.

If untreated, endometriosis can cause much discomfort and may result in
infertility.

Some Causes of Endometriosis

DELAYED CHILDBEARING

Women today frequently postpone pregnancy for an ideal time that suits them socially, economically, and emotionally. Pregnancy has become an option rather than a fact of life. Unfortunately, it's working against the natural female physiology to have your first child at age thirty-six.

A PREDISPOSING DIET

As an inflammatory condition, endometriosis is a disorder of prostaglandin metabolism. The tissue of the uterus is laden in prostaglandins, the balance of which to some extent is determined by diet. A diet laden with margarine and sugar and bereft of natural omega-3 oils, zinc, and vitamin C will tend to promote prostaglandin disorders.

BETTER MEDICAL DIAGNOSIS

The advent of fiberoptic technology and laparoscopic procedures in the early 1970s offered a less invasive way of visualizing internal tissues and making a definite diagnosis.

There is also a theory that levels of toxic organic chlorides like DDT and other pesticides in the environment may predispose women to endometriosis. These chemicals mimic some of the effects of estrogen. Sexually transmitted diseases and viruses are not considered risk factors.

Symptoms of Endometriosis

- Cramps five to seven days before periods
- Pain during intercourse
- Severe cramps with periods, that include abdominal cramps
- Chronic lower back pain or pelvic pain
- Heavy bleeding and clotting during periods
- Severe PMS symptoms, including body aches and low-grade fever

Treatment of Endometriosis

For years, the treatment that gynecologists cavalierly recommended for women with endometriosis was pregnancy. Since this is not practical for many women, medical treatment involves the use of hormones to stop menstruation and halt the inflammatory process. Birth control pills help endometriosis by simulating the hormonal condition of pregnancy.

Conventional surgical treatment involves laser removal or cautery of endometrial implants and laser myomectomy, which is the removal of these implants from the myometrium—the muscle layer of the uterus. Hysterectomy should be performed only in the most extreme cases!

Nutrient correction can also have a significant effect on endometriosis. Besides the recommendations for estrogen dominance syndrome, some useful nutritional supplements include

- Vitamin E, 800 International Units daily
- Borage oil or primrose oil, as a source of omega-3 and omega-6 fatty acids: borage oil, three 500-milligram capsules daily; primrose oil, six to eight 500-milligram capsules daily
- A calcium/magnesium supplement, with 1000 milligrams calcium and 500 milligrams magnesium daily
- Natural progesterone cream, to supply the hormone that counters estrogen-induced proliferation of the endometrium

An acupuncturist or practitioner of traditional Chinese medicine may be able to help with this condition. If symptoms are severe, a doctor should be consulted about the possible need for medical or surgical treatment.

Life After Forty

Some women these days are asking, "Is it safe to get pregnant when I'm forty?" For many, it is. This is just one example of how we've extended the range of women's reproductive functions. Our better knowledge of what exercise and diet can do to enhance longevity, combined with high-technology medicine, has really given women a new lease on life. It's part of the whole concept of life extension that we can extend our reproductive years.

Several of my women friends in their forties are now having a first or second child without it taking a terrible toll on their bodies. They've prepared themselves for it, they've exercised throughout pregnancy (which is a new notion), and they've taken strategic nutritional supplements.

For years, many women felt alienated from their reproductive organs, as if they had been appropriated by the medical establishment. Gradually, the tide has been turning. An important approach has been developing in our culture. It favors more natural childbirth, gentler and less invasive techniques for dealing with women's problems, and greater respect for women's reproductive organs that is borne out of true empathy and a greater knowledge. This comes on the heels of the sexual revolution that was taking place when baby boomers were first entering reproductive age. As important as the sexual revolution was the revolution in women's attitudes toward their own bodies. The idea became, "Inform yourself; take control of your reproductive health; use a mirror and examine yourself; open up this part of your anatomy to your own inspection; there's nothing to be ashamed of."

As baby boomers, we are the heirs of this revolution. It's an indication of the changing attitudes people have about medicine in general, which is that they want to be better informed and educated, and to be involved in the decision making process regarding their health.

Women no longer need to feel alienated from their reproductive processes. They can gain control of their health and opt out of some of the medical "battle zones" by increasing their knowledge, doing adequate self-checking, and using appropriate nutrient and natural therapies.

CHAPTER ELEVEN

Mostly for Men

A teenage driver in a souped-up Chevy waits for a light at an intersection. He leers at a passing blonde in a miniskirt and lets out a whistle. The light changes and he puts the pedal to the metal. The car lurches forward with a screech, leaving only tell-tale tire marks and the aroma of burnt rubber.

Olga, an Eastern European women's shot-put champion, steps up to the ring, her powerful squat body poised to explode. There is something uncannily masculine about the set of her jaw, her huge arms, her compact breasts, and her chiseled thigh muscles. She grunts as she whirls and propels the shot to a new record.

Back in the locker room at half time, an NFL pro guard rips his helmet off in disgust. His team trails 21 to 7. At 290 pounds, he is 30 pounds heavier than the average pro lineman was just a decade ago. Berserk with anger, he rams his massive fists into the metal locker in front of him, leaving it slightly dented. His teammates look around and shrug. " 'Roid Rage, I guess," they're thinking to themselves.

The preceding stories illustrate the dark side of the male hormone story. Testosterone peaks in adolescence, leading to typical aggressive behavior and sexual obsession. Now banned from Olympic competition, copycats of testosterone called anabolic steroids created awesome human anomalies like Olga. Despite vigorous campaigns against them and warnings to high school, college, and professional athletes, illegal use of anabolic steroids still abounds in the United States despite their dangerous and unpredictable effects.

But a new willingness to reconsider androgenic hormones is gradually creeping back into medicine. While some physicians have recognized their value for years, two recent New York Times articles thrust the issue into public focus. One article weighed the use of low-dose testosterone for women after menopause to enhance vigor and preserve libido. The other considered testosterone treatments for patients of both sexes with advanced heart disease, based on research performed by Dr. Gerald Phillips at Roosevelt/St. Luke's Hospital. Additionally, with all the attention being lavished on menopause, a new medical consensus is emerging that men suffer their own version of midlife hormonal decline, dubbed "andropause."

While in the main women have been given less attention by the medical establishment, the situation is reversed when it comes to menopause and andropause. We now have virtually institutionalized the practice of providing lifelong hormonal support to women, in the form of chemical copycats of estrogen and other hormones that sustain their youthful functions. This is based on the somewhat shaky but certainly ambitious premise that by doing so we will protect their hearts, protect them from bone disease, and slow down some aspects of the degenerative process — in short, provide them with rejuvenating therapy. While this premise is oversold (see chapter 10), we give virtually no recognition to the idea that a similar or analogous condition could exist in men. Why the double standard? Well, in women, menopause is an obvious event. It is heralded by striking symptoms, such as hot flashes and mood changes, and is proclaimed by the milestone of the end of menses.

In men, however, the process of hormonal change is more insidious. Men peak in their hormone production in their early twenties. From then on, hormonal production slowly declines. This is indeed accepted as a normal consequence of aging. We can scarcely imagine the consequences of men in their eighties having the same level of testosterone as teenagers, racing their cars at breakneck speed through the streets and terrorizing retirement villages across America. It could be rather calamitous.

But in men there is not a simple linear slowdown. Some men experience a rapid and decisive drop in hormone levels at a certain age, almost as if nature were engineering a kind of planned obsolescence; at the age of fifty-five they may have a rapid decline in testosterone production. And, as in women, there are really two hormonal shifts taking place — andropause and adrenopause. The testes and the adrenals are two sources of masculine hormones, with slightly different qualities in the way they energize, enliven, and invigorate. We do know that they both undergo decline, either independently or together. Unfortunately, the nuances of how important each is to the aging process have not really been explored by researchers. More studies have looked at andropause and the effects of changing testosterone levels.

What we do know about adrenopause is that it occurs in both sexes and describes a change in the secretion of hormones by the adrenal glands. Adrenaline is not a factor here, but there is a reduced secretion of hormones like DHEA. At the same time, the glands secrete higher levels of cortisol, a steroid that is catabolic, not anabolic. This means that it breaks down muscle and promotes fat accumulation. DHEA supplements may play a role in managing adrenopause, and stress reduction may aid in reducing cortisol production (see chapter 7 for more on DHEA and supporting adrenal function). The studies of aging adrenals don't offer clear prescriptions. There is much controversy about what the results mean and whether interventions are meaningful or desirable.

We know much more about andropause, which involves a decline in the production of testosterone by the testes. Testosterone is really the ultimate anabolic steroid. What is the role of testosterone in the body? It goes far beyond promoting aggression, body and facial hair, and male pattern baldness. Testosterone is anabolic, meaning that it promotes muscle growth. Loss of lean body mass is a major feature of aging in both men and women, and testosterone production offsets this loss.

Studies show that low levels of testosterone in both sexes predict susceptibility to abdominal weight gain, a pattern of obesity that is associated with heart disease, diabetes, and hypertension. A lower level of testosterone is one of the reasons women exercisers have difficulty achieving the perfect "washboard abdomen" look, despite ample situps and crunches.

Testosterone, like estrogen, is a hedge against osteoporosis. It also seems to be associated with better sleep quality, and its deficiency in senior men may account for the familiar sleeplessness of older age. Additionally, testosterone confers protection against autoimmune diseases like lupus, rheumatoid arthritis, scleroderma, and possibly multiple sclerosis. Decreased levels of androgens in women make them more susceptible than men to these diseases.

Are women totally bereft of this wonder hormone? Absolutely not. Testosterone occurs naturally in adult women at a level around one-tenth of that found in men. Moreover, women's adrenals pump out other androgenic hormones like DHEA and androstenedione — also under investigation as longevity hormones.

Curiously, certain lifestyle factors can promote or inhibit testosterone levels. Unhappily for some vegetarians, an ultra-low-fat diet limits testosterone production, since the cholesterol molecule is the building block for male sex hormones. Additionally, vigorous exercise promotes testosterone, but overtraining may diminish it. Sexual activity also boosts testosterone, but severe stress or depression may lower it.

The other source of significant male hormones are the adrenal glands. The adrenal glands produce DHEA (dehydroepiandrosterone), a hormone that enhances mood and immune response, has been found to help lupus and other autoimmune diseases, and in Europe is widely used to extend longevity, boost the immune system, and combat nervousness and exhaustion. Doctors can measure levels of DHEA in both blood and urine samples. DHEA is also found in women, but it is produced in higher levels — some three or four times higher — in men and appears to be a precursor to certain other hormones. A man's greater muscle mass seems related to both DHEA and testosterone.

There's some evidence that deficiency of DHEA can cause devitalization, lethargy, and a greater susceptibility to weight gain. In Italy, DHEA is a prescription medication, Astenyl, and is given to men and women who suffer from weakness, fatigue, or "neurasthenia." In general, though, it appears that women derive some of their hormonal vitality not from DHEA but from progesterone, which is an anabolic counterhormone to estrogen and serves some of the functions of testosterone in men. Unfortunately, only natural progesterone, which is seldom prescribed by gynecologists, provides an anabolic "kick."

LICORICE: A NATURAL ADRENAL TONIC

Certain herbs, especially licorice in the form of tea, can be used to boost adrenal function. Two or three cups a day will have a significant effect. However, licorice is such a potent herb that it really should be taken only under a doctor's supervision, and your blood pressure should be monitored. Every internist is aware of the danger of licorice consumption in patients with high blood pressure. This is because licorice has a powerful effect on the adrenal glands, slowing the breakdown of the mineralocorticoids and causing the body to retain sodium. Licorice's active ingredient is glycyrrhizin, a plant hormone that enhances the action of the adrenal hormones. For this reason, it's used in many Chinese herbal preparations designed to fortify kidney energy, or "chi."

Men experience a two-phased decline in normal hormonal vitality as they grow older, through the natural processes of andropause and adrenopause. Hormonally based fatigue, usually linked to declining testosterone levels, can and does strike men but too often is overlooked by physicians. Men usually don't undergo a decisive, life-altering event like menopause, but their hormones do slowly, insidiously decline. In some cases, abnormally low testosterone levels can cause debilitating fatigue and a low libido.

Fortunately, there is increasing support for the idea that the symptoms of andropause can be just as easily treated as the symptoms of menopause, and perhaps more safely. The method is testosterone replacement therapy.

According to Michael M. Dullnig, M.D., the idea of testosterone replacement is not new. In the belief that it would restore waning sexual function and vitality, extracts of animal testes were injected into elderly men as early as the 1800s. In one macabre scientific experiment in the early 1900s, the gonads of executed San Quentin inmates were transplanted into men with low libido. Benefits could hardly have been expected to occur because of the body's vigorous rejection of foreign tissue.

Safe oral and injectable preparations of testosterone have been available for at least fifty years, but only recently has widespread commercial access to accurate blood tests made the diagnosis of testosterone deficiency more than an educated guess.

The use of testosterone and related anabolic steroids is being considered for certain patients with AIDS and other wasting diseases like Crohn's disease and ulcerative colitis. Testosterone levels are often low in sick individuals, and supplemental doses help to restore weight, appetite, drive, wound healing, and resistance to infection.

Experimental studies are being conducted in the United States and Denmark to evaluate the role of testosterone in severe heart disease and circulatory conditions. Injections of the hormone given to both sexes have revived patients with failing hearts and severe angina and have even helped to avert toe and leg amputations. While this is no panacea, it is a promising new therapy that can help not only men experiencing andropause but many others who may suffer the effects of low testosterone production.

Low Testosterone

Many men may suffer from marginal or low levels of testosterone even before andropause, at which time the symptoms become more pronounced. Other factors can cause a decline in testosterone levels, including certain illnesses, such as orchitis, which affects the testes. Vasectomies can change the circulation and cause a lowering of testosterone as a side effect. Even extreme stress can work on the limbic system and affect the pituitary gland, resulting in lowered testosterone.

There's also some concern that environmental factors may be affecting sex hormone production across the whole population. It's well documented that the average sperm count of the American male has been dropping consistently over recent years. And there's evidence that our environment is increasingly estrogenic, with environmental toxins tending to induce estrogen production in men as well as women. This feminizing environment may be blunting the effects of testosterone in men, making them more prone to the changes of andropause.

Heavy drinking is likely to exacerbate the effects of andropause and the estrogenic environment, since alcohol distorts the processing of sex hormones in the body. This leads to the typical eunuchoid appearance of chronically alcoholic men, who have small testes, a reduction in male pubic hair, and an increase in breast tissue (but, ironically, often luxuriant thick hair with youthful hairlines). Men naturally produce a certain amount of estrogen, which is normally broken down by the liver but is not processed as efficiently in a liver strained by alcohol. The higher estrogen levels in alcoholic men or those with liver disease will cause symptoms like an increase in breast tissue. When estrogen excess coincides with decreased testosterone levels, the symptoms of both are exacerbated. In a typical scenario, a respectable middle-class executive, a hard drinker, begins to experience profound midlife changes, both psychologically and physiologically, as a result of too much estrogen and not enough testosterone at the same time.

While the classic effects of low testosterone are fatigue and low libido, there can be subtler effects as well, which do not always match the popular conceptions of what testosterone does in the male body. Good testosterone levels are related in men to general vitality, the kind of energy that makes you want to bounce out of bed in the morning and charge through your day. But this is not the same thing as the popular notion that high testosterone levels make men aggressive and hostile. In fact, some studies show that men with *low* testosterone levels display more volatile behavior. Men with low testosterone levels who are given supplements report feeling calmer and less anxious, with a greater sense of generalized well-being.

Men who are undergoing andropause may thus feel a general reduction of drive and stamina, or a vague malaise, which can translate sometimes to increased anxiety. Lowered testosterone levels can cause sleep disturbances, which can contribute to fatigue and anxiety. Testosterone also seems to have a direct confidence-building effect, so declining levels may contribute to a midlife crisis: men will start to feel rattled about things they used to feel very confident about. There are other possible psychological components: people expect to feel a certain way as adults, and when their hormones change, it can be disturbing. We do have this notion about the serenity that comes with aging. Some people will actually say, "Thank God I don't have to worry about things so much; it's a relief not to be thinking about sex all the time." But in the American culture that values drive and push so much, a loss of vitality can make someone feel weak and devalued, even losing their sense of identity.

There are other, more physical signs of decline in testosterone levels; again, these don't always match the popular conceptions. While lack of body hair may be associated with low testosterone, many individuals have heavy body hair and low testosterone. Conversely, balding isn't always an indicator of high testosterone levels. However, a change in body hair, especially a thinning of hair on the legs, can indicate declining testosterone.

Another physical indication is a change in body shape, typically the inability to lose a pot belly. Despite the look of those old cowboys you see at the rodeos, with their bellies hanging out of their jeans, the pot is not a "manly" characteristic. In the absence of other causes, such as Syndrome X (see chapter 6), an increase in abdominal fat is associated with lower testosterone. I have patients who tell me, "I'm eating better than I ever did in my life, a low-fat diet, and I exercise, but I can't get rid of this pot belly."

This is why body-builders use steroids, testosterone-like drugs, to achieve that cut-up look with the rippling abdominal muscles. The high steroid levels give them such an unnaturally low level of body fat that you can see their veins protruding under their taut skin. By contrast, low testosterone levels result in flaccid musculature, and either a tendency to put on fat or the opposite: a thin ectomorphic body shape in someone who has trouble gaining weight. The classic eunuchoid appearance of a thin upper body, fleshy thighs, and a flaccid belly is sign of low testosterone levels.

Testosterone also plays a vital role in maintaining bone mass and is partly the reason why men have greater bone mass than women and suffer less from osteoporosis. However, bone thinning is a real concern for andropausal males, and as men extend their longevity they can become prone to osteoporosis. While this remains largely a woman's disease, men suffer from it at about one-fourth the rate of women. It's possible that a judicious use of testosterone therapy, with its proven bone-enhancing effects, could change these figures.

Low libido is another typical sign of declining testosterone levels, though not always, since there is a strong psychological dimension to libido. But men do come in to my office worried about this. I'm opposed to using testosterone to promote sex drive if one has normal levels of the hormone. This is a harmful abuse, and not the same as a correction of a deficiency. But some men want this treatment. A high-powered businessman came in to my office once — a bon vivant, who ran a chain of hotels. He wanted the full "longevity program," with vitamins, minerals, and a diet and exercise prescription. At the end of the visit he leaned toward me and said, "You know, doctor, I have a lot of women in my life, and I want to be able to perform *very* well." I thought, "Uh-oh, here it comes." It turned out that his previous "holistic" doctors had prescribed testosterone for him, so I said, "I'll be happy to test you, but I don't want to provide you with excess testosterone if your levels are normal." He really wanted to push the envelope, but I don't see a place for this in good medicine. (Ultimately, his testosterone levels proved normal, and he shopped elsewhere for a less scrupulous "Dr. Feelgood.")

On the other hand, I've seen testosterone replacement work wonders with men who had a real need for it. One such patient was Jeff, a former fireman who had retired in his early fifties with the idea that he was going to really enjoy life after a very tough career. He was a health-conscious guy and physically fit, but he was experiencing a strange, diffuse devitalization and thought there was a problem with his circulation. I didn't really see such a problem, but he kept coming back, saying he just didn't feel good. I gave him a program of nutrient supplements, and monitored him, but whenever I asked how he was feeling, he would say, "Not much better." He seemed to be suffering from a kind of chronic, low-level fatigue that didn't improve.

Then it occurred to me that maybe there was a subtext to all this, and I asked him, "Is there a particular aspect of circulation you're concerned about? Is potency an issue here?" I hadn't thought to ask before, because his full head of hair made him look vital and healthy overall, and fairly youthful. Then he did say that he didn't enjoy his sex life the way he used to and that he just didn't feel his usual energetic self. Unlike many men, he wasn't going to resign himself to be in poor condition in his fifties. But my usual therapies of nutrients and diet changes hadn't been helping him.

With this new topic on the table, I said, "Let's check your testosterone." I was not surprised to find that he had a low testosterone level. I could tell him that he had a clear problem that was most likely very correctable and was certainly the key to his low libido and very possibly to his lowered vitality as well. With testosterone replacement, before long he was clearly a happy camper, regaining both energy and sexual confidence.

What interested me about Jeff was that he had had ample opportunity to have a placebo response to the other therapies, if there was indeed a psychological component. He was eager to undertake them, but he just kept complaining. Years ago, he was one my first patients to impress me with the insidious and subtle way in which andropause can manifest itself, and to suggest the potential value of testosterone replacement therapy.

Testing for Testosterone

Jeff's experience should also remind us that the normal battery of tests given in the doctor's office are pretty limited. Few doctors test men's hormone levels. Now I don't screen all men for this, but I do give the test when I suspect low testosterone may be causing very specific symptoms.

The best index of testosterone levels is the level of free, unbound testosterone in the bloodstream. However, testosterone levels fluctuate according to a diurnal pattern: they're highest in the morning, as evidenced by morning erections, which are not just related to sleep patterns but to the higher testosterone levels. There are other more unpredictable fluctuations, so when an initial test result appears normal but borderline, a second test might be useful.

I also test for DHEA levels as part of a workup for fatigue in men and women. There's also a replacement therapy for DHEA, but it remains controversial. It's a typical practice of holistic physicians to look at DHEA levels and supplement them. In my own practice I've found that DHEA therapy sometimes has subtle but definite effects, but often the effects are fairly modest. More typically, DHEA therapy is a way of providing androgen support to women when testosterone might create undesirable side effects, like increased facial or body hair or male-pattern baldness.

Testosterone Replacement Therapy

The artificial steroids that many athletes take have such a terrible reputation that a doctor who gives patients testosterone is immediately suspect. But there's a real difference between testosterone, which is a natural substance, and the anabolic steroids that athletes use, which are patented drugs and artificial mimics of testosterone. These can indeed cause the aggressive and hostile reactions that you hear about, and they can affect other body systems, causing enlargement of the prostate gland and problems with urinary flow. The artificial steroids can also raise cholesterol levels, unlike natural testosterone, which can actually improve cholesterol levels.

The question also arises whether testosterone use is safe, given men's susceptibility to prostate cancer, which is known to be hormonally stimulated. But clinicians experienced in the use of testosterone report no increased incidence in prostate cancer when patients are thoroughly examined before treatment. The advent of the prostate-specific antigen (PSA) blood test makes it easier to monitor patients receiving testosterone therapy. It appears that testosterone does not cause prostate cancer to develop in healthy men, although it may stimulate cancer growth if it is used once a tumor is well established. Nor does testosterone usually prompt urinary symptoms in men with enlarged or inflamed prostates; paradoxically, symptoms can sometimes be relieved when testosterone is initiated. Low-dose testosterone therapy prompted no prostate enlargement or increased PSA in healthy men aged sixty to seventy-five in a study recently performed at the Chicago Medical School.

An interesting question of medical philosophy arises: Is the specter of testosterone causing prostate cancer as real as the specter of estrogen causing breast cancer? Many doctors say that estrogen is a valuable therapy, that it's relatively safe, with only a 5 to 10 percent increase in cancer risk, which just means we should be careful and properly screen candidates for hormone replacement therapy. The same doctors will turn around and say that we shouldn't give testosterone because testosterone causes prostate cancer. But it doesn't *cause* prostate cancer, though it will exacerbate it in someone who already has it. Someone who has prostate cancer clearly shouldn't be taking testosterone. Now, some men have undiscovered prostate cancer, so if they take testosterone without careful prescreening or monitoring, it may kindle the preexisting prostate cancer. But even this is not clear, because there is some evidence that testosterone may not accelerate prostate cancer in the most common and early stages.

Just as with estrogen, proper screening is key. Before I give any man a trial of testosterone supplements, I do a very thorough check of his prostate: a manual examination and a PSA test. If there's any doubt, I send him to a urologist for a transrectal sonogram, which visualizes the prostate to make sure there's no sign of incipient cancer. If all that looks fine, he can safely go on a trial of testosterone replacement.

Of course, these men need to be monitored at frequent intervals, just like women receiving estrogen replacement therapy. I want to make sure that there's no sign of developing prostate cancer. Though in fact, with proper screening, I've never seen a case, and my European colleagues who have been doing this therapy for many years report that the incidence of prostate cancer in these patients is negligible. While some of the pronouncements in the press might lead to you expect an explosion of cancers related to testosterone replacement therapy, this has never been documented.

By contrast, I have seen that some men who have prostate problems, especially the younger ones with so-called chronic prostatitis, suffer from low testosterone levels and actually do better with testosterone supplements. So testosterone does have something to do with the health of the prostate, but it may not all be negative. Certainly, the very population whom we'd expect to have lower testosterone — men in their sixties and seventies — are the ones who tend to have enlarged and cancerous prostates. The link may be more subtle than is commonly thought.

The real problem of testosterone replacement therapy is that natural testosterone is very hard to administer. It's not absorbed well by mouth, and often it has to be given either through the skin as a patch or in a slightly modified injectable form. Depending on the objective of therapy, testosterone can be provided via injection (once weekly to once every six weeks), via sublingual capsules (two to four times daily), via a transdermal patch applied to the scrotum or to a nonhairy skin surface, or by rubbing a gel or cream into the skin. Skin patches (Testaderm, Androderm) and a gel (Androgel) have been approved by the FDA and can be prescribed by a doctor.

I try to avoid the methylated oral forms of testosterone, because long-term use can cause liver disease and ultimately liver cancer. This is why testosterone therapy has gotten a late start: unlike estrogen, the artificial oral forms are relatively toxic. They may also have adverse psychological effects, just as the synthetic female hormones used in estrogen replacement therapy can cause unwanted side effects like depression. I try to give the natural form of testosterone in gel application and to use a close-to-natural injectable form only for patients with profound testosterone deficiencies or those who have a real dislike of the gels and patches.

In conclusion, testosterone is a useful natural medicine that should take its rightful place in an innovative approach to medical problems. Judicious application of androgen therapy may be just the "spark-plug" necessary when diet, exercise, herbal therapies, and supplements prove inadequate to the task of restoring the body to optimal functioning.

Dealing with the Prostate

Sooner or later, most American men will have a rendezvous with the prostate gland. This doesn't have to mean prostate cancer, but two very common prostate problems can cause quite a bit of discomfort. The first, prostatitis, is an infection or inflammation that can affect men of any age. The second, benign prostatic hypertrophy (BPH), is a fancy name for the enlargement of the prostate gland that affects many men in their sixties and seventies. The main side effect is that the enlarged gland squeezes the urethra, making it difficult to empty the bladder and causing frequent, dissatisfying urination.

What is the prostate? It's a small gland about the size of a walnut that encircles the urethra and is mostly a factory for spermatic fluid. The prostate gland gives us the name for prostaglandins, which are chemical messengers that affect everything from inflammation to blood pressure. Embryologically, the origin of the prostate is similar to the origin of the uterus, and both those organs affect the metabolism of prostaglandins. The prostate gland produces lots of prostaglandins, but they are also produced in every tissue of the body. The prostate does not have a profound effect on general metabolism, though it may have an effect that is not currently understood or appreciated. Men who have the prostate removed don't have a significant change in their overall bodily prostaglandin levels. Unfortunately, the presence of all those prostaglandins in this small organ make the prostate gland reactive and finicky, so that an inflammation process that starts there can get out of hand.

Prostatitis — Who Can You Talk To?

This leads us to a very common but little understand and little discussed "men's problem": prostatitis. This is a catchall term for an inflammation of the prostate gland, which can cause a painful, burning sensation during urination and in fact can produce a fairly steady experience of pain in the groin. Men who have prostatitis in their late twenties or in their thirties are often struck with a sense that they're entering a degenerative phase. They recollect their father or grandfather experiencing prostate trouble — "plumbing problems," as they used to be called — but there's little connection at all between prostatitis and the prostate enlargement so common in older men.

What's unfortunate is that prostatitis afflicts men in unprecedented numbers, but most men experience it in isolation. While women very commonly and very easily share stories about their breasts, reproductive organs, infections, and symptoms, most men just don't talk about their bodies. It's difficult for many men to get beyond ordinary conversation to a discussion of their prostate, even with a close friend. They can be in agony and not talking to anyone and not getting much relief from the urologist. (This is changing with the recent establishment of a National Institutes of Health task force on prostatitis.)

Prostatitis may be one of the legacies of the sexual revolution. It often seems to start with a mild sexually transmitted infection, whether viral or bacterial, that makes its way into the highly sequestered prostate gland and sets off a cascade of inflammatory reactions that can persist for months or even years, long after the infection should have worn itself out. There aren't many blood vessels in the prostate, so it can be harder to get medications like antibiotics in there through the blood stream. It's not even clear that an infection is necessary to keep the inflammation going. Sometimes a urologist can isolate a bacterium from the prostatic fluid, sometimes not. Sometimes the inflammation will flare up with a change in sexual habits, such as a period of heavy sexual activity after long abstinence.

Urologists try different antibiotics, but they don't always work. One of my patients, James, told me of his own nightmare experience. He'd contracted a sexually transmitted disease after a one-night stand, and he was having the typical burning urination and was pretty much in pain all the time. He went to his internist, who prescribed a course of tetracycline. That didn't seem to help, so he saw a urologist, who prescribed a different antibiotic. That didn't help, either. Over the next two years, he ended up seeing about ten different urologists, who prescribed more antibiotics, different antibiotics, sulfa drugs, beta blockers to "relax" him, Valium, and even Librium, which gave him crying jags. None of them were able to isolate or identify an infectious agent, and some would go on and on about how "clear and normal" his urine looked. Several suggested that he should see a psychiatrist, but he was in daily, constant pain.

To add insult to injury, he had to keep bending over to submit to the standard manual exam of the prostate at each office visit. To perform the standard examination, a doctor puts on rubber gloves, daubs two fingers with Vaseline, and inserts them up the anus to manually palpate the prostate gland in order to check for pain or enlargement and sometimes to cause emission of some spermatic fluid for testing. James told me he'd had about enough of this for a lifetime.

Finally, in despair, he wrote a letter to one of the top urologists in the country, at a major New York teaching hospital, to ask whether there was anything that could be done. This doctor had the courtesy and refreshing honesty to write back, saying, "Unfortunately, medical science doesn't really know all that much about what causes this problem or keeps it going, and we don't have any sure-fire remedy for it. We know it's painful and upsetting, but fortunately, it often does seem to die out of its own accord."

My patient was so relieved to have this specialist "come clean," as it were, that he stopped hunting down new urologists and new medications, and resigned himself to waiting it out. Sure enough, the pain did slowly lessen over the course of another year, and a few years later it was just a memory.

That said, there are some steps you can take to alleviate the situation. There are more sophisticated tests now, and it's worth trying to get a bit of the spermatic fluid to culture for bacteria. Some urologists will advise the patient to increase sexual activity, on the theory that it is better to relieve pressure and release the prostatic fluid that may be harboring an infectious agent. Another doctor might dolorously advise reducing sexual activity, if someone is relatively active. Sometimes these maneuvers help. Alcohol and caffeine seem to increase the burning sensation, so they should be avoided. Physical stress, sitting for prolonged periods, and especially lack of sleep seem to make the inflammation worse, so simply slowing down a bit may help. Warm sitz baths sometimes provide relief.

For prostatitis, I prescribe Prostat, a flower pollen extract, which has been shown in European and Japanese studies to have a positive effect on the inflammation. I think it's important to consider this not just as an infection but as a inflammatory disease. A chronic inflammatory process can still be churning away, even in the absence of any virus or bacteria. Prostatitis can sometimes be allergic, and a food allergy profile may be worth doing. If the prostate is already inflamed, and thereby predisposed, it could react to an allergen in the diet.

Since the prostate is a rich source of prostaglandins, some of which play a part in the inflammatory process, inflammation is a special problem for this organ. The different types of prostaglandins mediate in a sort of yin-and-yang way in the body. The "bad prostaglandins" constrict blood vessels and bronchial tubes, produce inflammation, and may exacerbate symptoms of PMS in women. The "good prostaglandins" reduce inflammation, cause blood vessels and bronchial tubes to dilate. Accordingly, an imbalance in prostaglandin metabolism could easily set the stage for chronic inflammation of the prostate. I don't think anti-inflammatory medication is a good long-term solution, since in order to reduce inflammation it inhibits all prostaglandins — the good ones as well as the bad ones. If we could find a way to selectively inhibit the bad prostaglandins without inhibiting the good ones, we'd have a good therapy for prostatitis. ("Good" and "bad" are relative terms, of course, since inflammation and constriction of blood vessels are to some extent a useful response to a wound or an infection.)

One way to restore prostaglandin imbalance is to provide the precursors of the "good" prostaglandins, which are the essential fatty acids (EFAs), i.e., alpha-linolenic acid and linoleic acid. These are present in good ratios in flaxseed oil, which may therefore support the prostate in making the "good prostaglandins," the ones that reduce inflammation. The "bad prostaglandins" are derived from arachidonic acid, which is present in meat, so a diet high in meat and dairy products may contribute to prostate disease. Gamma-linoleic acid (GLA), found in primrose, black currant, and borage oil, may also help soothe the inflamed prostate.

In the future, I think we may find that some of the "bugs" that inhabit the prostate, if they're there at all, may be what's called "cell-wall-deficient organisms." They are very difficult to culture and difficult to eradicate, since most antibiotics kill bacteria by attacking the cell wall. Medical science may one day advance to the point of identifying and targeting them. But for now, any man who is struggling with prostatitis should console himself with the knowledge that this problem usually does die away with time.

The Aging Prostate

Most American men will need to face two issues as they head into their fifties, sixties, and seventies. They are prostate enlargement and prostate cancer, which are sometimes, but not necessarily related. It is very common to have prostate enlargement without cancer. In fact, prostate enlargement is virtually universal among North American men, while prostate cancer is not. Nevertheless, it's estimated that the vast majority of men may have "microfoci" of cancer: tiny clusters of cancer cells that are normally of very little consequence, because they are slow-growing. But some of them can develop down the line.

Prostate enlargement, or benign prostatic hypertrophy (BPH) is that annoying development that many men associate with their older fathers: the frequent urination pattern that would send them to the bathroom several times during dinner, or get them up repeatedly during the night. The enlargement that squeezes the urethra can kick in as early as the late forties, though it's more common in the fifties, sixties, and seventies.

While common in the United States, BPH is much less prevalent in some other parts of the world, so environment, lifestyle and diet clearly play a large part in it. Both prostate enlargement and prostate cancer are much less frequent in Japan, for example, apparently because of the higher consumption of soy, beans, and the cabbage family, all of which contain phytoestrogens (or isoflavones), which are cancer-inhibiting. Researchers have found much higher levels of these phytoestrogens in the blood of Japanese men than in Occidental men. They appear to have a blocking effect against prostate cancer and prostate disease in general.

Diet also affects prostaglandin metabolism, which may be important for prostate health. The arachidonic acid present in meats stimulates production of the "bad prostaglandins," while the American diet is generally deficient in the essential fatty acids (EFAs)—the omega-3 oils and the omega-6 oils—that promote the "good prostaglandins." The omega-3 oils are found in cold-water fish such as tuna, salmon, herring, trout, mackerel, sardines, and cod liver, as well as nuts like walnuts and seeds like pumpkin, which is also high in prostate-protective zinc. Omega-6 oils are found in vegetable sources, including primrose oil, borage oil, and black currant seed oil.

A common surgical treatment for enlarged prostate, is the transurethral resection of the prostate (TURP), which employs a kind of plumber's snake that goes up the urethra and shaves off part of the gland without removing it totally. New studies have suggested that this procedure should not be as casually employed as it once was, since it leaves a significant percentage of men with impotence or flow problems and even, rarely, leads to death.

Newer treatments like laser and microwave and freezing are in the wings, but prudence dictates that surgery not be used at the first sign of symptoms but rather saved as a last resort. A promising new therapy, transurethral needle ablation, or "TUNA," uses radio waves to zap prostate tissue, obviating side effects such as incontinence, impotence, or retrograde ejaculation. One heavily marketed prostate-shrinking medication, Proscar, works by blocking a hormone that can cause the prostate to enlarge. (The hormone is DHT, dihydrotestosterone, a major cause of prostate growth.) But Proscar doesn't work for everyone, and although the prostate may shrink, the urinary symptoms may not abate. Some men have seen an improvement in their urinary symptoms over two weeks to four months, but there can be serious side effects, including lowered libido or impotence, breast swelling, or allergic reactions. Prostate-specific antigen levels are altered, possibly masking the development of prostate cancer during treatment. Even more seriously, prostatic fluid transmitted sexually to a woman who becomes pregnant may cause genital abnormality in a male fetus. Some men achieve better results with blood pressure medications like Hytrin or Cardura, but these may cause side effects, such as dizziness.

An alternative natural therapy is extract of the saw palmetto. This can take a little longer to work, but it avoids the side effects of drugs. One study found that 160 milligrams twice daily of standardized extract of saw palmetto (*Serenoa repens*) caused an improvement in quality-of-life scores, urinary flow rates, and prostate size after a month and a half.[1] Another natural therapy uses extracts of the bark of *Pygeum africanum*, a tropical African evergreen tree, in a dosage of 50 to 100 milligrams twice daily. Several studies have reported on its positive effects.

Prostate Cancer

We have a new perspective on prostate cancer in the 1990s, which is both promising and troubling. The development of the prostate-specific antigen test has vastly increased our ability to detect cancer in the prostate long before it would become evident through manual examination or malignant enlargement. It should stand to reason that better detection would result in a vast improvement of statistics on prostate cancer, but it hasn't, and this has been quite distressing. Though our detection skills have increased, we unfortunately have not made any real advances in treatment.

The standard treatments — radiation or complete removal of the prostate — are not always effective, because a few cancerous cells can remain in surrounding tissue and spread to other parts of the body, usually the bones. On the other hand, in men over seventy, the vast majority of prostate cancers are relatively indolent. Someone with incipient prostate cancer may have a somewhat diminished life expectancy, but it could be as long as twelve to fifteen years, over which time most men of this age succumb to other causes of death. Surgery and radiation at this age may not ultimately slow the progress of cancer and may have other harmful side effects, which can themselves increase the chance of death. Accordingly, "W.W." — watchful waiting — is increasingly indicated. In fact, this approach is being used in such a variety of ailments that it's becoming one of the most popular "therapies" of the 1990s. If "W.W." were a drug, I'd say buy stock in it.

The PSA test is quickly becoming part of a standard blood workup that men get with their annual health exam. Its increasing sophistication, coupled with the lack of improved therapies, has generated a bitter controversy among medical scientists and clinicians. They ask whether the test is telling us more than we need to know? Some say, "How can you deny anyone this information about a potentially life-threatening disease?" Others respond, "What good does it do, since it won't change medical management and may just induce anxiety to no useful purpose." I think that the information should be made available and that it's worth having an annual PSA test after the age of fifty, or when symptoms warrant in a man under fifty. But the information should be used with appropriate restraint, by men who are aware that watchful waiting is a good option. Men younger than seventy whose PSA test result is positive might be advised to consider more aggressive treatment options.

Threats to the Family Jewels

Most men know about venereal disease and how to guard against it, but there are two threats to the male genitals that are less commonly known. The more serious is testicular cancer, one of the fastest-increasing forms of cancer and one that can attack even younger men in their twenties and thirties. The common form is called seminoma. It's unclear why this is on the rise, though it may be related to the increasingly estrogenic environment. My own anecdotal clinical experience, though it is not backed up by any statistics I'm aware of, is that all five men I've seen with seminoma *were all inveterate marijuana smokers.* (There are suggestions that estrogen-like effects occur with long-term marijuana smoking, such as the development of extra breast tissue.) The best safeguard against this is to do your own manual self-exam, just as women check for breast lumps.

A somewhat less ominous threat is the risk of the sexually transmitted human papillomavirus, or HPV, the major cause in women of cervical cancer. It is the reason women have the Pap smear test, named after Dr. George Papanicolaou, who invented it. The same virus can infect men and can exist on male genitals in the form of venereal warts. They may either be visible to the eye or be microscopic warts that are hard to detect. It's actually possible to examine the male genitals with a colposcope, which is usually used with women to examine the cervix. If your sex partner has a positive Pap smear, or you find visible warts on your genitals, it's worth having this checked out. It's important to know whether you have a transmissible disease, to prevent the transmission of the virus to women, in whom it's more dangerous, and also because the HPV virus is also a rare but plausible cause of a rare penile cancer. HPV infection is more common among uncircumcised men.

After the (Sexual) Revolution

Aside from the simply annoying or the somewhat more serious men's problems, there is one of another order that looms large in many men's lives. This is impotence, loss of libido, or sexual dysfunction. Since we know there is a strong psychological component to impotence or reduced libido, many men assume that it is emotional, psychological, or due to relationship problems. But they may be adding insult to injury, berating themselves needlessly or anxiously probing their psyches, when all along the problem can be attributed to any of several physiological problems that do not have obvious or definitive symptoms. If you're experiencing low libido or impotence, you should definitely rule out physiological causes before running headlong to a therapist or counselor.

What's remarkable about male sexuality is just how many different factors can affect libido, well beyond the issues of andropause and testosterone levels. A urologist can easily check for the common circulatory, neurological, and hormonal causes of impotence or low libido but may not think of heavy metal toxicity, as we'll discuss below. In fact, almost any devitalizing syndrome or chronic physiological dysfunction can lower libido, from Syndrome X to thyroid deficiency to heart disease to diabetes. Many medications affect libido; they include antihypertensive drugs (which are widely prescribed for high blood pressure), decongestants, and antidepressants, like Prozac.

Adam was a painter who worked in a machine shop for the New York subway system. His chief complaint was impotence — low sexual libido — which he said was affecting his marriage. From his occupational history, I thought he might have some degree of heavy metal poisoning, since he had been steadily exposed to heavy metals, toxic chemicals, and specifically welding byproducts. Indeed, he turned out to have high lead levels in his blood sample. While he didn't have some of the classical symptoms of lead toxicity, such as loss of appetite, constipation, abdominal pain, or paralysis, he did suffer from generalized weakness and malaise. I thought he might have a minor circulatory impairment, too. We undertook chelation therapy (see chapter 12), which would treat both his lead poisoning and any arteriosclerosis, and after chelation his measured lead levels were considerably lower. More important for Adam, he informed me that his marital situation was improving. The meaning is not so much that a chief symptom of lead toxicity is impotence, but that the general malaise and debility that come with an illness like lead poisoning did seem to contribute to his problem.

As mentioned, arteriosclerosis may cause reduced potency and can actually reduce blood flow to the penis. Men with diabetes typically suffer from impotence, first because they have poor circulation, and second because of autonomic nerve damage. This very common complication of diabetes can contribute to reduced potency even in younger people in their thirties and forties. Older men with diabetes who may also have arteriosclerosis and lowered testosterone levels will get a triple whammy.

In the standard workup for impotence or lack of an erection, a urologist will measure penile blood flow and perhaps perform an angiogram, in which a dye is injected to see how it travels through the bloodstream. Less invasive is the penile Doppler test, in which a ring with a sensor is placed around the penis to test for nocturnal tumescence. This is a high-tech form of the old postage stamp test, in which a roll of postage stamps was placed around the flaccid penis at bedtime and the checked next morning to see whether it had it popped or not. The intent, of course, is to indicate whether there is a physiological capacity for spontaneously occurring nocturnal erection independent of any psychological blocks or other factors that might be active during waking hours.

While we're discussing sexuality, it's worth while to mention vasectomy, which is becoming more popular, since it's the "ultimate" form of contraception, with a less than 1 percent failure rate. It's worth emphasizing that the 1 percent failure rate is real — pregnancies can occur. Since most people assume that vasectomy is 100 percent effective, someone in that 1 percent can have a real marital upset. Only a DNA test of the fetus will

REAL MEN HAVE CHECK-UPS

Male stoicism in the face of aches and pains is a positive trait, but when taken to extremes it can endanger health. Most of us have known guys who have bragged that they haven't seen a doc in five years. This is not so smart. The key problems that a checkup can detect are heart disease and sugar disease which can be revealed through an abnormal lipid profile in the blood, and prostate conditions. But you're not likely to suddenly uncover a life-threatening illness during an annual checkup. While there are instances of apparently healthy people being suddenly stricken with fatal illness, most serious and life-threatening disease is rarely silent in its onslaught. Colon cancer, while insidious, usually signals its advent by blood in the stool and weakness due to anemia. Heart disease rarely fells superbly trained athletes, but we all know it does afflict the sedentary and overweight. Prostate disease seldom spreads dangerously without accompanying urinary symptoms. Accordingly, the value of preventive checkups in otherwise well individuals lies more in predicting future disease and mitigating risk factors than discovering lurking assassins.

One key checkup that many forego is the annual eye exam, which provides an invaluable window into incipient disease processes. It can indicate potential heart disease by revealing chronic high blood pressure, and macular degeneration of the retina, which can lead to blindness. Annual checkups should include a digital rectal exam, starting from the age of fifty. This helps screen for prostate cancer by providing a quick check for blood in the stool and an evaluation of the size of the prostate. To screen for colon cancer, men should have a baseline sigmoidoscopy at fifty, which should be followed up with another one every three to five years. Men with an immediate relative who's had colon cancer should be tested more frequently.

convince some husbands that the pregnancy is due in fact to their own failed vasectomy, at which point the married couple may unleash a lot of stirred-up feelings against the vasectomist.

Some health risks are associated with vasectomy, including a possibly higher rate of prostate cancer, and I don't advocate it in most circumstances. By tying off those tubes you may change the circulation and hormonal flow in the area and create a problem, and there have been some clinical observations of lowered testosterone levels, though no studies have been done on this. Still, it may be the method of choice for a couple who doesn't believe in abortion and would be in difficult financial straits if other types of contraception, with higher failure rates, permit a pregnancy. Some suggest that the higher incidence of prostate cancer in vasectomized men is simply a result of their observing their physical condition more carefully and reporting changes more readily to a doctor. Men who have opted for this procedure are certainly less afraid of doctors and medical examinations and are less likely to ignore problems in this area.

The New Paradigm for Men

In the end, the real legacy of the sexual revolution may not just be that men and women have more sex, more regularly. There's also been a positive movement toward talking more openly about sexuality and reproductive issues, including physiological issues, and toward giving men's and women's sexuality and physiology equal attention. Men need to get on this bandwagon, start talking more openly about their reproductive physiology, and bring up issues they're concerned about with their doctors. Men who are experiencing changes in energy or libido in their forties or fifties shouldn't just assume they're entering a decline but should consult with their doctors about the process of andropause and the possibility of compensating for lowered testosterone levels. This is one of the real success stories of modern high-tech medicine that shouldn't be ignored.

CHAPTER TWELVE

The Heart of the Matter

Josef was an acclaimed classical musician with a hyperactive career. He had an amazing schedule: he performed regularly, often as a soloist; he had private students; he did benefit concerts for children, made recordings, appeared on television. He was a dynamo of energy. When he became my patient, I always wanted to say to him, "Just slow down a little." But when he first came to me, he had a more serious problem. He had been healthy and thriving until he reached his early fifties, when he suddenly hit a wall. It started with chest pain and evolved into an overwhelming sense of weakness. A cardiologist diagnosed cardiovascular disease. The arteries to his heart were pinched and blocked, and too little blood was flowing to the heart muscle. His heart was trying to keep him going, but with a reduced supply of oxygen and energy, it just wasn't working. He was running out of steam.

The cardiologist recommended a balloon angioplasty, in which a balloon catheter is inserted into the arteries of the heart, and air is pumped in to expand the balloon. This opens up the congested arteries and gets the blood flowing. Josef felt better and had less pain, but within three or four months the chest pain returned, along with the weakness. The specialist reminded him, "Sometimes this happens with angioplasties—the arteries close up again. We'll just have to do it again." So Josef went through the procedure once more and felt better for a while, but this time the arteries closed up again within an even shorter time, about six to eight weeks. The pain returned, he had to take medications that were making him feel extremely tired, and he was unable to keep up with his schedule of concerts and teaching. This was when Josef came to me for another opinion.

He faced a third angioplasty, or possibly bypass surgery, because the treatment just wasn't working. In fact, he was really confronting an enforced retirement or semiretirement, right at the peak of his career. The stress of the repeated medical procedures, and the heavy medications, were bringing him to a halt. He couldn't face the idea of more procedures or invasive surgery with uncertain results.

Many patients face a similar problem. Suddenly they just can't do things that are important to them, whether it's work and career or just taking a long walk through a park. They haven't (yet) been felled by a heart attack, but they are suffering from heart disease, and it's hitting them where they live.

The good news is that I was able to help Josef, like many other patients, get back to his life without surgery, through diet modification, vitamin supplements, and a treatment called chelation. The bad news is that too many Americans don't realize they have options other than surgery and medication when they have heart trouble, or that they can actually *prevent* heart disease through these same options.

We've all heard the statistics: heart disease is the "number one killer" in the United States. In 1996, sixty million Americans had some form of heart disease — more than one in four. In 1993, nearly one million died of heart disease, representing 42 percent of all deaths, or one of every 2.4 deaths. Total deaths from heart disease increased significantly in that year, perhaps because of the aging population, but also perhaps because people who had survived crises like heart attacks because of improved medical treatment were now dying of subsequent illness, such as congestive heart failure. Heart disease is the listed cause of death for four out of five Americans over sixty-five, but more than one-sixth of all people who die of heart disease are under sixty-five.[1]

What do these numbers really mean? Are we suffering from a modern scourge? Bare numbers don't tell the whole story. Heart disease probably shows a higher tally than some other ailments just because of the way the body works and the way death causes are recorded. Many ailments of older people, from diabetes to cancer to pneumonia, lead eventually to heart failure through one path or another. Heart failure may therefore be the final cause of death, though not the initial one. A harried medical resident in the hospital can find it much simpler to note "cardiac arrest" on the patient's death certificate than to go through the whole course of disease.

From another point of view, we might consider whether death of heart failure is really such a terrible thing. As the blues song says, "Everybody wants to go to heaven, but nobody wants to die." After a long, full life, heart failure may not be such a bad way to go. It can be quick and relatively painless, without the long-drawn-out suffering of some other kinds of illness. If your relative or parent should die of a heart attack at the age of eighty-five or so, while still active and engaged in life, that's probably something to feel grateful for. It's certainly better than long years of nursing homes, hospitals, and incapacitation.

Finally, there's a good side to the scary statistics. Heart disease has actually been declining steadily since the 1950s, when it was probably at its peak. The word has gotten out that changes in lifestyle can reduce the risk for heart disease, and lifestyles have been changing. There is less fat in our diets, more of us are exercising regularly, and there's been a revolution in attitudes toward smoking. Even better, there is now a real consensus that heart disease can not only be prevented but actually be reversed by changes in lifestyle.

We are entering the era of *reversal*. This is a major shift in our understanding of heart disease. Ten years ago doctors thought of heart disease as an inevitable, inexorable decline that could be slowed or arrested but never reversed. They scoffed at the idea of "curing" heart disease, especially by lifestyle changes, but all that has changed. We now realize that heart disease is a dynamic process, that it can wax and wane, and that reversal is indeed possible. As just one sign of the shift in attitude, several major health insurance companies have recently agreed to pay for Dr. Dean Ornish's program for treating heart disease through support groups; a low-fat, vegetarian diet; and exercise. (Other less rigorous diets may be just as effective in reversing heart disease, but more on that later.)

What *do* we need to be concerned about as our bodies move into the middle years? Is it enough to buy the low-fat, low-cholesterol products in the supermarket and go to the gym or go jogging once a week? Is heart disease on the way out, a relic of our parents' generation?

Well, it's not quite that simple, though we are in a better position than ever before to take intelligent preventive measures against heart disease. But there are still some issues we should be concerned about. One is quality of life. While it may not be such a tragedy to pass away from a heart attack at the age of eighty-six, no one wants to be at risk during the fifties or sixties. We don't want to wind up like Josef, suddenly cut off from his career and some of the things he loved most in life. Playing with the risks for heart disease is not just like gambling against the odds. A high-risk lifestyle can cause lots of premature suffering, from chronic chest pain, or angina, to a weakened condition in which normal physical activity can become painful, dangerous, or impossible. If the heart can't do its job, life can become very limited, well before advanced age. Fortunately, there are ways to avoid this, and we'll lay them out in this chapter.

Another major issue that we all have to face is the barrage of information, misinformation, scary reports, hopeful reports, and sometimes threatening language and rigid recommendations that we get from doctors, medical researchers, journalists, and government and private agencies. Should we drink two glasses of red wine a day to avoid heart disease? If we consume no-cholesterol mayonnaise, frozen "low-fat" yogurt and "polyunsaturated" safflower oil, will we live forever? Are medications really the best way to lower blood cholesterol? Which is the "good" cholesterol and which is the "bad"? Are we supposed to be eating monounsaturated fats, or polyunsaturated fats, or partially hydrogenated coconut oil? What about Jim Fixx, who helped start the whole jogging craze and then dropped dead of a heart attack while he was out running one day? It's not easy to sort all this information out and to compare the report we read in the paper today with one we read in a magazine two months ago. One thing we'll do in this chapter is provide some guidelines for making sense of the information overload.

Finally, there are serious issues concerning many of the standard medical tests and treatments for heart disease. Common tests include the annual blood test that measures cholesterol level and other substances, the treadmill stress test, and the high-tech angiogram X-ray that involves shooting dye into the heart. (See later in this chapter on recommendations for these tests.) Treatments range from powerful medications that lower cholesterol and reduce blood pressure to the types of invasive surgeries like bypass surgery or balloon angioplasty that have become so popular (and lucrative for cardiac surgeons and cardiologists) over the past two decades. The basic questions we must ask of all tests and treatments are the same: how safe are they, how necessary are they, and how well do they provide reliable, meaningful information or results? One crucial question is often left unasked: does the test or procedure have a positive effect on the eventual outcome? Will it help you live longer, live better, live happier? In this chapter we'll review the standard medical tests and treatments and look at some of the alternatives that are only beginning to be explored. By the way, don't forget Josef. We'll come back to his story later in the chapter. It was a real success story of alternative treatment.

This generation has a much better shot at maintaining cardiovascular health than our parents or grandparents did. A lot of folks in those generations had rheumatic fever and rheumatic heart disease, which can damage the valves of the heart, causing extra strain on the muscle and leading eventually to congestive heart failure. The steak-and-martini high living of the postwar period set many people up for trouble. More important, though, is the fact that we are now able to take control of this aspect of our health in a way that our parents couldn't, because we have better information. We need to take the intelligent approach without succumbing to diet fads, food industry advertising, the latest newspaper report, or, sometimes, to tests and treatments that are being pushed on us by medical professionals. To get started, let's take a closer look at what can go wrong in the system we want to maintain.

How Things Go Wrong

When we think of heart disease, we usually think of a crisis — stroke, heart attack, heart failure. Of course, none of these just happen by themselves. They are the end points of a progressive decline, which may or may not be apparent to the victim. The great shift over the past few decades has been toward a new awareness of the risk factors and the preliminary signs of progressive cardiovascular disease. We can now begin to identify the signs that the system is under stress, or has begun to deteriorate, even before we have any real symptoms. There are several possible dangerous end points, but the pattern of decline is similar for all.

By far the most common indicator for heart disease is arteriosclerosis, or hardening of the arteries (from *sclerosis*, a hardening.) This is the precursor for angina, heart attacks, strokes, and other problems. When the walls of the arteries harden, thicken, and lose their suppleness, they are no longer able to respond to the shifting pressures of the bloodstream. They can't expand to allow increased blood flow when it's needed by the muscles or other organs. The most common form of this problem is *atherosclerosis*, from *atheroma*, a fatty, porridgelike growth. It's the buildup of fatty substance on the interior walls of the arteries that starts the process of decline.

This begins with the buildup of fatty streaks on the smooth interior walls of blood vessels, especially the medium and large arteries that carry blood to the brain, heart, kidneys, and legs. The fatty streaks attract thicker deposits, called plaque. The rough edges of the plaque irritate the smooth lining of the blood vessels, causing scar tissue to form, and dead cells build up. This in turn attracts calcium deposits from the bloodstream, which increase the hardening and roughness. More scar tissue forms, and the arteries become increasingly hard, narrow, and inflexible. Blood flow decreases, and, because the heart is pumping blood through smaller, narrower arteries, blood pressure increases. The heart must work harder to maintain basic circulation, causing strain and weakening of the heart muscle. The narrow, inflexible blood vessels can no longer respond when muscles (including the heart muscle) demand increased oxygen and nutrients during exercise. Even minor physical exertion can lead to exhaustion and shortness of breath, as the heart tries in vain to push enough blood through the narrow vessels.

The roughened inner walls also become "sticky" and likely to attract clots, which can quickly grow large enough to completely block off all flow in the narrowed vessels. This kind of stationary clot is called a thrombus; if it breaks loose and travels through the artery to cause a clot at a different point, it's called an embolism. When a blood vessel is completely blocked, it is occluded. If the clot occurs in the brain, it's called a stroke. If it blocks off the flow of blood to the heart itself, it's called a heart attack. Once the flow is cut off, the tissue that is no longer being supplied with blood begins to die. In the brain, this leads to the kind of symptoms that we associate with strokes: paralysis, loss of speech function, coma. In the heart, the death of tissue is called a myocardial infarction. (The myocardium is the middle muscle layer of the heart. The tissue dies because it becomes infarcted, or "stuffed" with stagnant blood, which can't flow out because no new blood is flowing in.) A person can survive a heart attack, but part of the muscle is dead, and the newly weakened and damaged heart must work even harder to maintain the flow of blood to the rest of the body and to the heart muscle itself.

Once this kind of damage occurs, all bets are off. We can slow and even reverse the hardening and narrowing of the blood vessels, and cause the fatty plaque to dissolve away. But once heart or brain tissue dies, it's gone forever.

Well, that's a pretty scary picture. In fact, it's the picture that cardiologists use to sell their patients on all kinds of high-tech tests and procedures, from angiograms to bypass operations. To be fair, there are people who benefit from these procedures. But, fortunately, they aren't the only ways of dealing with the problem. As you read this chapter you'll learn about some other effective methods. To really understand methods for prevention and reversal, we have to ask the important question "What causes arteriosclerosis?"

The one idea that's made it into public consciousness over the last couple of decades as *the* culprit behind heart disease has to be cholesterol. The medical establishment, the federal government, and the National Cholesterol Education Project have all drummed it into our heads that we should watch the level of cholesterol in our bloodstream and avoid foods that will raise that level. The food industry has jumped on the bandwagon and mounted a billion-dollar advertising campaign to sell us low-cholesterol and cholesterol-free foods, with the idea that we're going to escape heart disease by consuming them.

Just how dangerous is cholesterol? Well, it's true that cholesterol is a major component of the fatty streaks that turn into fatty plaque on the inner walls of arteries. It's true that much research suggests that high cholesterol levels are associated with a higher incidence of heart disease. It's true that indigenous peoples around the world who eat a very low-fat diet have a much lower incidence of heart disease than we do in the industrialized West.

It's also true that other indigenous peoples, like the Inuit (Eskimo) of North America, can eat a diet that is super-high in fat and cholesterol and still have a very low incidence of heart disease. In fact, the scientific studies of the past twenty years show a very mixed picture of cholesterol. We know that there are different kinds of cholesterol, and current research suggests that different balances and ratios of fats and proteins in the blood may have much more to do with cardiovascular disease than simple total cholesterol level. Current research also suggests that the presence of "oxidized" cholesterol may be an important risk factor. When we consume cholesterol that's been overcooked, or stored too long, it can create free radicals, toxic molecules that react with the cells of the body and can damage their protective cell membranes. Low levels of antioxidant nutrients in the blood, which neutralize the free radicals, become another risk factor. There is some evidence that oxidized fats or even viruses can cause damage to the inner walls of blood vessels and thereby start the process of plaque formation. All in all, it's just too simple to say that cholesterol itself is the primary culprit. The picture is now much more complex than that.

For example, there is some evidence that the buildup of atherosclerosis may be partly related to infections and the immune system. Arteriosclerosis may begin with damage to the arterial wall, to the tissue called the *endothelium*. The damage may be physical, from prolonged high blood pressure.

Alternatively, it may be caused by an infectious agent or autoimmune reaction, or by free radicals or chemical poisons from pollution or cigarette smoke. Following the damage, blood platelets migrate to the damaged area, scar tissue and muscle tissue builds up, cholesterol is deposited at these spots, and there's a whole cascade of events that results in the formation of plaque. Researchers in Finland have traced the development of arterial plaque in some people to the presence of a certain type of *Mycoplasma*, a microorganism that may cause an immunological reaction to occur in the arterial wall and set off the buildup of plaque through a chain reaction. Different insults to the arterial wall may culminate in a single common process leading to arterial blockage.

Others have looked at the possibility that the herpes virus may damage the endothelium. There may even be an autoimmune reaction in some cases, in which certain cells of the immune system attack the body's own tissue, causing the initial damage to the blood vessel walls. Poor diet is also undoubtedly a factor, causing imbalances or abnormal composition of the cellular walls of the tissue that lines the blood vessels. Diet can change the proportion of omega-3 to omega-6 fatty acids in the cell walls; artificial *trans* fats from foods like margarine may also wind up in the cell walls and function abnormally. There's also the growth factor hypothesis: that some of the body's regulatory systems may break down and cause a proliferation of smooth muscle cells on the endothelium that acts as a starting point for plaque and contributes to hardening or constricting the arteries. We're now looking for whole new categories of drugs to treat this kind of disorder, which operates independently of cholesterol, and which may be the factor underlying the high failure rate of angioplasty.

These are some of the cutting-edge ideas about atherosclerosis. We can also pin down a handful of well-known risk factors that clearly contribute to heart disease and have a cumulative and interactive effect. They include smoking, obesity, high blood pressure, sedentary habits, and poor diet. Someone who smokes, *and* is overweight, *and* is sedentary, is pushing the envelope. The good news is that risk factors can be dramatically improved by changes in lifestyle, once you have the right information. Let's take a look at each of the risks, explain the current thinking on how they lead to heart disease, and investigate the ways of reducing them for prevention or reversal.

Risk Factors for Heart Disease

Many patients, like Josef, come to me for the first time with a diagnosis of heart trouble or cardiovascular disease already in hand. I look at the results of tests they may have had, and put them through a pretty careful examination that will probably cover some areas that haven't been looked at, especially blood nutrient levels. Sometimes these patients have already had conventional treatment or a recommendation for it. We look at that and consider alternatives, especially if they've been recommended for invasive testing or surgery. I bring up the costs, risks, and benefits of testing and procedures, and we take a close look at whether they are really likely to benefit the patient over time.

Other patients ask for a general health evaluation, or advice on improving their health. We go through a checklist, and one of the items on it is cardiovascular health. I look at cholesterol levels, triglyceride levels, body weight, cigarette smoking, blood pressure, diabetes, exercise patterns, and personality type (certain types are more at risk for heart disease), and I work up a complete cardiovascular profile. I ask the usual questions: "Do you have a family history of heart disease, a history of high cholesterol, diabetes; do you smoke; do you exercise?" but also "Do you take a multiple vitamin; do you take antioxidants?" I look pretty closely at diet and nutrition, because this is an area where many people have been misguided, or are just not following an optimal program.

Essentially I go through all the risk factors with any new patient, certainly with any patient who already may be suffering from symptoms of incipient or full-fledged heart disease. If it seems warranted, I'll do some of the more finely focused blood tests, such as the ones for fibrinogen and for homocysteine (more about these later). I can pretty quickly make an assessment about whether someone needs to start a program for prevention or even active treatment. Let's go through my checklist and review the current knowledge about risk factors and preventive measures.

Risk Factors: Cholesterol and Other Players

At the beginning of the twentieth century, the Russian scientist Arnitchkow discovered that he could induce heart disease — atherosclerosis — in rabbits by feeding them large amounts of cholesterol.* This was the beginning of the cholesterol hypothesis, which during the last thirty years has become the dominant explanation for why atherosclerosis develops. The medical establishment, and even the government, are firmly behind this. In 1987 the National Cholesterol Education Program (NCEP) recommended that everyone over the age of twenty have a blood test for cholesterol level and start a cholesterol reduction program if the count was 210 or over. Recently,

---

* The rabbits were also unnaturally fed huge amounts of vitamin D, which would tend to produce calcium deposits on arterial walls. In addition, there were later criticisms that the results were due not to the cholesterol itself, but to the fact that it was "oxidized," and so contained free radicals injurious to the arterial lining.

the goalposts were moved further — to 200. This includes a big percentage of the American population. For most people, total cholesterol goes up with age, so more and more people in our generation are entering the NCEP "warning zone."

During the past twenty years or so, the cholesterol theory has generated a huge market — in the billions — for drug companies, which now proffer drugs that lower cholesterol but whose benefit is questionable, except for people with very serious cholesterol problems, or those with pre-existing heart disease. For the general populace, it's unclear whether there's any benefit.

It has also generated a multi-billion dollar business for the food industry, which can advertise and sell "light" or "low-fat" or "fat-free" or "low-cholesterol" foods. This is an extremely effective marketing tool. It also encourages a lot of so-called preventive doctor's visits. Now, there's nothing wrong with preventive doctor's visits, but when you fixate on cholesterol as the end-all and be-all of prevention, you miss a lot. As Thomas Moore points out in his book *Heart Failure*, there's a great deal of economic impetus behind this cholesterol theory, and there's a vested interest in it: a whole medical-industrial-scientific complex that feeds on it. The focus on cholesterol may be masking some of the more serious risk factors in our diet, including large amounts of dietary sugar, refined flour, margarine, processed or heated vegetable oils, and food additives.

Here's the fuzzy logic behind the cholesterol hypothesis:

1. A high level of cholesterol in the bloodstream is associated with increased risk for heart disease.
2. Heart disease is America's major killer.
3. *Therefore*, if we reduce the level of cholesterol in our blood, everyone will live longer.

Here's how the hypothesis gets extended to diet and medications:

1. Foods high in saturated fats and cholesterol raise the level of cholesterol in the blood.
2. *Therefore*, if we eliminate saturated fats and cholesterol in our diets, heart disease will be eradicated.
3. *Or*, if changing our diets doesn't work, we should use drugs to reduce the amount of cholesterol in the blood, and *then* heart disease will be eradicated.

It's a compelling idea, especially for our generation. We want to take control of our lives and our health, and the notion that we can pinpoint something as simple and clear-cut as the level of a fat in the bloodstream is very attractive. We get our cholesterol level tested, just as we'd go to pick up a report card or get the results of an efficiency rating for our business. But the hypothesis is only that — a hypothesis — and it's too easy to base logical leaps and assumptions on it that just don't hold up.

In reality, there are so many factors that affect risk for heart disease, including genetic, environmental, and physiological factors, that it's nearly impossible to isolate one factor like cholesterol and precisely measure its effect. Other logical leaps are involved. For example, people with extremely low cholesterol may actually have a higher death rate from other causes besides heart disease. It's questionable whether medications to reduce cholesterol will be safe over the long term and whether their use will actually reduce the overall death rate. Actually, cholesterol is one of the most important compounds in the body. We couldn't live without it.

Cholesterol is a yellowish, waxy fat-soluble substance found in animal tissues, meats, dairy products, egg yolks, and some oils. There is cholesterol in every cell in the body, because it makes up an important part of the structure of cell walls. Cell membranes need to be made of materials, like fats and some proteins, that aren't water-soluble and don't have to be replaced all the time. There is a lot of cholesterol in brain tissue, where it "insulates" nerve cell membranes. Much cholesterol winds up in the skin, along with other fat-solubles, which make the skin waterproof and prevents excess evaporation of water from the body. A small quantity is used by the adrenal glands, the ovaries, and testes to form important sex hormones. Cholesterol is a precursor to cortisol, which the body produces in response to stress. It even mediates brain levels of the neurotransmitter serotonin, which is essential to normal brain function.[2] The biggest use of cholesterol in the body — perhaps 80 per cent — is in manufacturing bile, the liquid in the intestine that breaks down foods into usable components.

In short, cholesterol is really indispensable — we couldn't live without it. It's so important that the liver is set up to manufacture cholesterol out of simpler fatty acid components and turn it into bile. In fact, most of the cholesterol in the bloodstream is produced right in the body. Only a small portion comes from our diet.

Cholesterol is constantly being synthesized, broken down, and recycled in the body. Most of it is converted into bile acids, reabsorbed by the body, and recycled over and over again as bile. However, cholesterol is only one of the important lipids in the body and is not the only factor associated with heart disease. There are two other important lipids in the body: triglycerides, which provide energy to cells, and phospholipids, which are used in the structure of cell walls and in the insulating sheath that surrounds nerve fibers. All these lipids are made up of basic building blocks called fatty acids. The three major fats combine with proteins to make up particles called lipoproteins, which circulate through the bloodstream and transport the lipids to where they are needed in the body. Ninety-five percent of all the lipids in the blood exist in the form of lipoproteins.

Two major kinds of lipoproteins are associated with heart disease or health: high-density lipoprotein (HDL) and low-density lipoprotein (LDL). LDL has a very high concentration of cholesterol, which is of lower density than protein. We call it the "bad" cholesterol because it contributes to the formation of fatty deposits on the walls of blood vessels. HDL contains a high concentration of protein, about 50 percent, and relatively less cholesterol and phospholipids. We call HDL the "good" cholesterol because it may actually help keep arteries clear by scavenging fats from artery walls. In fact, the presence of HDL in the blood stream may be as important to cardiovascular health as the total level of cholesterol, or more important. A cholesterol count by itself is relatively meaningless if you don't know how much HDL is present in the blood.

How do cholesterol and the other fats affect our health? Well, there *is* a pretty clear statistical association between higher levels of cholesterol in the blood and increased risk of heart disease. (The association is less clear in women, and it's reversed in people over seventy-five, who sometimes show more heart disease with *lower* cholesterol.) The generally quoted figure comes from the 1984 findings of the ten-year Lipid Research Clinics Coronary Primary Prevention Trial, which found that for persons with high cholesterol, a 1 percent drop in cholesterol level was associated with a 2 percent reduced risk for death of heart disease.

However, there are several complicating factors. Let's look at some of them.

Conflicting Studies

When you look at the actual research studies that support the cholesterol hypothesis, a very interesting picture develops. Most new studies cite only the earlier studies that have supported the hypothesis and ignore others that did not support a close connection between high cholesterol levels and heart disease. Recently, a Swedish researcher named Uffe Ravnskov did an analysis of all the cholesterol studies over the past thirty years and found as many studies that did not support the cholesterol hypothesis as did support it.[3] Even in studies that showed some connection between *average* group cholesterol levels and death rates, people with low, high, and normal cholesterol levels were dying of heart disease.

Ravnskov also looked at studies that examined the effects of lowering cholesterol. He again found nearly as many nonsupportive studies as supportive ones. The longer trials (over five years) showed a significant number of people dying or developing heart disease soon after cholesterol-lowering treatment was started, perhaps because of serious side effects of cholesterol-lowering drugs. In fact, in two cases, researchers who tested cholesterol lowering as a prevention measure stopped their trials and didn't publish the full results because of side effects. The main side effect? Coronary heart disease.[4] Other studies have even suggested a possible carcinogenic effect of long-term use of cholesterol-lowering drugs.[5] Overall, the analysis showed that lowering "high" cholesterol made no difference in the rates of total deaths and deaths from heart disease. The study concluded: "the preventive effect of [cholesterol-lowering] treatment has been exaggerated by a tendency in trial reports, reviews and other papers to cite supportive trials only. . . . The impression of success presented to doctors is false because the numbers of controlled cholesterol-lowering trials in which total mortality and coronary mortality were reduced equal the numbers in which they were increased."[6]

Does this mean there is no connection between cholesterol and heart disease? No. It does mean that we should consider other factors just as seriously as we do cholesterol. We shouldn't rely exclusively on cholesterol-lowering treatments to prevent heart disease, and we should be especially cautious about using drugs to lower cholesterol. The candidates for such medications should probably be limited to persons who are known to have coronary heart disease and high risk factors.

Cholesterol, Aging, and Mortality

Some recent studies have shown that there is indeed a strong statistical correlation between cholesterol level and the occurrence of heart attacks. At the same time, there is such a wide range of cholesterol levels among people who have heart attacks that we can't use the cholesterol count to predict the risk for a specific individual. One study based on a group of doctors in the Boston/Cambridge area found that most heart attacks occurred in those with cholesterol levels below 200, including some with levels well under 150![7]

Also, the relationship between cholesterol levels and heart disease may change with age. One study found a positive correlation between high cholesterol levels and death of heart disease at the ages of forty, fifty, and sixty, but the correlation declined with age. At age seventy the correlation was statistically insignificant, and at age eighty there was a slight negative correlation! For those fifty and over, a higher cholesterol count was associated with *lower* death rate of causes other than heart disease.[8] The implication? We should probably be careful about recommending aggressive programs to lower cholesterol in men and women older than sixty-five or seventy. This study points to another issue: most of the studies of heart disease have used middle-aged men as subjects, and the national recommendations are based on this population. Fewer studies have been done of heart disease in women and older people, and we know less about how the disease progresses in these groups.[9]

Does Lowering Cholesterol Help?

The studies just mentioned point to questions about the third part of the cholesterol hypothesis: "If we reduce the level of cholesterol in our blood, everyone will live longer." There *is* clear evidence that reducing blood levels of cholesterol, even by itself, just by using lipid-lowering drugs, tends to reverse heart disease and reduce the extent of plaque in the arteries. This is part of the basis for Dr. Ornish's low-fat vegetarian diet, and the idea is that it will reduce mortality. However, one study of mortality rates found that the net result of lowering cholesterol would be to add just a few days to a few months to life expectancy, up to a maximum of twelve months in some high-risk cases.[10] Cost-effectiveness studies suggest that a lifelong course of taking expensive cholesterol-lowering drugs would place the price for an extra year of life for some individuals at several million dollars. While cholesterol-lowering medication costs the average individual less than $1,000/year, the use of these medications for prevention in low-risk populations means that hundreds of individuals use the drug with no impact on life span to achieve modest longevity increments in a small handful.

I think this puts into perspective some of the anxiety and Herculean efforts people go through to reduce their cholesterol levels. (Of course, these are statistical averages, and it's impossible to predict the effects of lowering cholesterol on an individual.) It's up to you to decide what those extra days or months of life would be worth. It *is* true that there is more to preventing heart disease than just extending life. We are all concerned with the quality of life as well, and life is certainly more rewarding and pleasant without the difficulties and restrictions that come with heart disease, even nonfatal heart disease.

As mentioned earlier, the National Cholesterol Education Program has recommended that everyone over the age of twenty have cholesterol levels tested and start a reduction program if the total cholesterol count is higher than 200. Still, there are many respected people in the medical profession who believe that the NCEP has gone overboard with its recommendations. Dr. Eliot Corday, past president of the American College of Cardiology and a member of the advisory council to the National Heart, Lung and Blood Institute, was one of those who argued against the recommendations for mass cholesterol screening of the adult population. He looked at the clinical trials of hundreds of thousands of people and came to the conclusion that there is no difference in mortality between people who are on a cholesterol-lowering regimen and those who are not. He comments, "We don't know what to do, but we spend billions of dollars. . . . They had no right to go out frightening the hell out of the whole world [about cholesterol] without having the facts . . ."[11]

Dangers of Low Cholesterol Levels

Here's an even stranger twist to the cholesterol story: low cholesterol doesn't necessarily mean you're in good shape. Recent studies have shown that while death of cardiac failure may be higher, on the average, among people with higher cholesterol levels, the rate of death of other causes actually increases among people with very low levels of cholesterol. The 6 percent of middle-aged adults with cholesterol counts below 160 have a higher risk of dying of a variety of causes, including lung cancer, liver cancer, respiratory disease, cerebral hemorrhage, alcoholism, suicide, and accidents.[12]

I'm not surprised, since I often see patients who have chronically weak constitutions, are susceptible to infections, and are generally devitalized. These people often have cholesterol levels as low as 120. I see patients with AIDS who have astonishingly low cholesterol levels of 80 or 90. Such low levels may indirectly predispose them to cerebral hemorrhage and chronic lung disease,[13] and they may be a marker for other problems. Since cholesterol is a precursor ingredient for the hormone cortisone, which is produced in response to stress and is needed for repairing damaged tissue, it's normal for cholesterol to rise in response to stress. It may be that lowering cholesterol levels with diet or medication does not address the imbalances that caused the cholesterol to rise in the first place, and may interfere with a natural adaptive response to stress or tissue damage.

There's another interesting way in which very low cholesterol levels may cause some of the high mortality rates we see in the form of alcoholism, accidents, and suicide. The fact is that cholesterol is an essential component of the brain. It's well known that the food with the highest cholesterol level is ... brains! Some researchers have proposed that cholesterol may have something to do with brain metabolism and that very low blood levels may have a neurochemical association with depression, violent death, and suicide. The idea is that lowering cholesterol below a certain threshold may actually change consciousness in some way.

HDL levels

The total level of cholesterol in the blood doesn't provide the whole picture of risk for heart disease. We also have to look at the proportions of HDL, the "good cholesterol," and LDL, the "bad cholesterol." HDL may prevent the deposit of cholesterol on arterial walls, or even remove cholesterol from arterial plaque. Dr. William Castelli, director of the Framingham Heart Study, has noted that just as many men and women who have a total cholesterol count under 200 have heart attacks as those with a total count over 300. He suggests that we should be much more concerned about low levels of HDL, and offers the ratio of total cholesterol to HDL cholesterol as the single best predictor of a future heart attack—much better than total cholesterol level. The Framingham studies show that people with total cholesterol of 250, considered in the danger zone, but with HDL of 75—a 3.3 to 1 ratio—actually have half the usual rate of heart disease.[14] Responding to such studies, the National Institutes of Health have increased the emphasis on measuring HDL levels in assessing risk. At this point, it seems that a total-cholesterol-to-HDL ratio higher than 4.5 to 1 puts you in the high-risk category.[15]

Two patients of mine offered an amazing demonstration of this principle. Bill was a police officer who had prided himself that he'd never had a total cholesterol count above 180. He thought he was in fairly good health, though he was stressed from work, as any New York City cop would have to be. He came to see me after he had his first heart attack at the age of thirty-eight. His records showed that while his total cholesterol had always been fairly low, his HDL had never been above 30: a 6 to 1 ratio, well into the high-risk group.

On the other hand, I've been monitoring another patient for some time now who is terribly concerned about her cholesterol level. Corinne is seventy-nine years old and a passionate folk dancer. She's out in Central Park every weekend with the folk-dancing group, and she dances the pants off all the younger people who are trying to learn the steps.

Despite her apparent good health, Corinne keeps coming to me because of her high cholesterol. Every year I see her, it gets a little higher. It started out at 260, but at that time her HDL was a hefty 85, so I said, "Don't worry about it." The last time I saw her she had reached a milestone: her cholesterol was 304, and her HDL was 110! I had never seen such a high HDL, but she doesn't have a trace of cardiovascular disease. My assessment is that at seventy-nine, she has passed through the window of vulnerability that afflicts people in their sixties and seventies with premature heart disease, and that her high HDL levels have protected her. Now she's at the age where high cholesterol does not really correlate with heart disease. So I tell her, "Don't start any programs to lower your cholesterol, and don't even consider taking medication for it. Just keep dancing, and don't try to change your diet. Whatever it is, it seems to be doing fine by you! Above all, don't start starving yourself!"

However, not all people with low HDL suffer from premature heart disease. HDL is actually a collection of particles of fats and proteins of different size and composition, and it may be that some of these subgroups have the significant effect. The latest research shows some interesting results that will probably be incorporated into a new and more sophisticated view of blood lipids over the next decade or so.

Eggs, Butter, and Cream: A Witches' Brew?

One spin-off from the cholesterol hypothesis goes like this: "If you reduce or completely cut cholesterol from your diet, you will reduce the amount of cholesterol buildup in arterial plaque." This has fueled the big push in marketing low-cholesterol and no-cholesterol foods. It's scared people away from high-cholesterol foods like eggs and butter, and created a market for margarine and egg substitutes. Now the theory would probably apply if you were to start eating great heaps of cholesterol and overdosing on vitamin D, or if you were — like Arnitchkow's subjects — a rabbit. The surprising fact is that in most humans, dietary cholesterol actually has a relatively minimal effect on the amount of cholesterol in the blood.

In fact, changes in dietary cholesterol usually shift blood cholesterol by no more than a few percentage points at the most. The rise is often accompanied by a corresponding rise in good HDL cholesterol. This is not surprising, since most of the cholesterol in the body is actually produced in the liver, and a feedback mechanism regulates production like a thermostat. Evidently, the amounts and proportions of other types of fats and oils in the body have a greater effect on blood cholesterol levels than the amount of pure cholesterol consumed. Moreover, people vary greatly in how they respond to dietary cholesterol. Some people are able to clear dietary cholesterol from the blood very quickly.

Probably the biggest bugaboos in the cholesterol scare are butter and eggs. A *New Yorker* magazine cover for Halloween week showed a witch cooking up an evil concoction of butter, eggs, and heavy cream. Butter and eggs have such a reputation that some researchers studied their effect on normal individuals without pre-existing high cholesterol or heart disease. The surprising results? Zero change in blood cholesterol level, whether the subjects were eating eggs or not, and no significant change in blood cholesterol in most normal individuals, whether the subjects were eating butter or low-cholesterol margarine. Most of the initial studies on eggs and blood cholesterol either had involved people with a very high intake of dietary fat, or were too short-term to reveal the long-term effects.[16] The conclusion? The dangers of eating eggs and butter have been highly overrated. You would have trouble committing suicide just by eating eggs and butter every day.

Triglyceride levels

If cholesterol by itself isn't the culprit, what about those other fats in the blood — the triglycerides? As you might expect, triglycerides are in the blood for a reason. They are the primary source of fat metabolism: the use of fats for energy. The triglycerides are also transported into the tissues for storage and transported back out for energy. As with cholesterol, it's too simple to say that high levels of triglycerides in the blood are bad and low levels are good. Triglycerides are a building block of very low-density lipoprotein, or VLDL, one of the "bad cholesterols," so that's one reason high levels can be a problem. But there may be "good triglycerides" and "bad triglycerides" as well. Triglycerides themselves can be made up of different kinds of fats, heavy saturated or lighter unsaturated, which have different associations with heart disease. Dean Ornish, the guru of reversing heart disease through diet, calls some of them the "fluffy triglycerides" — the less dense ones made up of unsaturated fats. These predominate with people who eat a low-fat, vegetarian diet, and Ornish claims they are much more benign than other types. The role of triglycerides in heart disease remains controversial, but high levels may be a marker for other problems that do lead to clogged arteries, such as insulin resistance, or Syndrome X.

Cholesterol Levels: How to Read Your Score Card

How often should you be tested for cholesterol and triglycerides? This is a hard one to answer. See your physician and have a cholesterol test if you haven't had one in three to five years. If the result is normal, don't buy into the hype of the annual blood test (though many HMOs are giving these with every annual checkup, whether you ask for it or not). If it's not normal, you'll need more frequent testing, but there is no strict indicator for how frequently you should be tested. This is something to be determined by evaluation of your specific, unique condition, and your doctor should provide you with a plausible rationale for any tests done. Don't assume that a yearly check up is mandatory.

Once you've had a blood test, ask for a copy of the printout listing all the results so you'll have an objective snapshot of your condition at one point in time. Save it even if your doctor says, "Your cholesterol's fine, nothing to worry about." Put it in a file, keep it as part of your own permanent health records, and keep track of any sudden or gradual changes over the years. If for some reason you need to change doctors, you won't lose track of the information.

What do all those figures mean? A typical blood test printout may have one or two pages of incomprehensible abbreviations or biological terms. Well, you already know a few things to look for, like total cholesterol levels, HDL and LDL levels, and triglyceride levels. I'll give you some rules of thumb about how to evaluate them. First, a caveat: the test results may not be all they seem to be. The figures are all down there in black and white, very specific numbers printed out from a computer, and it all looks very scientific and dependable. Nevertheless, they may not represent the most accurate picture of your blood levels. It's smart to look at any individual set of test results with a certain degree of skepticism, because there are too many variables that may significantly affect the scores of a given blood test.

For one, there is an inherent and accepted error rate for any laboratory results. Studies have shown that lab errors can be as high as 15 to 20 percent. Test results can also vary with recent eating patterns — even recent meals — and with recent exercise patterns, weight, illness, or medications. Studies have shown that individual variability can go as high as 25 to 40 percent — and that's on top of lab error rates. With just a 15 percent total variance, for example, your test results could range from 170 to 230 on two succeeding days. If you saw this shift between two yearly checkups, you might think, "Hey, something scary is happening." Still, it could mean nothing. If you see a level that indicates a drastic change, or your doctor recommends drastic treatment, it's good to get a second test to confirm the results.

The other blood levels can also vary widely from test to test. Triglyceride levels can vary by 20 to 100 percent. They are especially responsive to what you had for dinner the night before and your diet over the previous week. (These blood tests are always scheduled in the morning, after an overnight fast.) HDL readings commonly vary by 10 percent, LDL readings by 8 percent. If there's any significant change, get a followup test.[17]

Given that the tests aren't perfect, what kinds of numbers should you look for? The National Cholesterol Education Project suggests that a desirable total cholesterol level should lie below 200. They call the range from 200 to 239 "borderline high" or "moderate-risk," and above 240 is considered a high-risk level. The desirable LDL should fall below 130, the moderate-risk category is 130 to 159, and the high-risk category is 160 or above. As we've seen, though, any test result that moves you from one risk category to another should be followed up with a confirming test.

So, forget about the absolute numbers of cholesterol and LDL unless a number is so high that you need a confirming test. Instead, look at the ratios, especially the ratio of total cholesterol to HDL. If this ratio is 4.5:1 or greater, you should be concerned, and take some action to improve it. You can do this by either raising your HDL or lowering your cholesterol or both, and we'll talk later about how to do this. Optimally the ratio should be 3:1 or less. With a ratio of 4.5:1 to 6:1 you would be at moderate or intermediate risk, and anything higher is quite serious. Even moderate risk can threaten your life and health.

Besides cholesterol, look at your triglyceride level. This can vary a lot, but if it's over 120 you should think about changing the amount of carbohydrates in your diet. A high-carbohydrate diet can overload the body with glucose and push up the triglyceride level. I test for a protein called fibrinogen, which affects blood clotting, and sometimes for homocysteine, a protein that is a marker for risk of heart disease. (More on these later.) I like to work up a pretty complete cardiovascular profile for my patients so they can get more feedback on their situation.

The point is this: don't use cholesterol levels as a report card on your overall health and longevity. It's not like you're reading the lifeline in your palm. Cholesterol is simply one among several factors in a dynamic metabolic balance. Keep it in perspective.

At the same time, you can use cholesterol as one important clue to your cardiovascular health. If your level really is too high, you can bring it down, and bring down your risk of heart disease. We'll talk about this, but first let's look at the other fats in your diet.

Risk Factors: Fats in Your Food

After cholesterol, probably the biggest factor in most people's minds when they think of heart disease is dietary fat. In fact, this is one of the steps in the cholesterol hypothesis: To reduce risk of heart disease, don't consume cholesterol-rich foods, *and don't consume foods rich in other fats that lead to cholesterol buildup*. This has spawned a profusion of new low-fat food products with complicated labels that list strange-sounding ingredients. We're now reading the fine print on the labels, trying to figure out the percentages and amounts of fats: the unsaturated, the polyunsaturated, the monounsaturated, the partially hydrogenated. Is coconut oil supposed to be good or bad? What about corn oil, safflower oil, peanut oil, olive oil? What about these beneficial omega-3 oils we've been hearing about—what kind of food has omega-3? Is it necessary to give up red meat completely? What kind of fat are the French fries cooked in? Is chicken without the skin OK? If you eat only foods with polyunsaturated fats, can you eat as much as you like? Or should you try to cut out as much fat as possible from your diet, even the "safe" types? It's enough to spoil your appetite.

The conventional wisdom for some time now has been to avoid saturated fats, which are mostly found in meat and animal products, and to replace them with polyunsaturated fats, which include many vegetable oils like corn oil and safflower oil. This is because saturated fats raise cholesterol levels in the blood, while polyunsaturated fats, which are more metabolically active, do not. A diet that contains a high level of saturated fats can increase blood cholesterol up to 125 to 250 percent. If you want to lower your cholesterol level, it's much more important to reduce the amount of saturated fats in your diet than to worry about cholesterol in mayonnaise and eggs.

On the other hand, a diet rich in unsaturated fats will usually lower the blood cholesterol level by a slight to moderate amount. Though we don't know exactly why unsaturated fats have this effect, it's reason enough to prefer them to saturated fats. However, as with cholesterol, the picture is not quite this simple. Some saturated fats, such as stearic acid, do not generally raise cholesterol significantly. While polyunsaturated fats do tend to decrease cholesterol levels in the blood, they also decrease the level of the beneficial HDL.

The latest research in this area points to the benefits of the Mediterranean diet. It has long been noted that residents of Mediterranean countries like Greece and Italy have much lower rates of heart disease than those in northern Europe and the United States, even though the typical diet in these countries contains a large amount of fats and oils, especially olive oil. Olive oil contains high levels of monounsaturated fats, which were long thought to be less effective than the polyunsaturates in lowering cholesterol. However, recent research has revived interest in the monounsaturates, because monounsaturates like olive oil are just as effective in their cholesterol-lowering effect as the polyunsaturates. What's more, they do so without lowering levels of the beneficial HDL.[18]

What does all this mean, as you browse through the aisles of your supermarket, reading the labels? Well, the fact is that most fats and oils contain a mixture of the different types of fatty acids. The label on a bottle of peanut oil, for example, might tell you it has 14 grams of fat, composed of 5 grams of polyunsaturates, 7 grams of monounsaturates, and 2 grams of saturated fats. Since the saturated fats are so low, that makes it a pretty good buy. However, there is more to the fat picture than this. We need to look at two other factors — oxidation and hydrogenation — before we can lay out a complete prevention plan. And we still haven't considered *how much* fat you can safely incorporate into your diet.

Oxidized fats and cholesterol

If much of the risk of high fat or cholesterol in your diet has been overstated, there still is one way in which it can become especially dangerous. If you cook fats at a high heat, or overcook them, or use fats that have been exposed to air or left on the shelf for long periods of time, you are using oxidized fats. Fats combine very easily with oxygen in the air to form peroxides — compounds with extra oxygen. The long molecular chains of the fat peroxides then begin to break down into smaller, oxidized components, which easily generate free radicals. These are especially dangerous, because they are chemically active and combine easily with our own cells and body tissues, including the smooth lining of blood vessels. Once the vascular walls are damaged, they become susceptible to the fatty deposits that lead to clogged arteries.

Even if you have sworn off barbecued steak and deep-fried foods, you're not off the hook, because the light polyunsaturated cooking and salad oils oxidize very easily. Fat peroxides are common in highly processed foods and in foods that are heated, air-dried (like beef jerky), irradiated, and processed, like cheeses and evaporated milk. Fish oils are highly vulnerable because they are highly unsaturated. When ingested, the fat peroxides create free radicals. The consumption of oxidized cholesterol and oxidized fats has been linked very strongly with heart disease, and there is evidence that the oxidation byproducts — the free radicals — can increase the risk of cancer. The level of fat peroxides increases in the blood with age, whether because they are naturally produced in the body or because they are cleared from the bloodstream less efficiently. This increases the risk of heart disease during the middle years, but prevention measures can reduce this risk.[19]

The free radicals are so lethal that the body has evolved a system of defense against them: a collection of natural defenders called antioxidants. The body manufactures some of its own antioxidants, such as the enzyme superoxide dismutase, and absorbs others from food. As we've noted in previous chapters, many vitamins are natural antioxidants, including vitamin E, vitamin C, zinc, selenium, and the carotenoids. You can avoid much of the risk from free radicals by careful cooking habits and careful handling of oils, and by taking vitamin supplements. While most studies show clear benefits from taking various antioxidant supplements, one or two studies have seemed to cast doubt on this practice. However, there have been complicating factors in these studies, and the results are not all they appear to be. See chapter 16 for a closer look at this controversy.

INTELLIGENT MEDICINE TIP:

To avoid the dangers of oxidized fats, keep opened bottles of cooking oils tightly capped in a cool place or even in the refrigerator. Replace them if they smell rancid or you haven't used them up after several months. If you're going to fry or deep-fry, pick an cooking oil that's resistant to oxidation, such as peanut oil, and not one that's easily oxidized. Look at the chart in chapter 16 for a guide to which oils are better for frying.

Invented Foods: The Trans Fats

The history of margarine actually dates back over a century. Napoleon III, seeking a cheap source of nutritional fat to feed his armies, the peasantry, and the poor, announced a contest in 1867, inviting inventors to devise recipes. The winning concoction, a mixture of beef fat and skim milk, tasted so awful that it never caught on. ("Let them eat margarine," Napoleon III was reputed to have said, echoing Marie Antoinette.)

The advent of new industrial processes in the early twentieth century overcame a major obstacle to synthesis of more palatable butter substitutes.

Cheaper plant oils could now be rendered spreadable like saturated fats by a high-temperature process called hydrogenation, in which saturated bonds could be artificially created. The resultant trans-saturated hydrogenated margarines lagged in acceptance until given an impetus by global food shortages during World War II. Sales were jazzed up further in the postwar era when marketeers appropriated a health rationale for substitution of margarine for butter. Trans fats are used in many commercial baked products, including white bread, cookies, and cakes. Because of public concern about animal fat, the fast food industry has relinquished its practice of deep-frying burgers in beef tallow and substituted fast-oxidizing partially hydrogenated vegetable oils — a net loss for the heart-conscious public.

Trans fats are found in animal fat and dairy products in small amounts, but in different forms from the ones manufactured by the food industry. Even the natural forms have not formed a significant percentage of any diet that humans have eaten during thousands of years of evolution. There have been no long-term studies of the effects of artificially created trans fats on human health, but I think the conservative approach should make us wary of them. We just don't know enough about the effect of incorporating these artificial materials into the body, where they may become part of cell walls and affect delicate metabolic pathways.

Moreover, there is some evidence that trans fats can lower the level of HDL, the "good cholesterol," and raise LDL, the "bad cholesterol," in the bloodstream and thus increase the risk of heart disease. This meshes with studies that show an increased risk of heart disease among women who have eaten margarine exclusively for ten years or more. If you look closely at labels on margarines, cooking oils, and baked goods, you may see ingredients like "partially hydrogenated soy oil." Steer clear. Whatever benefits may be derived from using vegetable oil instead of animal fats are likely to be canceled out by the downside of trans fats.[20]

How Much Fat is Safe?

Fried chicken, sautéed broccoli, bran muffins, cakes and cookies, bread and butter, filet of sole, macaroni and cheese, fatty chicken soup, grilled cheese sandwiches, french fries, hamburgers, fetuccine alfredo, avocado salad, and salad dressing, to say nothing of cheesecake and strawberries with whipped cream — it's not surprising that Americans get nearly 40 percent of the calories in their diet from fats and oils, on the average. Too many foods in the "normal" American diet derive much of their flavor or character from fats and oils.

How much fat is really safe in our diet? Well, the official word from the National Cholesterol Education Program tells us that we should reduce our total fat intake to 30 percent or less of total calories and, further, that we should reduce our consumption of saturated fats to 10 percent or less of our total calorie intake, polyunsaturated fats to about 10 percent, and monounsaturated fats to 10 to 15 percent of total calories.[21] Dean Ornish prescribes a diet that derives no more than 10 percent total of all calories derived from fat, and exclusively polyunsaturated fat, for his heart disease reversal program. This is close to the percentage recommended in the now disfavored low-fat and low-protein Pritikin diet of a few years ago. There's no question that Dr. Ornish has been getting results with his program. What's not known is whether this is really a good plan for long-term health maintenance and disease prevention. Also, the diet may not be palatable enough to become practical for the vast segments of the American population at risk.

My recommendation? Try shifting your eating habits in the direction of the Mediterranean diet, which probably comes close to the 30 percent figure recommended by the NCEP but derives most of its fat calories from monounsaturated olive oil and relatively little from saturated fats. Avoid the saturated fats when possible, but also steer clear of the artificially doctored trans fats — the partially hydrogenated oils that crop up in processed foods and margarine. Avoid the oxidized fats as much as possible — the overcooked and smoky fried foods — since they may do more damage than cholesterol itself, no matter what kind of fat you're frying with. This is a good, basic game plan. Beyond this, current research is turning up a surprising fact. Some fats are actually good for you!

OLIVE OIL — A 5000 YEAR OLD WINNER

The Greek island of Crete has the highest olive oil consumption in the world and also the lowest mortality from cardiovascular disease. It's consumed in large quantities in other Mediterranean countries, which show a similar low level of cardiovascular disease. The benefits of olive oil may derive from its effect in reducing levels of harmful LDL cholesterol while not affecting the beneficial HDL.

Olive oil has been a staple in Mediterranean countries for five thousand years and has a pretty good track record. In contrast, we've studied polyunsaturated fats for only about fifty years and have no real data on the long-term, lifetime effects of a diet that emphasizes polyunsaturates. If you use more olive oil in your cooking, try to get the least-processed (and tastiest) variety: cold-pressed, virgin oil, which has been processed without heating or chemical additives. Remember, olive oil can suffer from oxidation like many other oils, so keep it in air-tight containers in a cool place, and use it for salads, cold dishes, and gentle sautéing, not high-heat frying.

Fish Oils and GLA Oils: The Alpha and Omega of a Heart-Healthy Diet

While most researchers were jumping on the cholesterol bandwagon, a few were taking a closer look at some of the diets of indigenous peoples that seemed to contradict the cholesterol hypothesis. In the 1970s, H. O. Bang and John Dyerberg were studying the diet of Eskimos in Greenland. The bulk of the calories in their diet came from marine life: seals, whales, walrus, and fatty cold-water fish like herring, mackerel, and salmon — all foods rich in cholesterol and fat. In fact, the Greenland Eskimos derived over 70 percent of their calories from fat! Yet, they had a very low incidence of heart disease, diabetes, and cancer. Of course, they got lots of exercise, and there was little or no sugar in their diet, but their diet contained nearly twice the fat content of the average American diet![22]

It turns out that most of the marine fish and mammals they ate are extremely rich in two kinds of oils called omega-3 fatty acids (eicosapentaenoic acid, or EPA, and docosahexaenoic acid, or DHA). These omega-3 oils, which are also found in wild game, like buffalo, have several beneficial effects on the body, including protection of the cardiovascular system.

Parallel research in the 1980s explored the protective effect of linoleic and linolenic acids, also called the essential fatty acids, which are found in various unrefined plant sources including flaxseed and the evening primrose. GLA, from certain omega-6 oils, has been found to contribute to an astounding array of beneficial effects, including diabetes protection, immune health, and alcohol rehabilitation.

Both omega-3 and omega-6 oils help form hormonelike compounds called prostaglandins, which are involved in the management of all cellular metabolic functions, including cardiovascular metabolism and blood clotting, and activities of the reproductive system, the immune system, and the central nervous system. Specifically, the fish oils and GLA work against heart disease by thinning blood, reducing the clumping of platelets, and lessening the constriction of blood vessels. They can be used as part of a therapeutic nutrition-based approach to reversing heart disease. In fact, the omega-3 oils and omega-6 oils are so essential to life that one could speak of a fat deficiency when they are too scarce in the diet, even in an obese person. Remember Grandma and her cod-liver oil? She knew better than we thought.

How should this affect your thinking about dietary fat? It would be a mistake to avoid all kinds of fatty foods indiscriminately. Nuts, for example, which are often cited as a high-fat food to be avoided, may not be as dangerous as was previously thought. In a group of vegetarian Seventh Day Adventists, the lowest rate of heart disease was associated with the highest rate of consumption of mixed nuts. The biggest nut-eaters were also the least obese![23] At the same time, some fats, like those in fish and marine life, and the fatty acids in olive oil, actually promote cardiovascular health. This is the basis for my Salad and Salmon Diet—a diet rich in fresh fish, greens, nuts, and vegetables, with olive oil or canola oil as the primary cooking oils (see chapter 16 for more details).

The Fiber Factor and Vegetable Proteins: Adjusting the Fat Balance

Most of us are aware of the different varieties of fats and oils in our diet. But did you know that the amount of fiber in our food can affect the balance of fats in the blood? Eating sufficient fiber not only is good for the digestive tract but can actually inhibit atherosclerosis. Oat bran and other water-soluble fibers, which include gums, mucilages, and pectin found in legumes, seeds, and some fruits and cereals, are able to selectively reduce the "bad" LDL cholesterol while not affecting the "good" HDL levels. Wheat bran and other water-insoluble fibers do not have this effect, though they do aid intestinal function. It's theorized that the water-soluble fibers may help build up that fatty acids that inhibit cholesterol production by the liver. They may also increase the excretion of bile from the intestine, preventing the recycling of cholesterol components back into the body. In one study, men with a high cholesterol level (over 250) ate 100 grams or more a day of fiber in the form of hot oatmeal cereal, muffins, or beans and showed a significant reduction in both total cholesterol level and in LDL levels. This quantity of fiber is far above the current health guidelines of only 20 to 35 grams a day.[24]

Another source of beneficial fiber can be found in a natural, gel-forming soluble fiber produced from husks of psyllium seeds and known as psyllium hydrophilic mucilloid. Some popular brands include Metamucil and Fiberall. This product is commonly used for help with bowel dysfunctions, but it has cholesterol-lowering properties similar to those of other types of fiber.[25]

Other studies have shown that vegetable protein, in particular soy protein, can also reduce the levels of total cholesterol and LDL. For some reason vegetable protein, and not animal protein, has this inhibitory effect.[26]

I don't like to give specific recommendations like "Do your duty and eat exactly one cup of bran for breakfast every morning" or to suggest that you should start counting the grams of fiber in your diet. That seems like a dismal exercise. I do recommend being conscious about whether you do eat significant sources of fiber. If not, think creatively about how you might add some in an easy or pleasurable way.

_____

If you add bran to your diet, look for oat bran and oat bran products rather than regular coarse wheat bran. If bran just isn't your thing, try supplementing your meals with a teaspoon of raw psyllium or flax seed. Replace some of the animal protein in your diet with protein from beans or soybeans. A good source of soybean protein is Japanese tofu or Chinese bean curd.

Other Blood Factors: Proteins, Nutrients, and Pollutants

The general hullabaloo about cholesterol and fats in the blood has tended to overshadow the effects of some other blood factors that may play an equally significant role in engendering heart disease. They include vitamin and other nutrient deficiencies, environmental pollutants that enter the bloodstream, and little-known factors like specialized types of proteins.

Fibrinogen

When preparing a cardiovascular profile, I like to test for fibrinogen, a protein that assists blood clotting. Fibrinogen generates little networks of fibers that link blood platelets to produce blood clots, making the blood "sticky." While this is beneficial if you've cut your finger, it's not so good if you already have buildup of plaque tissue in ever-narrowing arteries. Under these circumstances, fibrinogen can increase the risk of strokes. In fact, a high level of fibrinogen has been shown to be almost as powerful a risk factor as cholesterol. (This is why people who have had strokes are often given blood thinners.) Fibrinogen levels change with the season. Your blood is actually thicker in cold weather, which may cause an increased risk of strokes or heart attacks in winter. A high fibrinogen level can be brought down by exercise and by eating a diet that contains omega-3 oils, such as fish oil, which have a blood-thinning effect. Eating garlic, too, helps reverse excessive clotting tendencies.

Homocysteine

Homocysteine is an amino acid, a natural product of the synthesis and breakdown of proteins. It's normally processed by the body, but there's a rare and often fatal genetic disorder in which the body fails completely to process homocysteine. However, one person in ten has a milder form of genetic inheritance that prevents effective processing. When homocysteine builds up in the bloodstream it can increase the risk of heart attack, stroke, and blood clots in the lungs or legs; very high levels can triple the risk. We don't yet know why, but it may damage the cells lining the arteries. This is a risk factor completely independent of cholesterol—you can have low cholesterol levels and still be at high risk for heart disease or stroke.[27]

We can test for homocysteine in blood serum and urine, and the good news is that high levels can be brought down by vitamin supplements, especially vitamin B_6, vitamin B_{12}, choline, betaine, and folic acid. The recommended daily supplements for people with high homocysteine levels are:

Folic acid: 5 milligrams per day
Vitamin B_6: 100 milligrams per day
Vitamin B_{12}: 1000 micrograms (1 milligram) per day
Betaine: 500 milligrams per day
Phophatidylcholine (PC): 1000 milligrams per day

The test for homocysteine is easily performed but not commonly available. One reason is that it may not be reimbursed by health insurance, but another is that many doctors are just not keeping up with all the significant risk factors. This is unfortunate. The homocysteine test should be part of the basic cardiovascular risk assessment, and I encourage you to have it performed at least once if you are entering the high-risk years: over forty for men and over fifty for women.

Lp(a)—pronounced "L-p-little a"—is a little known but potent risk factor for cardiovascular disease. It is sometimes accompanied by high cholesterol and an adverse cholesterol-to-HDL ratio. But troublingly, it often presents itself as a single concealed risk factor for heart attack and stroke. High levels appear to encourage plaque development. Little can be done with diet or exercise to reduce Lp(a) since it has a strong hereditary component, thus making it a strong candidate to blame for the familial risk component of heart disease. But new research, some of it pioneered by the late Linus Pauling in the latter years of his career, indicates certain nutrients may help lower Lp(a):

- Vitamin C: 2 to 3 grams per day
- N-acetylcysteine (NAC): 600 milligrams three times per day

Necessary Nutrients—Striking the Right Balance

Such nutrients as natural minerals, metals, and vitamins can affect your cardiovascular health in complex and interactive ways. Some nutrients, like iron and vitamin D, may increase the risk of heart disease when consumed in excess. Others, like magnesium, signal increased risk when the body is deficient. Still others, especially the antioxidant vitamins C and E, and the carotenoids, actively guard against the metabolic conditions that lead to heart disease. The key to prevention and health is balance — making sure you get the right amounts of the right nutrients. Chapter 16 will offer good base levels of the key nutrients that affect cardiovascular health. Let's look at some of the most important ones.

Vitamins, Minerals, and Heart Disease

Studies based on laboratory animals have shown that low nutrient levels of vitamin B_6, vitamin C, copper, chromium, magnesium, and others are associated with buildup of arterial plaque, even if there is no cholesterol or saturated fat in the diet at all. The Nurses Health Study followed up 87,000 women for over a period of eight years and found that those women with the highest level of vitamin C in their blood had a 35 percent lower risk of heart disease than those with the lowest level of vitamin C. This may reflect the fact that women with a higher health consciousness may take vitamin supplements or vitamin-rich foods, but it may also be related to the antioxidant properties of vitamin C. There is also strong evidence that the other primary antioxidants, the carotenoids and vitamin E, also support cardiovascular health (see chapter 16 for more on this).

Vitamin B_6 is especially important for cardiovascular health because it's involved in metabolic pathways that actually remove cholesterol buildup. Monkeys who have been fed a diet complete except for vitamin B_6 have developed severe buildup of fatty deposits in their arteries, along with a high cholesterol level in the blood.[28]

THE CALCIUM/MAGNESIUM BALANCE

When researchers want to induce atherosclerosis quickly in animals for study, they feed rabbits a diet high in saturated fat from something like coconut oil and give them lots of vitamin D, which promotes absorption of calcium. Calcium is the mineral that builds up in arterial plaque and makes the arteries hard, stiff, and inflexible.

Calcium is necessary to promote growth and avert bone loss. Nevertheless, there is some concern that our current single-minded interest in calcium to prevent osteoporosis, and the heavy fortification of vitamin D in everything from milk to bread to breakfast cereals, may be setting us up for increased risk of atherosclerosis. The risk is increased by a gradual decline in the quantity of magnesium in our diets, a decline that's been continuous since the beginning of the twentieth century.

In an ideal diet, calcium is balanced by magnesium. The magnesium has a moderating effect on the parathyroid gland, which regulates calcium metabolism. Unfortunately, magnesium deficiency is all too common nowadays, because food processing and even agricultural practices tend to remove it from our diet. Magnesium deficiency tends to compound itself through a metabolic vicious circle: an excess of calcium causes stored magnesium to be increasingly lost into the urine.

Baby boomers may be at special risk, since they are the first generation to be raised on foods that are heavily fortified with vitamin D — a practice that began in the late 1940s. (There are few controls on *how much* vitamin D is added to foods like milk; studies show that it can vary from minimal to huge.) The emphasis on vitamin D and calcium as a public health measure has clearly had many beneficial effects: children are growing stronger bones and are actually growing taller than previous generations. Yet, there may be dangers unless we can supplement our diet with sufficient magnesium. Dr. Mildred S. Seelig, of Goldwater Memorial Hospital and the New York University Medical Center, is considered by many the foremost expert on magnesium in nutrition. Dr. Seelig suggests that the decline in magnesium in our diets, along with the increase in vitamin D, has had much to do with the sharp increase in sudden deaths from heart disease in the past half century and that magnesium supplementation is the best preventive remedy.[29]

INTELLIGENT MEDICINE TIP: _____

As a supplement, consider taking magnesium citrate, 150 miligrams twice daily, but cut back if you have the side effect of diarrhea!

IRON

Iron is crucial for health. It is an essential component of the red blood cells, which carry oxygen from the lungs to body tissues. When our diet provides us with more than enough iron, the excess is stored in the form of a molecule called ferritin, which is carried in the bloodstream. Iron is so important that the government requires some food manufacturers to add iron to their products. However, some studies have shown that high levels of iron in the body may increase the risk of heart attack. This may help to explain why premenopausal women are at a lower risk of heart attack than men of the same age: they are simply getting rid of excess iron during the blood loss of menstruation. It is theorized that excess iron may promote the formation of free radicals that can injure the walls of blood vessels. Free radicals also promote the formation of oxidized LDL cholesterol, which tends to prompt an immune reaction on the walls of coronary arteries. The implication? Adults, especially men, should avoid iron supplement pills unless they have a real iron deficiency. For men especially, giving blood is not just an admirable civic gesture; it may promote cardiovascular health by ridding the body of excess iron.[30]

ZINC AND COPPER

Animal studies have shown higher cholesterol levels and a tendency to build up arterial plaque when there is a deficiency of copper in the system. While copper deficiency is not that common in humans, it may be promoted by excessive zeal in taking nutritional supplements of zinc (more than 100 milligrams per day). Zinc and copper balance each other in the body, and an excess of zinc can reduce copper levels in the blood. Further, there is some evidence that excessive zinc supplementation may reduce levels of the beneficial HDL protein in the blood. Zinc supplements can be helpful in a good nutrition program, but it's probably wise not to exceed the 75 milligrams per day level.[31]

"Sugar Disease" and Your Heart

Most people nowadays know that diet is one effective way to prevent heart disease. Many have already made major adjustments in their diets to lower the cholesterol count. Still, many others are baffled and disappointed because they have switched to a low-fat, high-carbohydrate diet but are not getting the expected results. On top of this, they sometimes experience unpleasant side effects from their new diet, possibly including sudden exhaustion, mood swings, or irritability. This common experience doesn't mean you should give up on the dietary approach. Many of my patients drop their cholesterol counts by amazing amounts — not infrequently by over one hundred points — by following the Salad and Salmon Diet. Let's look at how the popular low-fat, high-carbohydrate diet can lead to trouble.

Alan was a forty-five-year old executive who came to me about his cholesterol problem. He said to me, "Doc, I can't understand it — my doctor told me that I had dangerously high cholesterol and that I was a bit overweight, and that I should try a diet, but if the diet didn't work, he could easily prescribe a drug or medication. I gave up hamburgers and french fries, and I gave up eggs and I switched to margarine. Everything that I eat is low fat, but my cholesterol, which was over 300, has only gone down to 285, and the doctor says that just doesn't cut it. He says that this is very common, and that people "make their own cholesterol" and diet doesn't have that much to do with it. He wants to put me on medication to lower my cholesterol, but I really don't want to go on drugs, Dr. Hoffman. Can you help me with this?"

I asked Alan for the details about his eating habits and saw immediately why he was having trouble. For breakfast he would have a raisin bran muffin or a "fat-free" muffin, or a healthy, high-fiber granola cereal, sweetened with fruit juice and with skimmed milk and banana over it, and a glass of orange juice. For lunch he'd have a bowl of pasta with some fruit as a dessert, and for dinner he might have fish or chicken, and baked potato with margarine, or whole wheat bread. During the day he would drink lots of healthy apple juice and other natural fruit juices, and eat a granola bar or trail mix with raisins for snacks. Alan had eliminated a lot of fat from his diet, but he wasn't losing much weight. Worse, he'd often feel tired and irritable and would snap at his wife or get argumentative. Sometimes Alan would feel his heart pounding and would break into a cold sweat and start worrying about a heart attack. He couldn't figure it out—why was this supposedly healthy diet not doing anything for him?

Alan's problem was what I call sugar disease, which we first discussed in chapter 6. In spite of his "healthy" diet, he was having too much juice, too much fruit, too many starchy vegetables, and too many flour products like pasta and bread, all of which were causing radical shifts in his blood sugar, resulting in his feelings of tiredness and irritability.

Alan's blood tests showed that he had low HDL (the good cholesterol) and very high triglycerides—in the 220 to 240 range. His internist had told him he didn't really need to worry about the triglycerides, that it was the cholesterol that counted, and anyway, that there were medications to bring down the triglycerides. We also did a glucose tolerance test for Alan to see how his body was dealing with sugar and whether there was any sign of diabetes. It showed a fairly normal blood sugar level, so we could reassure him that he was not diabetic. However, his insulin levels were very high. His body was producing excess insulin to deal with the sugar in his diet. This is a sure sign of Syndrome X, which is associated with heart disease.

I got Alan to eliminate high-sugar, high-carbohydrate foods and use our Salad and Salmon Diet. He couldn't quite believe what I was telling him. I said, "Just go on this cockamamie diet for one month, and we'll let the numbers speak for themselves. He kept asking me, "You mean I can eat six eggs a week? You mean I can eat chicken? I was even avoiding chicken; I was having that very rarely." Alan was practically phobic about oil and couldn't believe I was telling him to have olive oil instead of margarine, and that it was OK to eat oily fish like tuna and salmon. When I told him, "Those oily fish are good for you; salmon is good for you, because that's the right kind of oil," he was afraid I was telling him to go ahead and eat many of the things he'd been conditioned to avoid.

Nevertheless, Alan gave it a shot. As he came back, month after month, he saw his cholesterol steadily going down and saw that the diet was really working. After only six weeks, he was amazed: his cholesterol had dropped to 185, his triglycerides had dropped to 60 or 70, and his HDL had actually gone up a few points, so his cholesterol-to-HDL ratio was now in the near-optimal 4:1 area. What's more, he *felt* better — no more mood swings, no more sudden energy drops.

INTELLIGENT MEDICINE TIP: _____

Don't be beguiled into a false sense of security just because you're eating a low-fat, high-carbohydrate diet. Some fats and oils are essential to health, and excess carbohydrates and sugar can create problems of their own. Watch out for hidden sources of sugar and for flour-based foods and starchy foods that build up blood sugar too quickly.

The key indicator of Alan's condition was the high level of insulin he was producing — the hormone that enables the body to process blood sugar. Many people have this condition — we call it latent diabetes. They don't have the overt symptoms of diabetes, such as thirst and frequent urination, but they react abnormally to high sugar intake. Overproduction of insulin, is not pathological in itself, but it can be a harbinger of diabetes to come. As in Alan's case, latent diabetes is often associated with high blood pressure, high cholesterol, and high triglycerides. Like Alan, someone with this condition may also be suffering from fatigue, exhaustion, and irritation because of the wide swings in glucose levels and counteracting hormones like adrenaline. For a long time we've known that diabetes itself is a major risk factor for heart disease; we're now beginning to understand that this kind of latent diabetes also poses a risk.

Diabetes increases the risk of heart disease in several ways. First, the adult-onset form is usually associated with obesity and high blood pressure, which put extra strain on the heart and increase the risk of stroke. Also, it's been shown that insulin itself promotes atherosclerosis, the fatty buildup in the arteries. This is why we like to maintain people with insulin-dependent diabetes on the least possible amount of insulin.

People with latent diabetes have insulin resistance; that is, their bodies do not make effective use of the insulin it produces, perhaps as a natural reaction to the flood of excess insulin that responds to their high sugar intake. This condition is precisely the degenerative disease we've talked about in chapter 6 — Syndrome X.

INTELLIGENT MEDICINE TIP:

> There is some evidence that dietary factors other than sugar metabolism can affect insulin activity. Excess saturated fat and a dietary deficiency of the omega-3 or omega-6 essential fatty acids can induce insulin resistance, and a change in cooking fat and supplements with omega-3 fish oil have improved insulin action, corrected cholesterol imbalances in the blood, and caused latent diabetes to regress. This underscores once again the importance of having enough of the "good" fats and oils in the diet.[32] Be aware that smoking, too, increases insulin resistance.

What does all this mean for prevention? Well, the best we have to go on right now is that dietary habits seem linked to the development of Syndrome X, especially long-term overconsumption of sugar and simple carbohydrates. This is another case in which the conventional low-fat, high-carbohydrate diet can pose risks. A better alternative is the Salad and Salmon Diet outlined in chapter 16, which does not contribute to high levels of blood sugar and can especially benefit those with latent diabetic tendencies.

Excess Weight: The Triple Threat

"You really should get your weight down." This refrain is heard in countless doctors' offices and is part of the standard advice for preventing heart disease. Why? As long as the extra pounds aren't built from saturated fat and cholesterol, what's the difference? For one thing, excess weight usually is correlated with higher cholesterol levels. Beyond that, the extra weight is just an extra load to carry around, so your heart has to work harder. Excess weight actually does several additional things to increase your risk for heart disease. First, obesity changes the amount of insulin that your body makes. People who are overweight usually produce too much insulin because of insulin resistance — their metabolism doesn't respond effectively to the hormone. They suffer from the risks of excess insulin itself, and they start down the path that leads to incipient diabetes.

Also, someone who is overweight suffers from increased peripheral resistance: the heart has to pump a lot harder just to get the blood to circulate through all that fat tissue. The heart muscle tends to grow larger to pump harder to keep the blood circulating, and pushes up the blood pressure to get the blood out to the peripheral vessels. As obesity increases, the heart muscle is finally unable to grow any larger, is driven past its capacity, and simply start to fail — and the next stop on this route is congestive heart failure.

Up in Smoke!

When you bring up the risks of smoking, everyone thinks first of lung cancer, perhaps followed by emphysema, lip cancer, and throat cancer. But the serious risks that cigarette smoking poses to cardiovascular health are every bit as serious as the risk for lung cancer. Cigarette smoke is a complex compound, made up of not just nicotine and tar but of dozens and dozens of chemical compounds. Each can initiate its own pathway for inducing cardiovascular disease.

For example, nicotine narrows and constricts the blood vessels, at least temporarily, which may raise blood pressure. This can also change the flow characteristics of the blood so that there's more turbulence. The extra turbulence inflicts trauma on the arterial wall, and in response to trauma there is a buildup of calcified plaque, as a kind of scar tissue, until the hardened, narrow arteries of atherosclerosis result.

Cigarettes also deliver a lot of free radicals to the body. These are the active chemical agents that are also generated by radiation, sunlight, certain poisons, oxidized fats, or even chemotherapy. Once in the bloodstream, the first cells the free radicals come into contact with are the cells that line the arteries. Again, damage to these cells creates the sites where the buildup of calcified plaque can begin. The free radicals may also combine with LDL to create a more oxidized LDL particle, which is the most dangerous of all the particles. All of this ties in with the studies that show that antioxidants like vitamin C, vitamin E, and the carotenoids, which reduce free radicals, can retard heart disease. Popular medical writers sometimes say, "If you're going to smoke, take antioxidants." The problem is that smoking overwhelms not only your body's own natural antioxidants but any supplements you take as well. This is why some studies of antioxidants have shown no benefit of beta-carotene supplements to inveterate smokers. No matter how much of these antioxidants you take, you're going to get only partial protection. If you get a 25 percent benefit, that may be good, but it's not going to assure survival. You just might develop disease less quickly.

Another deadly effect of cigarette smoke is that it introduces a lot of carbon monoxide into your lungs, where it binds to the transport molecule hemoglobin in your red blood cells and prevents the hemoglobin from carrying oxygen. If you smoke, you reduce the oxygen-carrying capacity of the blood. (One of the signs of carbon monoxide poisoning is that the lips turn blue, because there's not enough oxygen circulating out to the peripheral body tissues. The body tissue literally starts to suffocate.) Carbon monoxide builds up to a high level in cigarette smoke, and when you take this into your lungs, the heart has to pump harder and build up more pressure to deliver more blood to the brain, the rest of the body, and the heart itself. This is compounded by one of the direct effects of nicotine itself, which is to increase the heart rate. If you smoke, you are overdriving the heart, loading on stress, and starting down the road that leads to an enlarged heart muscle and congestive heart failure.

The reduced supply of blood can cause other painful symptoms. Smokers with heart problems often suffer from intense pain in the calves when walking. This condition, called claudication, is due to reduced circulation in the legs, which may be caused by hardened arteries and is compounded by the reduced oxygen content of the blood. When they stop smoking, many people who suffer from this feel a great deal of relief because they're getting more oxygen to the tissue.

Drink to Your Health?

Every month or so we hear a new report on alcohol and heart disease. A glass of red wine every day reduces heart disease. Those who drink moderately have fewer heart attacks than nondrinkers. Well, this certainly plays into our complicated cultural relationship to this very powerful, legal, and socially acceptable drug. Alcohol as therapy — what could be more convenient? Various explanations are offered for the statistical results. It may be that alcohol in the bloodstream somehow inhibits atherosclerosis. One theory is that red wine makes platelets in the blood less sticky. Another is that the bioflavonoid-like compounds found in grapes and grapeseeds may have an antioxidant effect. A recent study suggested that a moderate intake of alcohol may keep HDL levels up.[33]

Well, alcohol or wine may really have the beneficial effects that show up in statistical samplings. At the same time, it's clear that there are many other ways to generate the same effects through good nutrition or nutritional supplements, without the clearly demonstrated risks and dangers of alcohol to the liver, to nutritional uptake from the digestive system, and to the nervous system. It's not clear that we want to make the French bargain: a reduced rate of heart attacks and a high rate of liver disease.

Alcohol does create some direct risks for other types of cardiovascular disease than arteriosclerosis. Because of its depressive effect, alcohol at first lowers blood pressure, which then rebounds to higher than normal levels, along with heart rate and body temperature. There is some evidence that alcohol may have a blood-thinning effect and may thus inhibit the formation of blood clots. This could explain why moderate drinking may reduce the rate of heart attacks. It may also explain why the risk of strokes due to cerebral hemorrhage goes up with alcohol intake, since blood thinners worsen this type of stroke, making the bleeding much more extensive when it occurs. While one or two drinks a day statistically reduce the risk of heart attacks, with more than two the risk of strokes increases drastically, especially in people over fifty. Alcohol in large amounts weakens all muscles, including the heart muscle, and a weekend overindulgence can also cause palpitations or irregular heartbeat. The "holiday heart" is a common phenomenon in hospital emergency rooms.[34]

What's the bottom line? One or two drinks a day probably cause no serious risks to the heart, though nondrinkers can acquire many of the statistical benefits of moderate drinking through good nutrition, imbibing purple grape juice, and supplements. If you have more than two drinks (or two glasses of wine, or two beers) a day, you're putting yourself at increased risk for stroke, to say nothing of such dangers as liver disease, breast cancer, accidents, and a possible dependence on alcohol.

Stressed Out? Heart Disease and the Type H Personality

Some years ago, researchers began to look into the correlation of personality type with heart disease. They identified what was called the Type A personality — active, aggressive, impatient, commanding, driven — exactly the sort of person who often rose to the top in business or a profession. People with this personality type, as identified through a personality profile questionnaire, did indeed seem to suffer higher rates of heart attack and stroke. By contrast, the Type B personality — more easygoing, patient, phlegmatic — seemed to enjoy a lower risk.

Since the first studies, however, researchers have refined this concept and are now talking about the Type H personality: H for hostile — or hopeless. When the A's were separated from the H's, the active, driven, demanding type often showed a very good profile of cardiovascular health. Jogging in the morning, on the go all day, and committed to a job or profession, the Type A person may be fielding a lot of stressful events and demands. But this in itself isn't a risk as long as he or she is getting some kind of aerobic exercise, following a good nutritional program, and satisfying the basic sleep requirements. Add the components of anger, frustration, or hopelessness and the risk for heart disease shoots up. The hostile demanding type, the person who is aggressive and angry, is running a risk. On the flip side, the one who passively takes all the blows the world has to dish out, resigned and hopeless, is also at risk. In particular, women who are passive, nonemotive, and self-abnegating, and who internalize the stresses of life, run the highest risk of heart disease. For these women, being more assertive can actually rescue them from heart disease.

This only reminds us of one of the most curious facts about stress: moderate stress is good for you. One study showed that working women have, on average, lower blood pressure than those who stay at home. In spite of all our anxieties about excess stress, many of them well founded, some degree of stress and challenge is needed to keep us in optimal mental and physiological tone. Even on the purely physiological level, you have to stress a muscle to strengthen it. You have to stress the heart with exercise to maintain the responsive capacity of the arteries and the health of the whole cardiovascular system. Only when we go beyond our capacities for handling stress, mentally or physically, does stress begin to cause damage, wearing down body and spirit. What the Type H studies may be telling us is that chronic anger and hostility are a warning sign that we are pushing ourselves or our social environment beyond the point of safety.

Birthdays and Mondays—and the High-Risk Hours

The Type H research is only one of many areas in which we find a correlation between heart disease and stress. Bachelorhood, cold weather, and life on the fast track all show statistical links to increased risk heart attack. One aspect of the research is careful separation of stress-related factors from other physiological factors. For example, cold weather may increase physiological stress, but it also correlates with a seasonal increase in the "stickiness" of the platelets in the blood, related to increased fibrinogen levels. This stickiness increases the likelihood of blood clots. Another direction is the study of "acute" risk factors as opposed to chronic ones. These are risks that strike on certain days or even certain times of day. Statistically, more heart attacks happen on Mondays than other days of the week. Rates of heart attack increase significantly during the days immediately preceding and immediately following birthdays. Are they due to the excesses of birthday parties, or to emotional stress? We don't yet know.[35]

In the 1980s, statistical studies revealed one of the oddest facts about heart attacks and heart failure: they strike people most often in the early morning, during the first few hours after waking. There is probably a stress-related component here, since blood pressure and heart rate both increase rather drastically as the body shifts from sleep to waking. Other physiological factors are peculiar to the early morning hours: increased stickiness of the blood, increased concentration of hormones that stimulate the heart, and increased incidence of "silent ischemia," a temporary, often painless, reduction of blood flow to the heart. Studies have shown that the longest and largest drops in blood flow to the heart take place between 3 A.M. and 10 A.M. — exactly the period when heart attacks are more likely. Here is a completely physiological factor, and we don't know yet whether it's a cause of heart attacks in itself or just one symptom in a longer causal chain.[36]

Family History: What Your Ancestors Left You

A new patient will sometimes dutifully report on a medical history that both parents died of heart disease. It turns out that mother died at, say, eighty-four of a heart attack and father at eighty-nine of a stroke. Well, that's not a bad history at all — both parents lived to a ripe old age and died quickly and relatively painlessly. We should all be so fortunate. On the other hand, if a parent had a heart attack before the age of sixty-five, or developed angina in his or her fifties, or had a bypass operation, or struggled with chronic high blood pressure, that's something to look at more closely. It's often hard, though, to tell exactly how to interpret a family history, since changes in diet and physical habits in the middle of the twentieth century may have put a whole generation at risk.

As the risk factors for heart disease become better known, and as people start on good nutrition and exercise programs, we'll probably avoid some of the patterns of our parents' generation. Still, there *are* genetic components to heart disease. In fact there are probably many of them, and we are only beginning to be able to pinpoint a few, such as genetic variations in the lipoprotein ratios, variations in hormone production, and the like. We have tests for some of these, which are mentioned elsewhere in this chapter. If there was early heart disease in your family, or you have a genetic marker for a higher risk group, this is not a sentence of doom. It just means that you may have to be a little more conscientious about nutrition, exercise, and managing your other risk factors.

INTELLIGENT MEDICINE TIP: _____

Take a close look at your family history and note any early onset of cardiovascular disease. Also consider diet patterns, smoking, and sedentary habits, which may have put family members at risk. If there was early disease not explained by the obvious risk factors, you may want to be tested for fibrinogen, homocysteine, and Lp(a) levels, as described elsewhere in this chapter.

The Pressure Cooker: Hypertension and Heart Disease

Hypertension, or high blood pressure, is not in itself an illness. Our blood pressure can normally rise to very high levels for short periods during each day. Chronic hypertension, on the other hand, is a major risk factor for heart disease as well as kidney disease. It's all the more dangerous because it's a "silent killer" — it produces no overt symptoms, at least in the initial to moderate stages. It's estimated that 40 percent of the adult population may suffer from high blood pressure and that at least half that number may go undiagnosed and untreated and be at risk for a whole array of deadly ailments.

What can go wrong? Even slight increases in blood pressure can cause the blood vessels to stiffen and become rough, creating sites for cholesterol plaque to build up. The hardened, narrowed blood vessels set the stage for angina, heart attacks, and strokes. High blood pressure increases the risk of a blood clot in the brain, or the chance that a weakened blood vessel will rupture and burst, releasing blood into the surrounding tissue, leading to a cerebral infarct. Heightened blood pressure can also cause small hemorrhages in the kidneys, eventually necessitating dialysis. Finally, pumping blood through the system at a high pressure puts a strain on the heart and may cause the heart muscle to enlarge, weaken, and eventually succumb to congestive heart failure, no longer able to pump out the blood returned to it by the veins. This is the type of heart failure that's more common among older women. The main risk factor for congestive heart failure is a history of poorly controlled high blood pressure. That's why it is hoped that improved methods of control of high blood pressure will enable us to reduce the incidence of congestive heart failure.

All this damage can begin silently, without symptoms. Only extremely high blood pressure will occasionally produce fleeting symptoms like headaches, ringing in the ears, light-headedness, or feelings of stuffiness in the head. The only way to track the risks is by testing, and building up a record of tests that will reveal any dangerous trends.

Hypertension is a disease of civilization. Indigenous peoples and those in traditional cultures with low-salt diets have little or no incidence of hypertension, and there is no increase in risk with age. In our high-stress Western cultures, flooded with salty snacks and processed foods, it's accepted as a given that blood pressure starts to climb at about age thirty-five or forty. Yet, much of this can be controlled by diet and lifestyle, and it's possible to avoid the lifetime sentence of diuretics and beta-blockers that are the most heavily prescribed medications today.

What causes high blood pressure? The frustrating answer is that most cases are classified as essential hypertension — a fancy medical term for hypertension that has no known cause. In fact, there is probably a complex array of causes, including genetic factors, environmental pollution, stress, salt intake, Syndrome X, extrasensitivity of peripheral arteries, and abnormalities in the hormones, that regulate blood pressure.

We do know much about how blood pressure is regulated and adjusted, and it's a marvelous, complicated system. Somehow the body must change and adjust blood pressure among various organs and body parts while always keeping the blood flow constant to the brain. This regulation adjusts the flow of blood to meet the needs of individual muscle groups and organs and compensates for changes in pressure in different parts of the body as we lie, sit, stand, and exercise. Overall, our blood pressure is changing constantly, reacting to physical activity, emotional stress, and even the time of day.

Three main factors that regulate blood pressure: the pumping force of the heart (and speed of the heartbeat), the constriction or relaxation of the peripheral arteries, and the total fluid volume of the blood. There is a complex system of feedback control, in which blood pressure is monitored in different parts of the body, and different systems are signaled to change the pumping rate of the heart, the constriction of the arteries, or the fluid volume of the blood to adjust the local or overall pressure.

The signaling systems include the nervous system, which can monitor pressure in the carotid arteries of the neck and send signals to the heart to pump more quickly or slowly and to individual blood vessels to contract or relax. This is done directly through nerve impulses and indirectly through the hormones and neurotransmitters of the sympathetic nervous system that are released during stress: epinephrine and norepinephrine. The nervous system can very quickly cause drastic changes in blood pressure in a matter of seconds. The nerve/hormone path is also the way in which psychological stress can directly raise blood pressure. There is a theory that some people live in a constantly heightened state of activation of the sympathetic nervous system and are constantly, unconsciously, pumping up their blood pressure.

Other systems control blood pressure more slowly, over hours or days, by raising and lowering the fluid volume of the blood. When blood pressure is high, the kidneys can lower it by removing water from the blood and releasing it into the urine. The kidneys also adjust the salt level of the blood. A high level of salt causes more water to be retained in the body, and the kidneys can reduce pressure by removing salt from the bloodstream and passing it into the urine. Even small amounts of salt in the diet can cause the body to retain water and blood pressure to rise. Finally, the kidneys control blood pressure through two hormones, renin and angiotensin, which cause blood vessels to constrict and the kidneys to retain salt and water — both factors that increase pressure. The main function of the renin-angiotensin system is to adjust for shifting levels of salt in the diet.

There's even a way in which the heart can work as a kind of gland to adjust blood pressure. Besides pumping blood, the heart produces a hormone, atrial naturetic peptide, which acts on the kidneys to make them release salt into the urine, thereby lowering the blood pressure. Cardiologists are looking into this with great interest in the hope of finding a natural substance that will accelerate the excretion of salt, as an alternative to current drugs.

Measuring Blood Pressure: The White Coat Effect

We measure blood pressure in millimeters of mercury (mm Hg), based on the concept of a force that will push a column of mercury so many millimeters high. It's like the system that's used in a barometer to measure air pressure. In the case of blood pressure, we measure the force exerted by the blood against a unit area of the blood vessel. Blood pressure pulses constantly, with each heart beat sending a surge of blood into the arteries and raising the pressure, which then falls to a lower level between the beats.

By the time it reaches the capillaries, blood pressure is evened out by the stretching and resistance of the arteries.

We measure both the surge pressure, called the systolic pressure, and the relaxed pressure, called the diastolic pressure, because the two figures together provide valuable information. A normal young adult at rest might have a blood pressure of 120/80, that is, 120 millimeters of surge pressure to 80 millimeters of relaxed pressure. In a young person, a reading of 140/90 is considered high; in a man forty to sixty years old, most doctors don't consider blood pressure high until it reaches, 150/90 or so. A diastolic (relaxed pressure) reading of 90 to 95 is considered on the edge of hypertension, no matter what the age.

One difficulty of getting a meaningful reading is that blood pressure can change drastically, even when you're at rest, especially in response to anxiety or even mild emotional stress. Hence the "white coat syndrome" — rise in blood pressure whenever a person is in a doctor's office, especially the blood pressure is actually being measured (by a professional in a white coat). This extreme sensitivity that everyone has to environment and expectations means that a single blood pressure reading does not tell us very much by itself. A diagnosis of hypertension can't really be made without a series of high readings on different days. Fortunately, research shows that blood pressure readings usually drop on successive visits to the same doctor or clinic. If a doctor suspects "white coat syndrome," you may need to learn how to take readings at home, under "low pressure" conditions. If I'm getting high readings from a patient in my office, I definitely get the person to obtain readings done in another setting.

Casual blood pressure readings present other problems as well, including error by an inexperienced medical assistant. The sphygmomanometer itself may be out of kilter; doctors usually purchase these instruments early in their careers and may or may not have them checked out and calibrated regularly. There are probably too many people who get a diagnosis of high blood pressure and a prescription for medication on the basis of a faulty reading. (On the other hand, there are clearly too many people who are going undiagnosed because they don't have regular checkups.)

If you feel that the stress of the doctor's office or clinic environment may be affecting your blood pressure readings, or if you want to confirm that several high readings are really telling you something, you can ask for ambulatory blood pressure monitoring, which enables you to find out what your blood pressure is over the course of a day as you go about your normal activities. You may discover that you do have some peaks of high blood pressure a few times a day and that you've been diagnosed with high blood pressure on the basis of those peaks, which might just happen to occur in stressful situations like your visit to the doctor's office. The rest of the time your blood pressure is normal or low. Unfortunately, ambulatory monitoring has not been very well reimbursed by health insurance, though it probably should be, given the wild variations that can occur in a spot-check of blood pressure.

Can Your Eye Doctor Diagnose Hypertension?

The sphygmomanometer is not the only means of detecting high blood pressure. One of the tell-tale signs of high blood pressure is an enlarged heart — the heart muscle gets bigger because it's working harder. If you're concerned about whether hypertension has begun to compromise your health, a chest X-ray, an echocardiogram, or an electrocardiogram (EKG) can reveal whether your heart is enlarged. Hypertension also affects the eyes; it can cause tell-tale changes or even little hemorrhages in the tiny blood vessels at the back of the eyes. An eye doctor can spot this right away and can confirm a diagnosis that you are getting from another source. In fact, eye doctors are trained to look for a distinctive picture that indicates extreme hypertension, the kind that would require immediate hospitalization.

Exercise Versus Aging: Stretch Those Arteries!

What happens to blood pressure with aging? For one thing, if plaque builds up in arteries, and the arteries stiffen and become less elastic, they are simply less able to respond to changes in pressure from the heart and from buildup in blood fluid levels. One's whole response and control system stops responding. Part of this is a natural process of aging: just as the skin becomes less elastic, so do the blood vessels.

Both the systolic "surge" pressure and the diastolic "relaxed" pressure can go up with aging, but the systolic pressure may increase more dramatically. I often see patients of eighty or so who have a systolic blood pressure of 150 and a diastolic pressure of 75. This is the typical picture when the arterial walls become stiff and inflexible, so they don't "give" in response to the surge of blood from the heart. Forty years earlier, the same individuals might have had blood pressure of 120/75 — the same diastolic pressure, but a much lower systolic.

There's one great way to compensate for this: exercise. If you intermittently stretch and contract your arteries, you can help keep them flexible. This is what happens naturally as you exercise — you raise your heart rate to high levels, your blood pressure goes up, and the arteries contract. Afterwards, your heart slows down, your blood vessels relax, and as your blood pressure goes up and down your blood vessels can stretch through a wider range, and your blood pressure can self-regulate more easily. Exercise "tones" your arteries as well as strengthening the heart. There is a synergistic effect between strengthening the heart and controlling blood pressure: after a time your circulatory system builds up a reserve, so that even with a low blood pressure you are pumping the amount of blood that your body needs.

Is Salt-Free Worry-Free?

Long before the rise of industrial civilizations, salt was a valuable commodity in trade, worth more than its weight in gold in parts of the world with few natural sources of salt. This is only one indication of our innate biological craving or need for some amount of salt in the diet. Yet, salt is not without its risks: probably the most popular notion about high blood pressure is that it's caused by too much salt in the diet. There's a clear mechanism for this: when we eat salty foods, we feel thirsty afterwards and drink more water, thus increasing the fluid volume of the blood. Salt in the blood causes the body to retain more water, so that the percentage of salt in the blood doesn't get too high. Even a moderate increase in salt intake can cause a measurable rise in blood pressure. When blood pressure is too high, the kidneys cause more water and salt to be passed into the urine, but if we keep eating more salt they have trouble keeping up. The reason diuretics are often prescribed for high blood pressure is that they work directly on the kidneys, causing them to pass more water and sodium into the urine and thus reducing the fluid volume of the blood.

There's no question that salt, or sodium, has an effect, yet people in Brazil and China, with high intakes of salt, do not usually have abnormally elevated blood pressure. Why not? Probably the best answer is that salt intake is just one of many complex factors that influence blood pressure. Salt is not the overriding factor, just as cholesterol isn't for heart disease. Other minerals, like magnesium, calcium, and potassium, affect blood pressure as well, and there are great genetic variations in how individuals respond to sodium and the other minerals. Some people seem not to be sensitive to sodium, and there are even some who have an inverse response to salt: when they restrict sodium intake, their blood pressure goes up! Some people with chronic low blood pressure have to maintain some salt in their diet, because it helps the kidneys maintain blood pressure within a normal range.

However, it is thought that excess sodium in the diet over a lifetime may have something to do with a permanent shift in metabolism toward higher blood pressure, so that just withdrawing sodium at a certain point may not be able to reverse the trend. High salt levels may set in motion hormonal or kidney function changes more or less permanently, so that after a certain point you can't just eliminate the salt and reverse those changes.

Still, about 50 percent of people with hypertension respond to a low-sodium diet with a drop in blood pressure. A low- or moderately low-sodium diet may be even more important for prevention to avoid getting stuck in the high-pressure pattern. This requires some extra attention, especially for those who eat a lot of processed foods. Most people get about 85 percent of their salt from prepared food and 15 percent from the salt shaker.

INTELLIGENT MEDICINE TIPS: _____

> Snack foods like potato chips and corn chips are notoriously high in salt, and so are many commercial soups and prepared dishes. If you find yourself craving two or three glasses of water after eating, something in the meal probably contained excessive salt. If you have a favorite Chinese restaurant, ask the cook to go easy on the soy sauce, which is very salty. In your own cooking, try using pepper or other herbs or seasonings for flavor. If you're using a traditional American cookbook, don't feel that you have to add salt to every dish just because the recipe calls for it.

Beyond Salt: Other Minerals and Blood Pressure

The three minerals besides sodium that have the most significant effect on blood pressure are calcium, magnesium, and potassium. Different individuals have different degrees of response to these, but many people, perhaps about 40 percent of the population, respond to supplements of these minerals with a drop in blood pressure. It's interesting that a vegetarian diet, the kind prescribed by Dr. Ornish's plan, is inherently high in magnesium and potassium, and low in sodium. In green plants, every chlorophyll molecule has a core of magnesium, just as every hemoglobin molecule in animals has a core of iron, so green vegetables inherently have a lot of magnesium. Plant foods also have a much higher potassium-to-sodium ratio than animal foods, including dairy products, so vegetarian diets sometimes do the trick for people with high blood pressure.

PREVENTION TIPS: _____

> If you have trouble getting enough green vegetables into your diet, you might try a calcium/magnesium supplement. A supplement combining 1000 milligrams of calcium with 400 milligrams of magnesium would be a good ratio, and amount. Over-the-counter potassium supplements generally don't provide much potassium, so a good bet is to eat high-potassium foods: lots and lots of green leafy vegetables. Vegetable juice is better than orange juice, which is high in potassium but also high in fruit sugar, which may lead to sugar imbalance and Syndrome X. For the same reason, greens are better than high-potassium but high-calorie bananas and citrus fruits.

Circulation and the Kidneys: A Hormonal Short Circuit

The kidneys are crucial organs for regulating blood pressure, and researchers have observed a typical decline in kidney function, especially after the age of fifty. With age, the kidneys take longer to filter and pass on the blood that circulates through them. There's often a little fatty buildup and narrowing of the arteries that further reduces circulation. The result of this reduced circulation through the kidneys is a rise in blood pressure.

How does this come about? One of the oldest experiments in physiology was to clamp off one of the renal arteries in experimental animals, thus clamping off blood flow to one of the kidneys. In response to reduced blood flow, the kidney sends a hormonal signal to the to the whole body to clamp down all the blood vessels. This is a natural protective response intended to maintain blood pressure in the case of injury and excessive bleeding. When circulation is reduced in the kidneys with age, the kidneys perceive it as a threat and send out the hormonal signals to increase blood pressure to protect against a nonexistent blood loss and blood pressure drop. It's an adaptive mechanism when you're injured and bleeding, but it's a feedback loop that runs amok with age. As blood vessels narrow and blood pressure rises, the arteries choke off more circulation to the kidneys and become more susceptible to atherosclerosis. The kidneys then send out more signals to raise the blood pressure, so a vicious circle may have begun.

One risk factor for this kind of kidney decline is excess protein in the diet. Over a period of years, or a lifetime, a high protein load is thought to cause the kidneys to deteriorate more rapidly.

INTELLIGENT MEDICINE TIP: _____

> Avoid extra-high-protein weight-loss diets. They can disrupt the metabolism in several ways besides putting a strain on the kidneys. The steak and hamburger overload that was a sign of prosperity in the 1950s may have contributed to the high rates of heart disease in our parents' generation. If you do like meat, consider limiting your meat meals to one a day, or cooking with meat as one element in a recipe or a meal but not the main course.

Lowering Blood Pressure: The Beneficial Oils

We have already looked at the benefits of omega-3 oils in thinning the blood, lowering cholesterol, and reducing atherosclerosis. Another way they prevent heart disease is by lowering blood pressure, apparently by causing arteries to gently dilate. This has been demonstrated with fish oil and with flaxseed oil, which is a vegetarian source of omega-3 oil. Adding these oils to the diet can induce a reduction of up to 5 points in blood pressure, which for some people may be all that's needed.

Other studies of the effect of saturated and unsaturated fats on blood pressure have come up with some fascinating results. In one study, people with normal blood pressure were given a low-fat, high-carbohydrate diet, low in saturated fats, with total fat amounting to 22 percent of calories. The results? A drop of 2.3 points systolic and 4.7 points diastolic blood pressure. In the same study, another group was given a diet with the same low level of saturated fat, but rich in olive oil, *with fats amounting to 41% of total calories.* The remarkable results? *The second group showed almost the same drop in blood pressure:* 2.7 points systolic and 4.4 diastolic. This supports the other studies that demonstrate the benefits of olive oil, a monounsaturated fat and an ancient food source, for cardiovascular health.[37]

PREVENTION TIPS: _____

My Salad and Salmon Diet, rich in omega-3 oils, and the Mediterranean-type cuisine—low in carbohydrates and rich in olive oil, seafood, and fresh salads and vegetables—both show promise for controlling blood pressure.

Garlic: A Folk Remedy that Works

In the 1920s, researchers at the prestigious Sandoz Pharmaceuticals in Switzerland conducted several analytic and clinical tests of garlic. They isolated a component of chopped or crushed (or chewed) garlic, allicin, which turned out to be a powerful antibiotic. Allicin and another component called ajoene also have remarkable effects on the cardiovascular system. They not only reduce blood pressure but also reduce cholesterol and prevent the kind of blood clotting that triggers heart attacks. At least a score of studies throughout the 1970s and 1980s have reported on these and other beneficial properties of garlic in the major medical journals.

PREVENTION TIP: _____

Three to ten cloves of garlic a day are needed to induce the beneficial effects for the cardiovascular system. However, the garlic cloves must be crushed, chopped, bruised, or chewed to release the full effect. You might want to try some of the popular garlic-rich Italian and Asian dishes. If you're worried about the famous odoriferous side effect of consuming garlic, do as the Europeans do and take your garlic in concentrated odor-free capsules.

Pollutants and Heavy Metals

There are some serious environmental risks for high blood pressure in the industrialized world. One common heavy metal pollutant is lead. Sources include water, paint residue in old housing, and lead-fired crystal and pewter cups. Studies have shown that blood and bone lead levels are significantly higher in many people with high blood pressure and that this is one of the most persistent statistical indicators, along with family history and excess weight. In industrialized nations, lead may be even more of a risk than sodium![38]

Another common heavy metal pollutant is cadmium, a toxic metal used in many electrical and mechanical appliances, batteries, rubber and plastic, insecticides, photographic materials, and semiconductors. It's also found in paints — cadmium red is a traditional pigment that artists now often avoid. Cadmium is known as a cumulative poison, a poison that builds up in the body over many years, and it accumulates mainly in the kidneys. Since the beginning of this century, environmental pollution in Europe alone has caused a fiftyfold rise in the concentrations of cadmium in the human kidney, where it can cause permanent, irreversible disease. Cadmium buildup in the kidneys, even at moderate levels, can also lead to high blood pressure, which contributes to heart disease. About 10 percent of the general population of Belgium suffers from cadmium levels that are high enough to harm the kidneys. We would expect similar levels in the highly industrialized regions of the United States.[39]

Cadmium levels can be roughly estimated by hair analysis and can also be identified through blood testing or urinalysis.

Coping with Pressure: Stress and Hypertension

You have an argument with your boss or a near-accident driving home. Maybe you received some exciting *good* news: you've just been promoted to a new and more responsible position at work, or your offer on a new home was accepted. Well, all these kinds of stress can affect your blood pressure. It can go up within a few seconds, but remain high for some time. In fact, there's a name for this: neurogenic hypertension. A strong stimulation of your sympathetic nervous system, releasing hormones like adrenaline and norepinephrine, can temporarily raise your blood pressure to an acute level for several days, after which it usually returns to normal.

This is a temporary effect, but there is some evidence that repeated episodes can lead to chronic high blood pressure. Further, there is evidence that excess norepinephrine in renal arteries can directly damage kidney tissue.

Fortunately, we can learn stress reduction techniques that may counteract some of the normal physiological responses of speeded-up pulse and increased blood pressure. Among my own patients, I've seen individuals who have consciously set out to modify their high-stress lifestyles and to take up meditation or yoga, and these practices have actually decreased their blood pressure as measured in my office.

It's In Your Genes

As we've noted, there is a purely hereditary component to heart disease in general and high blood pressure in particular. There are huge individual variations in response to salt, response to stress, and other environmental influences. While we all share the same basic systems, everyone's individual body chemistry and metabolism is unique.

One of the most persistent patterns of hypertension, which probably has some genetic component, is the high incidence of hypertension among the African-American population. This has been ascribed to demographic factors, since the diets of poverty are generally high in saturated fats, sugar, and salt. There may be a sociological component: a response to the stress and frustration of living with racism. There is probably a genetic component as well. In many interior parts of ancient Africa, the diet was probably very low in salt. In fact, the basis of the early caravan trade in the sub-Sahara was that salt was traded for gold, and Africans who mined gold were happy to trade it for salt, which was such a rare commodity and such an exciting culinary delight. In northern Europe, however, salt was plentiful, and salting was the most common way of preserving foods. You can read accounts of medieval life in which salt meat was a dietary staple, and this persisted to the time of the great English and Spanish sailing fleets. It's possible that Europeans may have been genetically selected over centuries to accommodate a higher sodium intake.

INTELLIGENT MEDICINE TIPS: _____

Take into account the effect that as an individual you may have an especially sensitive or insensitive response to risk factors for high blood pressure. If you belong to a racial or ethnic group that shows a high overall risk, take special care to monitor your blood pressure.

Choose Your Poison?

Alcohol consumption (more than 2 ounces a day) and cigarette smoking are associated with higher blood pressure. Caffeine addicts who drink six to eight cups of coffee a day (or as many diet colas) are increasing their heart rate and blood pressure, putting extra strain on the cardiovascular system, and setting themselves up for an exaggerated nervous response to stress, which can lead to chronic high blood pressure.

Medications for Hypertension — How Safe Are They?

Drugs to control hypertension are the most widely prescribed medications in America today. They range from diuretics, which reduce blood pressure by reducing the fluid content of the blood, to beta-blockers, which put a brake on the heart so that it can't pump too hard and build up pressure. They are all very effective in lowering blood pressure and thus reducing some of the dangerous outcomes of chronic hypertension. What's less clear, however, is whether they actually lead to improved health and a lower overall mortality rate.

In fact, some of the first studies that looked for long-term benefits from these medications found, paradoxically, that more people died when their blood pressure was lowered through drugs than when they were left alone. One of the first of the very large studies on the effects of preventive health intervention in the 1980s was the Mister Fit study (a loose acronym for Multi-Center Risk Factor Intervention Trial). The researchers got a group to stop smoking and take blood pressure medication to reduce their risk factors. They found that some of the people who took blood pressure medication didn't live longer but actually had a higher mortality rate. These results suggested that there might be some problems with the long-term use of the medications.

In fact, the antihypertensive medications have revealed several dangerous side effects. The diuretics, for example, deplete the body's store of magnesium and potassium, which are precisely the substances that sometimes are helpful for lowering blood pressure. Further, these minerals also help prevent arrhythmias, which may explain a higher incidence of what was called "sudden death" in the Mister Fit treatment group. "Sudden death" is one of those understated medical terms for an inexplicable phenomenon that leaves no signature — you don't know why the person died, because no physiological clues are left behind. However, an arrhythmia of the heart is known to be one of the causes. This is why when people take diuretics, they're advised to also take potassium supplements, and magnesium supplements, which are just as important, because magnesium helps to reduce arrhythmias and also to keep the potassium levels high. Another problem with diuretics is that they raise cholesterol levels but lower HDL levels. These are serious considerations, above and beyond the simply annoying side effects, such as fatigue. While diuretics used to be the favored drugs of first resort, and are extremely cheap into the bargain, they've now fallen in popularity.

Another common type of blood pressure medication is the beta-blocker,

REDUCING BLOOD PRESSURE: THE OPTIMAL PROGRAM

- First make sure you have a real problem that shows up over several readings, in different settings.
- See an eye doctor, who not only may be the first to identify hypertensive damage to your circulatory system, but can actually help assess its severity and whether it is a chronic problem.
- Start an exercise program to stretch those arteries and reduce excess body weight.
- Use the nutrition options: fish oils and GLA oils, calcium/magnesium supplements, green leafy vegetables for potassium.
- Avoid the dietary risk factors. Reduce salt in your diet, avoid excess fats that increase body weight and excess sugar that can lead to insulin imbalance, avoid excess protein that can cause premature aging of the kidneys, avoid excess caffeine that can lead to chronic nervous stress.
- Don't smoke cigarettes.
- Have a blood test to check for heavy metals, especially lead and cadmium.
- Take up a stress-reduction program: meditation, relaxation techniques, or yoga.

which operates by inhibiting the speeding-up of heart rate that comes with exercise or stress and therefore keeps blood pressure from rising. Beta-blockers are popular, but they do cause tiredness and a heavy, limp feeling. This is more serious than a matter of discomfort. If you are taking a beta-blocker you may feel less like exercising. Moreover, the beta-blocker will reduce the benefit even if you do push yourself to exercise. The main benefit of exertion is that it challenges your heart to pump faster, which strengthens your heart muscle and enhances your circulation. With a beta-blocker your heart muscle often *can't* pump faster to meet the increased demands of exercise. In addition, many of the beta-blockers, though not some of the newer ones, have a deleterious effect on your lipid profile: the balance of cholesterol, HDL, and LDL in your blood.

Nor is excessive lowering of blood pressure always beneficial. Below a certain pressure, the heart is less able to fill the blood vessels leading to crucial organs, and blood flow is compromised. This results in tiredness, wooziness, and shortness of breath, and it may conceivably cause potential harm to the brain or other organs.

This leaves us with quite a range of risk factors that come along with antihypertensive medication. Using drugs, we can change one parameter — lowering the blood pressure — but we be creating new risks: making the patient tired, sedentary, or depressed; affecting his or her sexual desire; perhaps depleting minerals, increasing cholesterol count, and impairing circulation.

Medications have undoubtedly saved lives, but except when blood pressure is consistently elevated, I think it's always better to try the nondrug therapies first. Some studies show that fully 40 percent of patients receiving high blood pressure medication have normal blood pressure when they're given a "drug holiday" and stop taking their medications, even if no lifestyle interventions such as diet modification, exercise, stress reduction, or nutritional supplementation are undertaken. That 40 percent turns to 80 or 90 percent when natural interventions are provided in lieu of drugs. Try a change in diet, try nutritional supplements, test for the presence of heavy metals like lead or cadmium, exercise to keep the arteries flexible, take up a stress-reduction program. If possible, use the body's own chemistry and natural responses before you use drugs that tamper with fluid metabolism and heart rate.

Exercise: The Best Prevention Strategy

Over the past twenty or thirty years we've made remarkable discoveries about the benefits of exercise for everything from strengthening bones to keeping the body limber and enhancing the immune system. Professional athletes train to build strength or endurance or to improve performance. Many of us unconsciously associate exercise with building muscles, running faster, or playing a better game of tennis. Actually, one of the most important benefits of exercise has nothing to do with muscles or competition. It's the power of exercise to tone and optimize the cardiovascular system, improve the circulation, make the blood vessels stretch and give, and build up the heart's capacity to deliver life-giving oxygen and energy throughout the body.

Along with good nutrition, exercise is one of the best ways to slow the decline of the cardiovascular system and reduce the risk of heart disease. Many studies have shown that exercise reduces the incidence of heart disease and reduces mortality. Exercise can help reduce pain from angina. It can reduce risk factors like high blood pressure, glucose intolerance, and insulin resistance and can even improve the health picture in the face of continued risks, like smoking and obesity.

Almost any kind of exercise will do, as long as it's *aerobic* exercise, which makes a big enough demand on the cardiovascular system to push it close to its capacity. In one British study, which lasted for nine years, groups of middle-aged men with no history of heart disease undertook four different exercise patterns: (1) frequent vigorous aerobic exercise at least twice a week, through a sport or a fast walk cycle, (2) less vigorous exercise at least once a week, through a sport or fast walk of longer than half an hour, (3) occasional vigorous exercise in one to three sports activities a month, or brisk walks of less than half an hour, and (4) no vigorous exercise. While both the first and second groups showed lower mortality rates in general, only the first group, exercising vigorously at least twice a week, showed a reduced rate of death from heart disease. The exercise was beneficial whether or not the participants had exercised before the study began, and it helped even those who smoked, had high blood pressure, or carried too much weight. The British study also confirmed what others have shown: that exercise has a dose-dependent effect—the more you exercise, the better the results.[40]

Other studies have shown that consistent, moderate exercise is the safest way to improve cardiovascular health. It has a strengthening, toning effect and reduces the risk of heart attack, whereas infrequent, very strenuous exercise can actually increase the risk. In other words, taking a long, brisk walk two or three times a week is doing you good, while going out to shovel snow or chop wood once a month can be risky behavior.[41] The key is to take it gradually. One Canadian study showed that even people who suffer from angina, who are normally advised against strenuous exercise, could build up slowly and gradually, over the period of a year, to a fairly intense calisthenic workout using the Canadian Air Force Program for Physical Fitness. They started with just eleven minutes a day of workout. The same study showed that the exercise program improved the capacity of the heart to respond to physical stress and was just as effective as beta-blockers in reducing the symptoms of angina.[42]

How does exercise perform these miracles? Well, the common conception is that you need to exercise your heart muscle itself. In fact, high blood pressure and narrowed, hardened blood vessels can actually overstress your heart, making it work too hard. Exercise helps reduce the strain by lowering blood pressure, perhaps by requiring the arteries to expand and relax over a wider range, making them more flexible. It also raises HDL levels. Though we may not know all the ways exercise helps, study after study clearly associates it with a reduced risk of heart disease. The interesting thing is the speed with which the body responds to exercise, or lack of it. You can lose the benefits fairly quickly, like the college athletes turned couch potatoes who show up at their twenty-fifth reunion, overweight and already at risk for heart attack. Conversely, you can gain the benefits fairly quickly if you embark on an exercise program, even if you've never ever been a jock.

How to Exercise for a Healthy Heart

How much exercise is good exercise? No matter what form of exercise you perform, you want to know that you are exercising in your *target zone*, which means that you've raised your heart rate to the point where you are getting an optimal aerobic workout. Exercising harder than this won't provide any additional benefits for your heart, and less won't give you the maximum protective effect.

How do you determine your ideal rate of aerobic exercise? All of us have a typical resting pulse, which may range from 50 to 90 beats per minute. The average is usually in the low 70s. Each of us also has a maximum rate — a speed beyond which our hearts cannot physically beat. Most people's maximum heart rate is about 220 beats per minute — minus their age. Therefore, if you're thirty years old, your maximum heart rate is probably about 190.

One way to determine a maximum target pulse range for your aerobic exercise is to use the following formula:

1. Determine your maximum heart rate (220 minus your age).
2. Determine your resting pulse. Find your pulse in your wrist, count the beats for 30 seconds, and multiply by two.
3. Determine the difference between your maximum rate and your resting pulse, and take 70 percent of that number. If you are more than 20 pounds overweight, smoke, or have recently had surgery or an illness, take only 60 percent of that number.
4. Your target zone — your ideal aerobic rate — is your resting pulse plus the 70 percent figure above.

   Example: A healthy forty-year-old has a maximum heart rate of 180. This person's resting pulse is 80. The difference between those two is 100. Seventy percent of 100 is 70. Add 70 to 80 and you get 150. The maximum target rate for this person would be about 150.

This formula applies for ages thirty to fifty, but it breaks down at higher ages. If you're sixty or above, living life in the fast lane and competing with fit middle-aged people, endless math calculations are absurd. You don't have to slow down as much as the formula recommends, if you've been exercising over the years. You may want to cut back a little, but the important thing is to follow your body's own cues and the suggestions of your physician.

When you are exercising aerobically, your breathing may increase, and your breaths may come more rapidly, but you will not feel out of breath. As you build up to your aerobic target zone, you should be able to sustain exercise at this level for 20 to 30 minutes or longer. Aerobically fit individuals can sustain this rate for an hour or two. In fact, the art of preparing for a marathon is actually to extend your aerobic capacity so that you can run in your target zone for the length of time it takes to traverse 26 miles — perhaps 3 to 5 hours.

One way to determine whether you are exercising at your aerobic capacity is to buy a pulse meter, a gadget that's become extremely popular. It can be worn on the wrist and chest, costs $35 to $150, and can be bought in many sporting-goods stores. When I was training for the marathon, I'd run for 2 to 3 hours at a time, and I wasn't sure how fast I should be running by hour two or three. The pulse meter allowed me to monitor my heart rate and keep it in my aerobic range. I found that at the beginning of my training it was as great an exertion in hour three to run *half as fast* as I did in hour one. Using a pulse meter, I was able to sustain my training exercise at a constant level, rather than beginning with a jackrabbit burst of enthusiasm and putting myself into aerobic "debt," requiring my muscles to function in the absence of sufficient oxygen. I didn't have to berate myself for dragging along like a tortoise, because I was still hitting my aerobic pace. Gradually, I extended my aerobic threshold.

Advanced Exercise Techniques: "Going for the Burn"

If you push yourself beyond your aerobic target, you are forcing your muscles to function with insufficient oxygen. This is called *anaerobic* exercise, and it's what people talk about when they say they are "going for the burn." Anaerobic exercise can build endurance and a finely sculptured body, but it can also lead to extreme fatigue and injury, especially for weekend warriors. There are other types of exercise: interval training, which alternates aerobic and anaerobic training, and pulsed exercise, which can help those who have chronic illness or fatigue. There are stretching techniques like yoga, and strength-building techniques like isometrics. All of these have their uses and their benefits, but the conventional wisdom is that these do not directly contribute to cardiovascular health. Still, at least one study has shown that strength training, through weight lifting, has comparable effects to those of aerobic training in reducing risk factors for heart disease. Both the strength training and the aerobic training improved glucose metabolism and reduced the hyperactive insulin response that's associated with Syndrome X.[43] Still, aerobic-type exercise is probably the safest and most sure-fire approach to reducing the risk of heart disease.

Whenever you start an exercise program, remember that the key word is *gradual*. If you are getting out of breath and your heart is racing, you are pushing beyond the point of beneficial aerobic exercise, so back off until your breathing is no longer labored, even if you are breathing more rapidly than normal. Don't worry if you don't get up to the target pulse rate right away — you are still getting beneficial aerobic exercise.

INTELLIGENT MEDICINE TIPS: _____

> For your basic minimum prevention program against heart disease, your best bet is to exercise aerobically at least two or three times a week, for 20 to 30 minutes at a time. You can get the benefits through many forms of exercise: brisk walking for half an hour or longer, running, bicycling, swimming, dancing, calisthenics. Figure out your target pulse rate and use it as a guide. Use a pulse meter if that makes it easier.

Troubleshooting: Symptoms and Diagnosis

The focus of this book is on prevention, but maybe you've experienced chest pains from time to time and secretly wondered whether you have a heart condition. Or maybe you've felt your heart racing and wondered whether you should have some tests. Or maybe your doctor has told you that your cholesterol or your blood pressure is way too high, and if you can't bring it down with diet, you can always take medications to fix it. Maybe you've even been advised to have an angiogram, a test to look at the condition of your coronary arteries. Dealing with symptoms, or with the medical system, can be stressful and confusing, especially when specialists or cardiologists tell you that you've got problems or that your chest pains don't have anything to do with heart disease. This part of the chapter will help you deal with the medical system and provide some information about the common tests and medical procedures that you may be offered or pressured to undergo, as well as some of the alternatives.

Most people have had a pain or strong sensations in their chest at some point, even if it's just the feeling of a racing or pounding heart associated with stress or a sudden shock. Well, when you're twenty and you get a chest pain, it's not usually alarming, but when you're forty or forty-five and have chest pain, it makes you think pretty hard. This is really a major issue for baby boomers.

A patient of mine, Iris, forty-one years old, was at home on a Saturday afternoon preparing a gourmet dinner when she suddenly began to feel chest pain—a sense of immense weight pressing on her chest, with pain radiating down to her fingertips, particularly to her left hand. She felt congestion in her throat and shortness of breath, and she had a sense of impending doom, that she was going to drop dead. Now, these are all the classic symptoms of a heart attack, and that's exactly what she thought: "I'm having a heart attack; I've got to get to the hospital."

The fact is that they're also the classic symptoms of a panic episode, as we've seen in chapter 5. This is an involuntary meltdown of the autonomic nervous system—all of a sudden everything stops, there's a lot of physical sensation, and everything gets very scary.

Iris went to the emergency room, the physicians started running tests and established that she was *not* having a heart attack, and before she knew it, she was back out on the street without really understanding what had happened. This is a common scenario for people in their thirties or forties. Emergency room staffers see it all the time, and they often don't sit down and try to explain what happened. It's often hard for the patient to understand, because the symptoms are so powerful.

By the same token, this does *not* mean that you should ignore chest pains, chest pressure, or even other unusual visceral pains, because there really might be a heart problem. I remember an incident very vividly that demonstrates this. It was during my own internship, and I was working in the emergency room. One night a forty-year-old man came in — very charming, articulate, well dressed — complaining of a bad stomach pain. "Maybe I have an ulcer," he said. "I've had heartburn in the past." Otherwise, he seemed fine, and was chatting away with us. We did the usual tests, and we did an EKG to check his heart, which is standard procedure. We were startled to see that his EKG was wild looking! Sure that it was a mistake, we did the EKG again. It still looked bad.

"We think you may have heart trouble," we told him. He protested that he wasn't a smoker, he ate a healthy diet, he exercised. He really didn't want to hear this. He was in the midst of trying to convince us that he just had heartburn when he started turning ashen. Before he knew it, he was in the coronary care unit with a major heart attack at age forty.

Pain is a funny thing, especially visceral, internal pain. We don't always interpret it correctly, and it can be quite difficult to accurately pinpoint its source. Visceral pain radiates, and heart attack pain radiates typically to the left arm, and down to the ring finger and the pinky sometimes, on the left hand. So if you are having sudden, overwhelming chest pains, chest pressure, or internal pain, get it checked out right away. If it turns out not to be a heart attack, count your blessings, thank the doctors, and go home and look into what may be happening with your autonomic nervous system.

This being said, there *are* cases in which heart attacks are not correctly diagnosed. This may especially happen to women who may not completely fit the classical profile for cardiovascular disease, which is based on studies of men. Make sure an EKG is taken, and if you go home and still feel pain or weakness, get a second opinion.

Angina and Other Causes of Chest Pain

A recurring or chronic chest pain, angina, can also be a sign of heart problems. This is a warning sign of future trouble and possibly of future heart attacks. Angina typically occurs with exertion: climbing a hill, climbing stairs, or doing unusually strenuous exercise. It's typically worse in colder weather — shoveling snow can trigger chest pain. However, angina sometimes occurs during rest or emotional stress. You should see your doctor if you have chronic chest pain, and your doctor will try to put this in context. A good doctor will look at your cholesterol history and ask you if you smoke, if you exercise, if you have diabetes, if there is any heart disease in your family history. He or she will go through all the coronary risk factors, eyeball you to see whether you're overweight, and then decide whether to do an EKG or a stress test. (More about these below.)

Still, several things besides heart trouble can cause chronic chest pain. One pattern that shows up very often, especially with women, is chronic chest pain that feels like angina. Along with doing an EKG, an examining doctor will press the rib cage and find that there's a great deal of tenderness in the chest wall, which can come from inflammation around the cartilage where the ribs join the sternum. This is a condition called costochondritis; it's a form of arthritis and can cause a lot of chronic discomfort.

Another problem that can cause chest pain is mitral valve prolapse, a disorder of one of the valves of the heart. It can stir up a whole range of symptoms, including chest pain and breathlessness, and it can accompany other disorders, including irritable bowel syndrome, panic episodes, and migraines. The mitral valve prevents backflow of blood into the chambers of the heart, and some people have a slight congenital variant of the normal valve structure. When you listen to the heart with a stethoscope you can hear a murmur, a sort of whooshing of blood, and this is a sign of possible mitral valve prolapse. It can be confirmed with an echocardiogram — an ultrasound reading of the heart — and is often the underlying cause of phantom sensations in the chest, breathlessness, and even panic episodes. People who have this tend to be mercurial types, with a lot of variations in energy levels and moods.

There are other causes of angina-like pain, including lung problems, severe heartburn, and some kinds of stomach problems. I'm also convinced that the old-fashioned feeling of heartache really exists, as a kind of pain or pressure or heaviness in the chest that's associated with grief, depression, or anxiety. A good doctor will consider all the possibilities. If there's no solid evidence of an alternative explanation, it's important to follow up on the possibility of heart disease.

Testing for Heart Problems: How Useful?

There are many very sophisticated tests for heart disease and some very simple ones. They can all be valuable in providing you with information about your cardiovascular health and in identifying serious problems. However, they can also serve as stepping stones for a kind of escalation of the testing process, which can lead toward the prescription of medications and procedures that are of questionable benefit. Cardiology is not just a medical specialty; it's a big business that generates millions of dollars of revenue for hospitals, surgeons, and pharmaceutical companies. A good doctor will apply some judgement in determining which tests are really necessary and how to use the information they provide.

Blood Pressure

We've already talked about testing for blood pressure, which is probably the most common test applied to your cardiovascular system. You might get a blood pressure test every time you go to a clinic, certainly every time you get a checkup. What you get is a "snapshot" of your blood pressure on that particular day, at that particular moment. You might go out, walk around the block, have a cup of coffee, come back, and get a completely different reading. While chronically high blood pressure is definitely a risk factor for heart disease, the trick with blood pressure readings is to be able to draw some conclusions from these snapshots about your long-term, habitual blood pressure.

The Electrocardiogram, or EKG

The heart has its own system for generating rhythmic electrical impulses and conducting them to different parts of the heart muscle to cause contractions. The electrical impulses spread to nearby tissues, and a small proportion of them even spread to the surface of the skin. If we place electrodes at different points on the skin, we can read these very faint impulses and amplify them to make a drawing or graph of their rhythmic patterns. This graph is called an electrocardiogram, or EKG. (The process was invented by a Dutchman, who spelled *kardio* with a *k* instead of a *c*.) The pattern of impulses recorded as an EKG can provide a lot of information about the heart. Abnormal patterns show up if the heart muscle is not receiving enough blood flow or if part of the muscle has been damaged in a heart attack. A doctor should be able to look at an EKG and tell whether you've had a heart attack, and even which part of the heart has been damaged.

It's worth mentioning that this is not a fail-safe method of identifying heart disease. You can have a "normal" electrocardiogram and drop dead as you leave the doctor's office. Usually, though, the EKG will spot gross abnormality as well as minor irregularities: certain characteristic patterns that are associated with poor circulation in the heart (coronary artery disease) and with arrhythmias (abnormal patterns of heartbeat).

When to do an EKG is currently under debate, because cost containment-minded insurers have recently challenged doctors' perogative to perform "routine" EKGs unless there is other strong evidence of a heart problem. So, generally, the test should be used to confirm the hypothesis that a person has cardiovascular disease. On the other hand, someone who is about to embark on a rigorous program of sports or exercise should probably have an EKG done because it could spot some of the anomalies that might indicate a risk of sudden cardiac arrest and death.

Some insurance companies and HMOs may also like to do a baseline EKG, so that if you ever wind up in an emergency room your normal EKG will be on file as a point of comparison, to show whether there's been any damage to the heart. The whole approach to doing EKGs is very much in flux now, partly responding to economic interests of the doctors who do it, partly to cost containment measures, and partly to medical/legal factors.

My own approach is that I don't perform EKGs routinely on patients before the age of forty who are not about to embark on arduous exercise. After forty, I think a routine EKG every five years is reasonable, and it's certainly indicated if there are any symptoms of chest pain, or angina, or palpitations, or a finding of high blood pressure that might strain the heart.

The Stress Test

The EKG is a little like a blood pressure reading — it provides a snapshot of your heart patterns at one short period of time. It describes how you function when you're at rest. The stress test overcomes this limitation by looking at the behavior of your heart while you are exercising, and putting it under stress. It usually involves exercising on a treadmill, while the doctor or a technician monitors your blood pressure and EKG patterns and observes you for any chest pain or shortness of breath.

Sometimes a person who is elderly or handicapped, has lung problems, or is in poor physical condition can't exercise hard enough to challenge the heart. In this case, we give a substance that causes chemical constriction of the arteries and replicates the stress conditions of exercise.

A stress test provides an even more accurate picture of cardiovascular health than the EKG, and it will confirm or contradict a diagnosis of heart trouble. If you have been sedentary for years, have a history of smoking or high cholesterol, and are about to embark on a program of heavy exercise, your doctor may want to do a stress test to see how your heart will perform. On the other hand, if you are gradually building up your exercise program, you are really performing your own daily stress test by building up to the level of heart rate that could create breathlessness or chest pain. If you have some risk factors for heart disease, or even if you've just been sedentary for a long time, you should always start out gradually with your exercise anyway. The stress test would really be superfluous. Its real value is in pinning down reasons for chronic pain or checking out the heart condition of somebody with serious risk factors.

A refinement of the stress test, the thallium stress test, gives an even more subtle picture of possible heart disease. It involves injecting thallium, a radioactive isotope, into the bloodstream and observing exactly where the blood flows into the different parts of the heart muscle, to identify areas that may be poorly supplied with blood and to indicate coronary artery disease. This is particularly valuable when a chest pain is hard to pin down — is it rib cage pain, an ulcer, the esophagus, or the heart? A regular stress test result might be normal, but the more sensitive thallium stress test could reveal that there is some ischemia, or lack of circulation.

Coronary Angiograms

The current standard in testing for heart disease is the angiogram, also known as cardiac catheterization. This is an expensive, high-tech test that's done in an operating theater by a cardiologist. Dye is injected directly into the main coronary artery, and X-ray pictures are taken that show the dyed blood making its way through the arteries that supply blood to the heart. It's possible to see how well blood is getting to the heart muscle, whether any areas are undersupplied, and how constricted the coronary arteries may be. It's a very popular test among cardiologists and generates income for specialists and hospitals. This test will confirm a diagnosis of heart disease already made, it. Unfortunately, there is a subjective component to interpreting test results. Different radiologists can interpret the same tests quite differently: one will say the patient has 80 percent blockage of the arteries; another will say 50 percent. The future may give us more objective ways of analyzing angiograms, perhaps through computer analysis. Right now this is a test that can produce equivocal results.

A more serious issue about angiograms is whether they really help us treat patients any better and whether they contribute anything to the patient's long-term health. I think there's a real question about the way the medical system is "selling" these tests and procedures. People get put on the cardiac conveyor belt, and it just carries them along from procedure to procedure. Now I certainly don't mean to say that angiograms and surgery are pointless and people should just be given a vitamin. Still, we do about four times as many angioplasties and coronary artery bypass grafts as the Canadians and the British, and we don't have any better statistics in terms of coronary heart disease mortality. Our highly touted "best medical system in the world" is not producing better results through all these procedures. Studies comparing accessibility of high-tech medical care from region to region across the country show that the decision to test is the most important determinant of the decision to treat with angioplasty or bypass, and that patients' insurance coverage and the number of cardiologists and cardiothoracic surgeons in their locale are the biggest influences on who gets care.

Tests and Alternative Tests

Some expensive but useful high-tech tests are available that are relatively noninvasive. The Ultrafast CAT scan will reveal the degree of calcification of coronary arteries. It's a static snapshot, but a series of CAT scans will suggest whether coronary disease is advancing. The PET scan shows actual heart metabolism. It's a flow test that tags glucose with a radioisotope marker, and it shows where the heart cells are alive and metabolizing and where they're not.

A good prelude to expensive PET scans and angiography is one fairly simple test that any doctor can do. It involves checking the blood pressure at various points along the legs to find out whether the circulation declines on the way to the feet. If it does, there is a very high likelihood of hidden heart disease, because people who have blockage of the arteries in their legs have a much greater frequency of problems with their heart. This is called a plethysmogram test, and I do it for many of my older patients to screen them for heart disease. It can be supported by a Doppler test, which can show blockages in the arteries of the legs or the carotid arteries in the neck (where it can also indicate risk for stroke). These tests are part of the burgeoning science of noninvasive diagnostics of the circulatory system. Such tests are important, because they can highlight early development of atherosclerosis, before it becomes advanced. They are not tests that you can just infer risk from, like the cholesterol test. Because they are noninvasive, they don't put you in the hospital setting where specialists are waiting to do surgery.

Other Problems, Other Tests

Not everyone with heart problems has atherosclerosis, or has atherosclerosis alone. Several tests can indicate other kinds of problems. The echocardiogram produces an image of the chambers of the heart and can help with the diagnosis of congestive heart failure, which tends to be an older person's problem. It's usually the result of chronic high blood pressure or repeated heart attacks that have damaged the heart muscle. Compromised blood flow could also result in arrhythmia, an abnormal heartbeat, running first slow and then too fast, or in an irregular rhythm. You can hear it with a stethoscope, and it will also show up on an EKG or on a Holter monitor, which records the heartbeat for 24 hours or more at a time.

Treatments: The Good, The Bad, the Alternatives

If tests do show some heart disease, a whole array of treatments is available, ranging from simple diet-and-exercise plans to fancy drugs and high-tech surgery. Let's look at some of what's out there, including both the conventional medical treatments and some of the alternatives.

"Medical Management" and the Drugstore

When doctors use the term medical management, they mean drug therapy as distinct from surgery. All too often, drug therapy starts with cholesterol-lowering drugs, and we are witnessing the advent of a lucrative cholesterol-lowering industry. Many doctors are going overboard on drug therapy. I recently saw a young woman in my office who had a cholesterol count of 237 and an HDL of 45. The ratio may not have been perfect, but her doctor had recommended Zocor, a cholesterol-lowering drug, before even talking to her about diet and exercise.

These drugs do have an effect. Studies show that they can be used in reversing heart disease. Whether that reversal occurs at a cost to other organ systems is not really clear. There are rare side effects in some patients, including liver damage, muscle degeneration, muscle pain, and, rarely, sleep disturbances. When hundreds of thousands of people, perhaps millions of people, are taking these drugs, many of them will experience the side effects. We don't know enough about their long-term effects, over years and years. These drugs are often used in preference to low-tech, free therapies such as diet change. They are easy for doctors, who don't have to spend as much time talking to their patients, and they are backed by a big marketing effort.

How have cholesterol-lowering drugs become so strongly positioned? Doctors have been successfully pitched with medical studies, some partially financed by the very companies that manufacture cholesterol medications. One oft-quoted study concluded that it was possible to modulate cholesterol only about 5 percent with dietary modification, whereas a popular "statin" drug could produce a 15 percent reduction. In my practice, however, I have patients who routinely drop their cholesterol by 80, 100, or 120 points — way over 15 percent. Why do studies show such poor results of diet change? The diet they used was the American Heart Association diet for cholesterol reduction, which is a low-fat, cholesterol-free diet, but with minimal restrictions on carbohydrate intake or on sugar intake. This is not the diet I prescribe.

I think there is no question that a low-tech, low-cost approach to cholesterol management is nearly always preferable to cholesterol-lowering drugs.

Some people have hereditary problems that cause unusually high cholesterol, and they are the ones who can benefit from those drugs. They should
not be popular drugs; they should be used very sparingly for rare genetic
syndromes and the like. They should be sold to perhaps 200,000 Americans
at most, not to the millions who are taking them today. A good diet, good
nutrition, and exercise not only are just as effective in improving your
cardiovascular health but are good for every system in the body. The side
effects and long-term effects are only positive.

Crisis Management with Drugs

Another group of drugs that don't have anything to do with cholesterol is
prescribed for heart patients. They include nitrates, beta-blockers, and
calcium channel blockers.

Beta-blockers, commonly prescribed for hypertension, work by preventing the heart from building up to a pace that will increase blood pressure. As
we've noted, they also have problematic side effects, and prevent the
cardiovascular system from gaining the benefits of exercise. To someone
who is recovering from a heart attack, they provide a safety net, but long-
term use has problems. One British study of people with stable angina
showed that a careful, gradual program of exercise was just as effective as
beta blockers, after one year, in correcting angina — the exercise was reversing the heart disease, not just masking it.[44]

Nitrates are also prescribed for people who are recovering from a heart
attack or who have severe pain from angina. Nitroglycerine comes in long-
acting pills or patches and in quick-acting sublingual (under the tongue)
doses. It works by dilating the blood vessels and can be a useful safety valve
to protect against severe angina, if you are embarking on a long-term diet-
and-exercise reversal program. It is among the most effective drugs available, though it's no substitute for nondrug reversal efforts.

Calcium channel blockers make up another class of blood vessel dilators,
which are prescribed for high blood pressure and for angina. They will also
prevent vasospasm, sudden contractions of the blood vessels, which cause
nearly as many heart attacks and strokes as blood clots, especially in people
with constricted arteries and high blood pressure. Low magnesium levels
and high levels of the stress-induced hormones in the bloodstream can
increase the risk of vasospasm.

Calcium blockers work because calcium is a messenger substance that
can induce spasms, and blocking the calcium messenger keeps the blood
vessels dilated. The drugs have few side effects, though they sometimes
cause constipation, dizziness, and fatigue.

An alternative approach is to use magnesium supplements, because calcium and magnesium both compete for the same receptor sites in smooth

muscle. When calcium lands in those sites it induces spasm, but magnesium doesn't. If high enough levels of magnesium are maintained in the blood, the magnesium will land in those sites in place of the calcium and prevent the spasms in the same way that calcium blockers do. This supports the idea that magnesium supplements can play a role in preventing heart disease. Calcium/magnesium supplements normally come with a higher proportion of calcium, about two to one. When I am treating a patient with advanced heart disease, though, I reverse the normal ratio and give, perhaps, 800 milligrams of magnesium with 300 to 400 milligrams of calcium.

It's not unusual for doctors to prescribe all three categories of drugs for someone who has suffered a heart attack or is having severe angina. They may also prescribe aspirin, which acts as a blood thinner and prevents blood clots. A beta-blocker slows down the heart to reduce its oxygen demand, nitroglycerine dilates the blood vessels, a calcium channel blocker will prevent spasms, and aspirin will prevent clotting. This combination is usually very effective in a crisis and will provide a temporary safety net until the patient can begin a diet-and-exercise reversal program.

Surgical Procedures

Cardiac surgery is a big business that generates a lot of income for specialists and hospitals. There are two principal procedures that take place in the operating room: balloon angioplasty and coronary artery bypass.

Balloon angioplasty is not strictly a surgical procedure, though it's done in an operating room. The cardiologist inserts a balloon catheter in a cardiac artery and pumps up the balloon so that it expands and dilates the constricted artery. The catheter is then deflated and removed. The problem with angioplasty is that the artery can constrict again. This is called reocclusion, and there's about a 50 percent chance of its happening within the first year. The rate of reocclusion is so high that cardiologists have convened emergency conferences to look at the problem. The search is on among pharmaceutical firms for the ideal drug to prevent reocclusion. Oddly, one of the few things that've been demonstrated to have any effect in preventing reocclusion has been fish oil, which helps, but not in a spectacular way. However, there are other reasons why fish oil can help prevent heart disease, as we've seen.

The other option for the cardiologist is bypass surgery, which uses small grafts from a long vein of the leg or an artery of the chest to bypass obstructed arteries in the heart and thus to supply peripheral coronary arteries beyond the blockages. Bypass surgery can relieve the pain of angina and extend life if the coronary arteries are not too damaged. If only a single artery is obstructed, a cardiologist will usually try angioplasty. Bypass surgery is appropriate for two types of patients: those with multiple blockages in several arteries, posing at least the theoretical risk of heart attack, and those who have a lot of pain that the drugs can't alleviate. If someone is suffering a lot of chest pain, can't walk around town, and can't make love, then bypass could make a material difference. Diet and exercise may effect some reversal, but it may take several years before quality of life is improved.

A sure sign of the impending need for bypass is "pump failure." When people with this condition exercise or put stress on the heart their blood pressure falls instead of going up, and their heart may actually reduce its output. They may not feel pain while exercising, but the heart may not keep up. This is a very ominous sign, and these people are at high risk for death. They are also good candidates for bypass surgery.

Surgery can be a lifesaver to someone who has a severe heart problem that can't be managed through drugs. On the other hand, if the problem can be managed with medication alone, that buys time for a reversal program.

But the medical establishment mounts enormous pressure on patients to go through with these procedures. It usually starts with an angiogram test, the first step on the conveyor belt to more procedures. Heart patients feel threatened and vulnerable, and they tend to agree to the surgery that the cardiologist recommends, even though it may not ultimately improve their long-term prognosis. Not too many cardiologists will stop and say "Don't just stand there — do nothing."

The truth is that angiograms, angioplasty, and bypass surgery are not always in the best interests of patients. There have been interesting studies of the long-term effects of these procedures. In one followup study of patients recommended for angiograms, but who did not have them, the mortality rate was remarkably low, and only 3 to 16 percent were later judged to need angiograms or further testing. The study concluded that angiograms could be deferred for medically stable patients with predictable symptoms during exercise and without a significant drop in blood pressure during a stress test.[45]

Other studies of the long-term benefits of bypass surgery show that it usually relieves the symptoms of angina, but even the bypass grafts tend to constrict and close up over time unless the patient undergoes a radical change in lifestyle. One study compared a group of patients who underwent surgery for angina to a group that had only medication therapy. Though the surgery seemed to be more beneficial at first, the differences began to diminish after five years. Eighteen years after treatment, the survival rates were roughly equal.[46] Another major study criticized the system whereby patients are referred and treated, noting that often it's the same physician who does the diagnostic angiogram, recommends the surgical procedure, and finally judges its success. Nicolas Danchin in an article in *The Lancet* noted that angioplasty itself has "ballooned" from a few dozen cases in the late 1970s to several hundred thousand currently, with a huge increase in health costs, and doubtful benefits for the long-term outlook or well-being of the patients.

Danchin noted that the heart can actually sustain some degree of occlusion or blocking off of smaller arteries, without a heart attack being precipitated. To a certain extent, the heart can compensate by rerouting capillaries around the blockage, a process called collateralization. Danchin suggested that correcting the occlusion could remove the impetus toward this natural rerouting of the capillaries, and that there were very limited data on the effectiveness of angioplasty. While the data seem to show initial improvement in exercise tolerance in some patients, there is a definite risk that the procedure itself can trigger a heart attack. The study concluded that the procedures might help symptoms but showed relatively little long-term health benefit, and it suggested that cardiologists and surgeons drop the "scare techniques" they used to sell these procedures.[47]

Reversal Alternatives: The Diet Plans

It's Dr. Dean Ornish, of course, who has really popularized the idea of reversing heart disease through diet and has even convinced some of the major health insurers to cover his program. Dr. Ornish's plan has three main components: a vegetarian diet that is very low in fat, guided exercise, and an active support group in which others on the plan meet together and discuss their commitment, their progress, their difficulties, and so on. I think the real genius of his plan is the support group. It's not easy to make major changes in diet and lifestyle, and most doctors don't even expect their patients to do that. They think it's just too hard, and they move quickly on to medications and procedures. I think one reason for Dr. Ornish's good results is the good psychological support.

I take a similar approach with my patients. I give them a detailed diet plan, talk over their exercise plan, and have them come in so I can monitor their progress. I *work* with them, and I see people go through amazing turnarounds. They drop their cholesterol levels by amazing amounts, they give up smoking, they start and maintain active exercise programs, and many adopt yoga or meditation.

There are some differences in what I prescribe for reversing heart disease. With my Salad and Salmon Diet I encourage more of the beneficial oils in the diet, especially fish oil and olive oil. I play down the very high levels of carbohydrates, because there are risks involved. Too much carbohydrate can lead to glucose overload, insulin resistance, and Syndrome X. Unlike Ornish, I also add nutrient and vitamin supplements to the prescription because of the abundant evidence that nutrients like antioxidants, magnesium, and essential fatty acids can play a role in preventing or reversing heart disease.

There are many nuances to the issue of diet and nutrients, and we've got to accept that this is a complex area with no simple, ideological answers. Dean Ornish contends, for example, that the best diet is one that is high in complex carbohydrates, devoid of oil, devoid of animal protein, because that is what will lower the cholesterol. However, I've noticed a certain phenomenon in people who are following a very radical vegetarian diet. They will definitely lower their cholesterol, but their HDL will drop to a pretty low figure too. Their triglycerides will remain intermediate — sometimes at 160 or 180, sometimes overtaking their cholesterol. This is the result of a very high proportion of carbohydrates in the diet.

It has been shown, however, that certain types of vegetable protein, such as soy protein, have cholesterol-lowering effects. It may be that a vegetarian diet, which relies heavily on protein from legumes, is beneficial not only because it's lower in fat but because the protein itself does something favorable to the metabolism of fats. We've got to remain open-minded about this very complex issue of diet and cardiovascular health. We have to keep following the research and avoid being ideological about it. I too used to support the idea of a diet that is very low in fats and very high in complex carbohydrates. But I think we know more about this now, and more about the value of specific supplemental nutrients. Intelligent medicine draws on everything we know.

This is why I propose the Salad and Salmon Diet as the model diet for cardiovascular health. It is a diet that does emphasize complex carbohydrates from whole grains. It deemphasizes flour products, even whole-grain pasta and whole-grain bread, because their glycemic index is high — they raise blood sugar levels very quickly and generate a lot of insulin, which leads to problems. It also deemphasizes fruits, which contain a lot of sugar, for the same reason. It includes the beneficial omega-3 oil and the monounsaturated oils, like olive oil. It emphasizes lots of vegetables, to provide fiber, which can work in several ways to reduce heart disease. Finally, I think the Salad and Salmon Diet is a little easier for some people to switch to than a strict no-fat vegetarian diet; it does contain some animal protein, and some oils. This doesn't mean everyone should be on the Salad and Salmon Diet, but I think it is the best approach for people with cardiovascular disease or risk of disease.

Whatever your diet choices, there's one element that ought to be some-how included, and that's fiber. As noted earlier in the chapter, dietary fiber is associated with lowered cholesterol levels. Remember that cholesterol is a primary component of bile, secreted into the stomach? Well, fiber tends to act literally as a sponge for cholesterol in the bile, soaking it up so that it will pass through the GI tract and be excreted rather than absorbed back into the bloodstream through the intestinal wall.

Nutritional Supplements: A Key Support System

Throughout this chapter we've accumulated tips about nutritional supplements. Here's a master list summarizing the supplements that are key in preventing heart disease.

Vitamin C	Helpful in preventing arteriosclerosis. Recommended: 1000 milligrams daily.
Mixed carotenoids	Excellent antioxidants shown to reduce the likelihood of arteriosclerosis. Recommended: 25,000 International Units daily.
Vitamin E	Extremely helpful for reducing the stickiness of platelets and improving blood flow. It also tends to slow the progression of arteriosclerosis and may have something to do with reversing it. Recommended: 400 to 800 International Units daily.
EPA Fish oil	A natural blood thinner. Recommended: two or three 1000-milligram capsules twice daily.
L-carnitine	A natural agent for helping to promote energy production in the cardiac muscle cells. Recommended: one 500- to 1000-milligram capsule twice daily.
Co-enzyme Q10	Another catalyst for energy production in the cardiac muscles. Recommended: 100 to 400 milligrams daily.
Calcium	With magnesium, helps control blood pressure. Recommended: 400 milligrams daily.
Magnesium	Plays a role in preventing arterial spasm. Recommended: 400 to 800 milligrams in chelated form daily; or magnesium citrate, 200 milligrams twice daily.

Chelation — An Alternative Treatment

One of the most dramatic ways of reversing advanced atherosclerosis is chelation. It doesn't work with every patient, but it often gives remarkable results. Added to diet changes, exercise, and nutritional supplements, chelation can greatly accelerate the reversal process. A chelator is a substance that tends to pull minerals and metals out of the body. Since calcium deposits are a major factor in the hardening of arteries with atherosclerosis, anything that removes the calcium deposits will start to improve this condition. How does chelation therapy work? A solution of vitamins, minerals, and a chelator is infused into the bloodstream through an intravenous drip. The chelating substance picks up the calcium from the arterial plaque, and it's passed out of the body in the urine. The chelator also picks up heavy metals like lead and cadmium, that may be generating free radicals or affecting kidney health and blood pressure. Patients usually undergo twenty to fifty chelation treatments over several weeks or months. Each treatment lasts several hours, during which patients can read or watch a movie.

Remember Josef, from the very beginning of this chapter? He was the busy classical musician who had been crippled at the height of his career by severe atherosclerosis. With frequent chest pain, and with his career nearly at a standstill, Josef had already undergone two angioplasties and was grudgingly considering bypass surgery when he came to me. I was literally his last resort.

I set him up with a diet and supplement plan and proposed chelation therapy as an alternative to surgery. He gladly agreed to try it. Initially, he didn't feel any better, even after six or eight chelations. I told him to persevere — that we were trying to fix a condition that had been building up for years. By the twelfth or fourteenth chelation he was feeling so much better that he was able to reduce his other medication. Josef was very happy with this, because he was taking nitrates, beta blockers, and calcium channel blockers. The medications were making him tired all the time, and he was taking such high dosages that his blood pressure sometimes dropped to the point where he felt dizzy and weak. Josef continued with the chelation, and after thirty treatments he was feeling splendid. We didn't completely discontinue medications; he continued to take low-dose calcium channel blockers to prevent coronary artery spasm. However, we were able to taper him off the fatiguing nitrates and beta-blockers. Now, after a total of about forty-five chelations, he regularly comes in once a month, and he's resumed his high-powered schedule, teaching privately, performing regularly, and doing volunteer concerts for children. I still ask him to slow down a little.

To back up the chelation therapy, we also modified Josef's diet and gave him a regimen of vitamin supplements. Interestingly, his cholesterol had never been that high, averaging around 185, but he did have a very low level of HDL, which had been overlooked as a potential cause of problems. His cholesterol was originally about 185, but his HDL was only about 24 — a ratio of almost 8:1. We got his cholesterol down to about 165 and his HDL up to about 38, for a 4:1 ratio. He's also lighter. Though he wasn't really heavy to begin with, he's now shed 12 to 15 pounds — a spry fellow, full of energy. He is doing really well, with much less medication, and he's very happy to have gotten off the conveyor belt that was putting him through the repeated medical procedures and leading toward surgery, with a new scar to confirm his membership in "the zipper club." Those procedures, and the likelihood of surgery, were stopping him in his tracks and were quite likely to have pushed him into retirement.

FACTS ABOUT CHELATION THERAPY

Chelation therapy must be performed by an experienced practitioner. Since the chelator is excreted by the kidneys, the possibility of kidney damage is a concern and the procedure must be closely monitored. Minerals and nutrients may also bind with the chelator, so their levels must be carefully checked and controlled through supplementation. Chelation must be done slowly over 3 to 4 hours. Too much fluid at too fast a rate might cause an increase in blood volume and a fluid overload, which could be a problem, particularly in patients with serious heart disease. Oddly enough, the magnesium in the chelation bottle might cause the opposite: a drop in blood pressure. That's why all patients must be closely supervised.

To safeguard against possible problems, blood and urine tests are taken before chelation to check kidney function. Cardiac function is evaluated through a stress test and an echocardiogram. After every few chelations, blood tests are repeated. The patient is advised to eat a good meal before the treatment, and blood pressure is monitored before and after each infusion. At least 16 ounces of water must be drunk during the treatment to flush the kidneys.

You can find a doctor certified in chelation techniques by calling ACAM, the American College for Advancement in Medicine, at (714) 583-7666. They can be reached by mail at 23121 Verdugo Drive, Suite 204, Laguna Hills, California 92653, or view their website at www.acam.org

I've seen chelation work wonders in many other patients. One was Bill, seventy years old and retired, who was enjoying his daily walks until he began to feel severe pain in his calves while walking. This kind of pain, claudication, is the result of poor circulation in the legs due to constricted arteries. The pain got so bad that Bill couldn't walk more than a block at a time. Now Bill knew he was developing circulatory problems. He had been seeing a vascular surgeon, who had monitored him repeatedly over the years and noticed a modest but steady deterioration in the blood flow to his legs. At Bill's most recent visit, the specialist had observed a striking dropoff in circulation — a rapid deterioration. This doctor suggested that Bill begin to think about either angioplasty or a bypass graft to the arteries in his legs.

Bill didn't like the idea of surgery, and he came to me for alternative therapy. I prescribed a change in diet, since he did have a high cholesterol level, and also prescribed some specific nutrients, including vitamin E, fish oil, and magnesium. Bill also started a chelation program, and after about fifteen sessions he noticed he could walk a little farther. By the thirtieth chelation, Bill could walk long distances without pain, and by the fortieth treatment, he told me he was virtually free of leg pain. He was able to spend his afternoons in pleasant walks all over the city, visiting museums, and walking through the parks.

After several months, Bill reminded me that he was due for a checkup with his vascular surgeon. I encouraged him to go see the doctor, but I said, "Look, don't mention that you've undergone chelation therapy and let's just see what he has to say. I'd like to know if the subjective results that you feel are matched by his objective evaluation." One afternoon I got a call from the vascular surgeon, whom I happened to know. He sounded very excited over the phone. He said, "I've got Bill here; he says that he's been seeing you. What the heck have you been doing with him?" I said, "Why do you ask?" He said, "We're seeing the darnedest thing here. We really never see this. He had virtually complete occlusion of his blood vessels, and now he's got substantial flow. We were looking at a steady, progressive deterioration in his circulation, and now it suddenly looks as if it's actually getting better." I said, "That's really interesting—I've been doing chelation therapy." The doctor got so excited about this that he accompanied me to a conference on chelation therapy and copresented Bill's case to a group of five hundred interested doctors. Since then he's become very supportive of this therapy and refers patients to me.

A Look to the Future

The good news is that the rate of heart disease continues to drop as more and more Americans become aware of the importance of diet and exercise in prevention. We can look to the future for more sophisticated and more accurate blood tests to check for the different fats and lipoproteins in the blood, and to identify subtle risk factors, including genetic factors. Within ten years or so, you should be able to go into your doctor's office and get a blood test that will not only tell you your current risk profile but also identify your genetic predisposition to cardiovascular disease, whether high or low.

While high-tech medicine has clear contributions to make in this area, it seems that right now the low-tech approach of diet, exercise, and lifestyle adjustment is much more effective in preventing and reversing disease. I expect that as more researchers look into the nuances of diet and nutrition, we will be able to use these tools in an even more sophisticated way. Even now there is much we can do, both to prevent and to reverse heart disease, without expensive surgical procedures. The key element is your willingness to get involved and take a proactive stance. I like to say that the most important organ for heart health is your brain: how much attention and intelligence you're ready to bring to bear on the reality of the risks to heart health in our culture and environment, and how ready you are to develop a rational life plan that will minimize those risks.

CHAPTER THIRTEEN

Breath of Life:
The Respiratory System

Do I risk getting emphysema like my aging mother, even though I don't smoke? If I smoked but stopped, am I still likely to have serious lung problems? Do the lungs deteriorate as part of the aging process? Can I get asthma in my forties? How much should I worry about environmental pollutants if I drive on the highway and breathe in diesel fuel every day? Will the fumes from fresh paint and a new carpet at the office affect my lungs? These are the kinds of question my patients sometimes ask, reflecting their concern with maintaining healthy lungs. Fortunately, we do not generally deal with life-threatening diseases in this area, except for those who smoke.

In the nineteenth and early twentieth centuries, respiratory diseases provided one of the main exit scenarios for both old and young. People frequently died of pneumonia, tuberculosis, and influenza, all of which have been largely conquered. The respiratory system has been a site of major advances and success stories in modern medical science, and is now a battleground of diseases that are bothersome but usually not killers.

What do we need to be concerned about, then? Smokers are still setting themselves up for the few lethal diseases that do attack the lungs: emphysema, which so weakens the lungs that they can no longer oxygenate the blood, and lung cancer. We are still relatively helpless in the face of allergies, but we are discovering more useful therapies. Asthma, often set off by allergies, is another problem. Worse, we are discovering new strains of old diseases, such as TB, that are resistant to all the antibiotics commonly in use and can be treated only by combinations of several extremely expensive, synthetic drugs.

Unless you are struck by a lethal disease, you normally are not aware of any lung damage because of the body's natural reserve system. Smokers, for example, may not notice any physical changes until they lose 50 percent of their lung capacity. Similarly, only extreme environmental exposure produces measurable changes in pulmonary function.

Conscientious nonsmokers should take note that a poor diet can also produce lung disease. A recently published study shows that a diet high in saturated fats correlates with a higher risk of lung cancer among women who do not smoke, either actively or passively. (High levels of saturated fat in the diet correlate with other types of cancer as well.)

There are other nutritional aspects to healthy lungs. In fact, we can offer here the supplementary "recipe" that supports healthy epithelial tissue, which includes the tissue of the mouth, throat, and skin. Note that these dosages are not in addition to those given on page 408, but contained within them.

- Vitamin C: 1000 milligrams per day
- Vitamin E: 800 International Units per day
- Mixed carotenoids: 25,000 International Units per day
- Vitamin A retinol: 25,000 International Units per day (but no more than 5000 International Units daily in case of pregnancy)
- Selenium: 100 micrograms twice daily
- Zinc: 30 milligrams twice daily
- Folic acid: 1 milligram twice daily
- Flaxseed oil: 1 tablespoon twice daily

Respiratory Diseases

The idea of the respiratory tree explains the similarity of many respiratory diseases to one another. We can visualize the respiratory system as an upside-down tree, with its roots in the sinuses, the trachea or windpipe as the trunk, the bronchi as the two main branches of the lungs, and the many branching bronchioles as the smaller internal branches of the lungs, bearing the "leaves" of the alveoli, which are little air sacs where oxygen diffuses into the blood and carbon dioxide diffuses out. In the normal adult, the total surface area of the lungs is huge: some 50 to 100 square meters, or about the floor area of a 25-foot by 30-foot room. The surface tissue of the air passages and the lungs is all physically connected, from the sinuses to the bronchi to the inner lining of the lungs. Bacteria and viruses can easily travel from one part of the tree to another, spreading infection. Gravity can pull a postnasal drip of infectious material into the lungs, causing bronchial infection or pneumonia. Colds, flus, sinusitis, bronchitis, and pneumonia are thus interrelated and often intercausal. A chronic mucous congestion can create the perfect trap and incubation environment for bacterial growth. The congestion keeps the mucous membranes inflamed, thereby reducing the local immune response. This explains how someone can have chronic sinusitis and asthma at the same time, both of which have allergic, infectious, and inflammatory components. The two most common respiratory infections are sinusitis and bronchitis.

Sinusitis is a chronic inflammation of the nasal passages. It can cause fatigue, headaches, and eye and teeth problems, and can lead to serious bacterial infection. Problems with the upper teeth can precipitate sinusitis, which can in turn bring on a bacterial infection in the lungs. Sinusitis can also be a frequent cause of bronchitis, because it acts as a nursery for certain bacteria that drop into inaccessible recesses of the lungs and create infections.

Bronchitis is an inflammation, either acute or chronic, of the bronchial tubes or part of them, caused by infection or occasionally allergies. Just as sinusitis can lead to bronchitis, bronchitis can lead to pneumonia, which is an inflammation or infection of the lungs themselves. Pneumonia is now a kind of historical anachronism, and we generally see it only in cases of extreme immune suppression, medical neglect, or environmentally caused lung damage. "Galloping" pneumonia can so weaken the whole system that it becomes susceptible to other bacterial infections. But this is rare. On the other hand, all of us have to deal with that most persistent and annoying of respiratory diseases, the common cold. Not just a nuisance, a cold can be the precursor of more serious infections, so it makes sense to start here with a long-term approach to respiratory health.

Why Can't We Cure the Cold?

It's the old nagging question: if we can put a man on the moon, why can't modern science find a cure for the common cold? The common cold and flu are still on the frontiers of medicine, right up there with the some of the more serious illnesses. While there's not a lot of funding for research into the common cold, incredible sums of money are spent on developing and advertising cold remedies, many of which are of limited or no value. In fact, some conventional treatments may have long-term debilitating effects. Decongestants in the form of nasal sprays are among the worst offenders. People who use sprays may develop a condition known as medically induced chronic rhinitis, or rhinitis medicamentosa. The nasal mucosa become dependent on the decongestant agent and become soggy and swollen when they don't get it. People can develop a physical addiction to the spray. These decongestants can cause mucous tissue to weaken, actually increasing susceptibility to bacteria. The drying action itself is counterproductive. During an infection, the sinus membranes actively secrete mucus to slough off infectious agents. Decongestants, whether oral or spray, can actually prolong the course of a viral infection by drying out these membranes. I do a daily radio show, so I'm tempted to use decongestants on occasion to avoid the nasal tone that's a dead giveaway for a cold. But I've sworn off them for good because the congestion returns in greater force when I stop using them.

My first step with patients who have chronic or lingering colds is to explore possible causes of the disease: the chemical or pollutant environment of the patient, history of allergies and infections, general immune health. Doctors often prescribe antibiotics rather freely in these cases, on the theory that the original cold virus has weakened the system and opened the door for a bacterial infection. It's important to note, however, that antibiotics have zero effect against viral infections and that every antibiotic treatment increases the risk of antibiotic resistance in the body, which can come into play when an antibiotic is needed to fight some much more serious illnesses. It's true, though, that a pocket of chronic bacterial infection can seed the lung and persist unrecognized, causing repeated chronic infections. I've had good success with antibiotic therapy in specialized cases, but this is not something to undertake lightly. If there has been "bad weather" in the respiratory tract—an allergic component, pollutants, smoking, or a virus—a patient has no business using antibiotics.

For chronic colds, I investigate whether the patient is iron-deficient, is allergic to dust or milk, or consumes too much sugar. Elevated sugar intake can raise the blood sugar, which can weaken the activity of phagocytes, the cells that pursue and devour foreign invaders like a cold virus. Often people think they have a healthy diet, but they are loading themselves with sugar by drinking too many fruit drinks or eating oat-bran muffins sweetened with fruit juice and raisins for breakfast every morning.

Also, I check to see whether the patient may have an overgrowth of intestinal yeast, which could cause a cycle of respiratory infections. Some researchers believe that *Candida*, a common yeast that travels in the human intestine, can release substances that the body finds foreign and therefore trigger a wide range of allergic symptoms. Connecting *Candida* to the common cold is unpopular in the medical profession because *Candida* growth is promoted by the use of antibiotics, steroids, antacids, and hormones, all of which are mainstream treatments. Diet and natural or prescription antifungals can correct the yeast problem. (See chapter 9 on the gastrointestinal tract for details on treating *Candida* infection.)

Zinc has recently been discovered as a means to shorten the duration and reduce the symptoms of the common cold. This effect was discovered by accident when a doctor in Austin, Texas, switched zinc lozenges for the zinc capsules he had prescribed to a three-year-old girl to correct a zinc deficiency. The child suddenly ceased having her chronic symptoms of a constant runny nose and frequent colds. A followup study in Texas gave zinc lozenges or placebos to 146 volunteers with colds. Those taking the placebo averaged 10.8 days of infection; those taking the zinc lozenges averaged 3.9 days with reduced symptoms. Twenty percent of the subjects recovered completely within one day!

DOSAGE FOR COLD SUPPRESSION: 180-milligram lozenges of zinc gluconate (each containing 20 to 23 milligrams of elemental zinc), up to twelve tablets a day until symptoms cease, or up to 7 days.

Finally, our attitude toward antibiotics and respiratory infections is shifting. Some cases clearly call for massive doses of antibiotics, but in many cases I prescribe "WW," the "watchful waiting" method, which is becoming the byword for how we deal with a lot of medical conditions. Over and over again, statistical analyses of various treatments and therapies show that conservative management, or simply doing nothing, correlates with a long-term health outcome that's as good as or better than more invasive treatments. Antibiotic therapy runs the risk of creating yeast infections, diarrhea, rashes, allergic problems, and increasing resistance to antibiotics. Simple bed rest is a powerful tool against all kinds of respiratory infections and can often give better results, without lingering side effects, than other treatments.

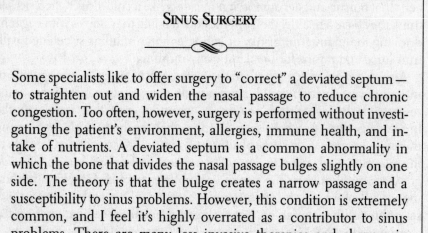

SINUS SURGERY

Some specialists like to offer surgery to "correct" a deviated septum — to straighten out and widen the nasal passage to reduce chronic congestion. Too often, however, surgery is performed without investigating the patient's environment, allergies, immune health, and intake of nutrients. A deviated septum is a common abnormality in which the bone that divides the nasal passage bulges slightly on one side. The theory is that the bulge creates a narrow passage and a susceptibility to sinus problems. However, this condition is extremely common, and I feel it's highly overrated as a contributor to sinus problems. There are many less invasive therapies and changes in lifestyle that should be explored before surgery is undertaken that may be of questionable benefit.

Allergies

Every spring and summer finds millions of Americans carefully tracking the pollen count just as they do the weather report, staying indoors with windows shut on beautiful days, suffering itchy eyes, runny noses, and congestion. People know it when they have respiratory allergies—or do they? While hay fever is a high-profile allergy, millions more people may suffer from unidentified allergies that contribute to chronic nasal congestion, frequent colds, bronchitis, or asthma outside the pollen season.

As we've noted in chapter 4, allergies are caused by an overactive immune response. The immune system reacts to something that isn't otherwise harmful, called an allergen, and starts producing large numbers of antibodies. The typical antibody that's released in an allergic reaction is a special type, immunoglobulin E, or IgE. IgE signals other cells of the immune system to release a compound called histamine. Histamine is a normal component of cells, but in the allergic reaction it circulates in high amounts through the bloodstream, where it constricts small muscles around air passages, increases the flow of mucus, and causes some blood vessels to contract and others to relax and leak fluid into tissues. Hay fever brings about a runny nose and fluid in the windpipe, and the resulting coughs and sneezes are an attempt to expel the allergens from the breathing passages. With asthma, constricting muscles in the windpipe can choke off the flow of air.

The first medical reports of allergic reactions came out of nineteenth-century industrial England. Allergies are, possibly, a byproduct of the Industrial Revolution and the polluted air that came with it. A polluted environment contributes to a person's overall sensitivity to allergies, making symptoms worse if not directly inducing an allergic reaction. A British study has demonstrated that nitrogen oxides and ozone, the main components of automobile exhaust and also byproducts of burning natural gas, increase the production of symptom-causing immune compounds and may increase susceptibility to allergens. The result is more sneezing and coughing. Automobile exhaust is just as dangerous as pollen, if not more so, for people with allergies. Japanese studies have observed that children living near heavy traffic and diesel truck exhaust have a higher rate of allergies than do rural children.[1] People who have hay fever and asthma suffer when exposed to any irritant, whether it's cigarette smoke, perfume, or cleaning fluid. Here in New York City, doctors and hospitals in the South Bronx have observed skyrocketing rates of asthma among children and adults, which are ascribed to general air pollution and to interior pollutants like smoke, dust mites, roach parts, and roach poison in cramped, overcrowded urban apartments. Nitrous oxide is another common indoor pollutant. A recent study shows that nitrous oxide levels are highest in kitchens with gas stoves and that this correlates with a higher risk of respiratory problems in women, who presumably spend more time in the kitchen than men.

The rising use of environmental pollutants could begin to explain why the incidence of asthma and the number of deaths from asthma have surged more than 60 percent throughout the 1980s. African Americans are three times more likely than others to die of an acute asthma attack. We don't yet know whether this is due to unknown genetic factors, the possible overuse of bronchodilators, medicines, increased environmental pollution, or poor access to health care.[2]

The Common Culprits — and How to Foil Them

Housekeepers and sufferers from allergies and asthma all have a common problem: dust. Add to that mold, lint, dust mites, cockroaches, grass, cigarette smoke, gas stoves, and diesel fuel, all of which commonly cause allergic, hay fever, or asthmatic symptoms.

DUST AND DUST MITES

House dust contains a potent mix of potential allergens: carpet fibers, insect parts, pet dander, pollens, molds, bacteria, lint, skin flakes, and perhaps the most inflammatory of all — dust mites. These microscopic creatures, which look like invaders from outer space when magnified, were discovered as major culprits in allergies only in the 1960s. They are the single most common agent that precipitates attacks of childhood asthma. Up to 80 percent of asthmatic children have positive test results for dust mite allergy. Mites require humidity and warmth to grow. They feed on animal and human skin flakes (the average human loses up to 1.5 grams of skin every day), dust, and other particles. Their life cycle is 30 days. Each mite produces ten to twenty waste particles per day. These microscopic fecal pellets usually bring on allergic responses, causing chronic illness. Often found in mattresses, upholstery, carpets, quilts, pillows, and almost all textile products including toys, they also like the sleeping areas of house pets. Research shows that dust mites are becoming more prevalent around the world. The move to energy-efficient but poorly ventilated homes is one probable reason behind the increase.

MOLD

To those who are susceptible, molds can also cause nasal congestion and watery eyes. If you're allergic to mold, you should also try avoiding breads made with yeast, cheese containing mold cultures, vinegar, and mushrooms. Fermented beverages like wine, beer, and cider can also cause nasal congestion.

Environmental molds in old carpets or bedding, air conditioner systems, humidifiers, poorly ventilated closets, damp attics and basements, and compost heaps can also cause problems.

INTELLIGENT MEDICINE TIPS:

Use dehumidifiers, fans, and ventilation to decrease the humidity that provides ideal growing conditions for mold. Keep relative humidity below 40 percent and temperature below 70 degrees. Mold grows in damp, humid areas. Dust mites, too, like humidity and warmth. By keeping humidity at a healthy level, you prevent excess mildew, mold, and musty odors.

To remove dust, dust mites, and mold, thoroughly clean all carpets, upholstery, and beds, including mattresses and pillows. Remove carpets and heavy drapes from the bedroom. Encase mattresses and pillows in zippered, plastic, or allergen-proof covers. Wash all bedding in hot water, 130°F or above. Neutralize dust mite residues with nontoxic compounds such as tannic acid and benzoyl benzoate.[3]

POLLEN AND AIRBORNE MOLD

Airborne pollen from weeds, flowers, shrubs, and grasses is the best-known allergen, but many people are allergic to eating grass. Nobody in their right mind eats grass, do they? In fact, we commonly eat domesticated forms of grass, such as wheat and other grains. Someone who is highly sensitive to the allergens in grasses may suffer nasal congestion from eating wheat bread or corn products.

Alternaria is a mold that colonizes grain elevators and triggers many cases of asthma in people who live in farming areas. This mold can proliferate on any kind of dead plant material, even if dry. New farming practices and chemical spraying tend to leave crop residues in fields that used to be either burned or plowed. Modern harvesters blow dust and the *Alternaria* spores sky-high, sending them over large distances. When *Alternaria* levels soar in the fall, we often hear of sudden deaths caused by asthma.[4]

INTELLIGENT MEDICINE TIP:

Keep windows and doors closed during pollen (or *Alternaria*) season, and use a room air purifier to provide maximum protection from airborne allergens and pollutants. Seal windows with tape to stop infiltration from outside.

ANIMAL DANDER

Most people know it if they're allergic to furry or feathered creatures. Cats produce a substance in their saliva that can be a powerful allergen, which they spread over their bodies as they groom themselves. Feather dust can trigger allergic reactions, and so can urine from small pets like rabbits, hamsters, and guinea pigs. Animal fur and other animal allergens affect people selectively — you may be allergic to cats but not to birds, for example. People who are allergic to animals usually can't be around them, but keeping a pet out of the bedroom, using an air purifier, and applying a nontoxic grooming treatment to the animal may reduce the symptoms of mild allergies.

ROACHES

Some people living in urban areas have a definite sensitivity to cockroach allergens, which can increase the risk of asthmatic attacks. The little buggers have been here longer than we have, but someone with chronic respiratory problems should definitely try to keep them under control.

INTELLIGENT MEDICINE TIPS: _____

> To control cockroaches, keep all foods in sealed containers. Remove all food waste from the home. Maintain plumbing to reduce leaks and condensation on pipes, which becomes a water source for roaches. Use boric acid as a roach control in kitchen cabinets and under appliances and sinks.

SMOKING

Even passive smoking greatly increases vulnerability to allergies. It can cause transient or lifelong allergic reactions. I am amazed when someone comes in complaining of chronic sinusitis and then says, "Oh incidentally, I smoke. Do you think that's affecting things?" When it comes to smoking cessation, I demand unconditional compliance from my allergy patients.

Asthma

A man in his forties came into my office recently complaining that he couldn't shake colds and was always coughing. Even the slightest chemical odor made his nose run. The final straw, he said, was a visit to his neighbor, whose cats made him so uncomfortable that he had to leave practically as soon as he sat down. That night he could barely sleep because his lungs were so constricted. I asked him whether he had had asthma as a kid. He said, "Yes, but I thought I'd outgrown it." I gave him an inhaler and said as sympathetically as possible, "Welcome back to the asthma cycle."

This is an unfortunate but typical scenario of someone who suffered from asthma as a child and overcame it as a teenager, only to have it resurface as a problem in middle age. Those early years of being in and out of the emergency room, missing school, and being highly allergic can set someone up for a later susceptibility to colds and infection as the immune system weakens with age. The hormonal changes of the teenage years often strengthen the immune system, so that many can "outgrow" their asthma. Yet, the aging process and continual exposure to adverse environments can reawaken a person's susceptibility to asthma or to chronic obstructive pulmonary disease (COPD), which is similar to emphysema. There is probably a genetic component to asthma as well. Study groups have identified two chromosomes as locations for genetic mutations that signal the body to produce excess IgE antibodies in the blood. Some scientists believe that the gene mutation explains why some people are more susceptible to asthma and allergies.

What is asthma? Doctors define it as inflammation of the lungs that is associated with increased mucus production, and constriction of the tiny airways that lead to the oxygen-absorbing areas of the lungs, and increased sensitivity to chemicals, allergens, and cold air. But diagnosing asthma may not be a simple matter. Sometimes it requires special pulmonary function tests in which the patient breathes into a special apparatus before and after medication is administered.

Asthma has been around for a long time. Therefore, with the inexorable march of medical progress we should be steadily advancing toward eradication of the disease, right? Wrong. The number of Americans with asthma increased 60 percent over the years 1983 to 1993. Of the U.S. population, 4 to 5 percent has asthma, which equals 10 to 12 million cases. The disease appears to be becoming more severe, reflected in higher hospitalization and death rates. Between 1983 and 1987 there was an average of 463,500 hospitalizations annually for asthma. The asthma death rate has increased from less than 2000 per year in the United States in 1978 to more than 4500 per year in 1993. The cost of treating asthma patients in the United States was estimated to be $6.42 billion in 1990.[5] This trend is increasing worldwide, with statistics showing that asthma is getting worse precisely in those countries that should have the best medical care: the United States, Canada, Australia, and New Zealand. Why the gloomy figures?

Some might surmise that it is our worsening air quality that is responsible for the increases in asthma incidence and death. Yet, statistics indicate that because of the Clean Air Act, the levels of air pollution in our major metropolitan areas are actually declining. So while air pollution and chemical exposure play a major role in asthma, we can't conclude that the increase in asthma problems is due simply to deteriorating air quality. Some argue that smoking is responsible for our worsening asthma statistics. But here, too, research indicates that the number of smokers is declining overall, despite still-high smoking levels among teenagers and young women.

The increase in asthma statistics has remained a curious anomaly without apparent cause — that is, until recently. Research scientists now think they have an answer to the mystery, and that answer strikes directly at the heart of modern medicine and the type of therapies doctors commonly choose.

If you or a loved one has asthma, you know that the mainstay of asthma therapy is the use of inhaled bronchodilator medications. They go by various names, including Proventil and Alupent, and are designed to open constricted lung tubules. Indeed, most people with asthma welcome the temporary relief these inhalers give. Like other doctors, I was taught in my medical training that the use of potent medications was essential for asthma management. The notion was deeply inculcated that patients should never undermedicate, which would leave them vulnerable to acute asthmatic attacks that could land them in the emergency room.

People with asthma, however, know the side effects of bronchodilator use. Puffing again and again on their inhalers to obtain relief, they note rapid heartbeat, tremor, and anxiety. Parents of children with asthma often claim that their children exhibit hyperactivity and decreased attention span.

The intriguing answer to the riddle of increased asthma incidence and death may lie in a recent article in *The Lancet*, Britain's most respected medical journal. The authors of this study looked at eighty-nine persons with moderate asthma and compared the use of bronchodilators in people who used the inhalers only for the relief of symptoms versus those who used the inhalers routinely. The authors found that in only 30 percent of cases was asthma better controlled during routine inhaler treatment, while in 70 percent, control was better during treatment with the inhaler for symptom relief only. Surprisingly, the less frequently the medication was used, the better the asthma symptoms were controlled.

The authors of the study concluded that "the trend toward use of regular, higher doses of longer-acting inhaled treatment may be an important causal factor in the worldwide increase in asthma." They went on to state, "Physicians who manage patients with asthma are therefore confronted with the uncomfortable possibility that the mainstay of their treatment may be harmful."[6]

A similar debate surrounds the use of other well-known asthma medications. A debate has arisen recently over the use of Theo-Dur, a long-lasting oral medication for asthma. Critics charge that Theo-Dur and medications like it can easily produce debilitating psychological symptoms as well as dangerous cardiovascular problems like heart arrhythmias and heart attacks. Drawbacks also accompany the use of oral aminophylline and theophylline preparations, so that many asthma specialists now prefer inhaled steroid sprays for first-line treatment.

Unfortunately, the situation may be little better where steroids are concerned. While inhaled steroids offer some measure of relief, oral steroids, which are often used to manage more severe cases of asthma, are associated with dependency, thinning of bones, psychosis, diabetes, ulcers, cataracts, weight gain, and other unpleasant side effects. While they are preferable to pills taken orally, because of reduced risk of side effects, new studies suggest that inhaled steroids may stunt the growth of children, and contribute to higher incidence of glaucoma. Another drug used is Intal (cromolyn sodium), which works on the mast cells, located just outside the capillaries, which explode open and release histamines into the bloodstream. However, while admittedly producing few side effects, Intal is weak and does little to halt the inexorable progression of asthma.

Recently, the immune suppressive agent methotrexate has been introduced as an alternative to steroid treatment. It's interesting that we're now using methotrexate, a chemotherapy drug newly appropriated to fight rheumatoid arthritis — another kind of inflammatory disease. This reflects a shift in our approach to asthma, which we once thought of as basically an allergic disease. Now we're coming to regard it as an inflammatory, immune-modulated disease with an allergenic component. New leukotriene-modulating drugs are the latest advance in asthma treatment. These medications are rarely employed alone, but rather are intended to boost the effectiveness of old standby sprays and pills. While gaining popularity, it is unclear at the present whether they will materially affect long-term outcomes.

The fact is that the medical profession, by its own admission, is facing a crisis in the management of asthma. While mainstream medicine continues to try out new pharmaceutical agents, perhaps with new unpredictable side effects, it is worth surveying the wide assortment of alternative therapies that really work for asthma.

New Methods for Fighting Asthma

In the spirit of preventive medicine, I first encourage my patients to avoid situations that can irritate the respiratory system: passive smoking, environmental pollutants, dust mites, chemicals, and mold. As we discussed in the allergy section, mold allergy is becoming increasingly appreciated as an asthma precipitant. Asthma sufferers can use "mold plates" to identify the presence of troublesome molds at home. Home and office tests kits for pesticides and chemicals have recently become available and will soon revolutionize air quality control for sensitive patients.

At the same time, research is under way to improve on the old questionably effective system of allergy shots, which must be painstakingly administered over long periods of time — sometimes years — and require careful supervision by doctors because of the ever-present danger of severe allergic reactions to the shots. These newer measures include techniques for administering antigens via oral solutions or nasal inhalations as well as "souped-up" allergy vaccines that require less frequent administration. One such therapy that I have used successfully on asthma patients is called EPD, for enzyme-potentiated desensitization.

Physical therapy can play an important role in treating asthma. Relatives and home care attendants can be schooled in the proper methods of "clopping" and postural drainage. Extensive training in these techniques for nursing care personnel in the Netherlands has kept asthma mortality rates there well below those of adjacent countries. To experience this effect, lie prone on the edge of a bed or sofa with your head leaning over the edge to allow gravity to mobilize secretions. A physical therapist or cooperative spouse or friend then vigorously "clops" you on the back to shake loose the stuck mucus plugs, which can then be coughed out and expectorated.

Physical training can also help adapt the lungs and circulatory system to the demands of limited breathing capacity. Rigorous swimming is well suited to people with asthma because of the special respiratory dynamics of intermittent breathing; recent studies show that mild carbon dioxide retention tends to relax the airways. This is also the basis of the "pranayama" breathing techniques used in yoga, which may also help the asthma sufferer. The idea here is to develop a regular slow rhythm of breathing. To try this, count slowly 1-2-3 as you inhale, hold your breath for counts 4–5, and slowly exhale for counts 6–10. Adjust the counts as needed for comfort.

Nutrient therapy can also offer remarkable benefits. New research points to the antihistamine effects of vitamin C. In fact, all the antioxidants, including vitamins C, E, and A, along with mixed carotenoids, zinc, and selenium, can help reduce the inflammatory condition of asthma. Chief among nutrients important to people with asthma is magnesium. Intravenous infusions of magnesium can halt even some of the most severe exacerbations of emphysema under emergency room circumstances. Magnesium apparently acts as a natural bronchodilator, relaxing the smooth muscle that lines the tiny tubules that bring air to the lungs so that it doesn't go into spasm. (Many people with chemical sensitivities turn out to have a magnesium deficiency). Vitamin B_6 is another important vitamin for asthma control; paradoxically, it is depleted by theophylline-type asthma drugs. Vitamin B_{12} can provide relief to asthma sufferers through its ability to activate the body's chemical detoxification pathways.[7]

In my office, I sometimes use an "asthma drip," an intravenous "cocktail" of nutrients that are particularly helpful. It contains vitamin C, which acts as a natural antihistamine; pantothenic acid, a B vitamin that supports adrenal function; magnesium, which is helpful in patients with chemical sensitivities; zinc; and selenium.

Molybdenum, a trace metal and important nutrient, participates in the body's vital sulfite oxidase pathway, helping the body break down and eliminate sulfites, which commonly trigger asthma attacks. Environmental physicians can use lab tests to determine whether adequate molybdenum is present in the body.

To treat respiratory problems, the Europeans use another nutrient and superb antioxidant, N-acetyl-cysteine (NAC), which is an activated form of an amino acid. NAC, which breaks up mucus, is used in solutions that wash the lungs of patients with cystic fibrosis and can be taken orally as a supplement. The Europeans sell it as a drug, while we sell it along with vitamins and nutrients. (Paradoxically, several important nutrients available in health food stores here are sold as drugs in other countries, not because they're dangerous but because they're effective and are reimbursed by the government or the health care system.)

The Holy Grail of current asthma research is to come up with drugs that modulate the leukotriene system. Leukotrienes are the chemical messengers associated with inflammation and smooth muscle tone. Although leukotriene-modulating drugs are new, we have long manipulated the body's own leukotriene production through using the essential fatty acids, including the omega-3 oils and gamma-linolenic acid (GLA). GLA is a fatty acid that modulates the synthesis of prostaglandins, a group of hormones, some of which promote inflammation and swelling of tissue and some of which inhibit it. Primrose oil, borage oil, and black currant seed oil are all good sources of essential fatty acids. Primrose was valued by the American Indians as a treatment for respiratory problems. Recent studies have linked the consumption of fish, which are rich in omega-3 oils, to freedom from respiratory diseases.

Herbs can also be helpful in asthma management. A traditional Chinese herb, ephedra, is a mainstay of asthma treatment in Chinese medicine. Typical Western herbs include pleurisy root, yerba santa, and lobelia. *Ginkgo biloba*, commonly thought of as an antiaging nutrient, has specific antiinflammatory effects in asthma.

Acupuncture, the ancient Chinese healing art, has been proven in numerous studies to be helpful in mitigating the symptoms of asthma. In China, departments of pulmonary medicine, while adopting modern techniques of pharmacological management, are never without the attendance of skilled acupuncturists. I find that acupuncture can be useful in the treatment of patients trying to stop smoking as well as in the treatment of asthma.

One therapy recently proposed for asthma is the use of *intravenous gamma globulins*, or IgG. This was very naively headlined on a TV program as "a new cure for asthma that has changed the life of many." What the show didn't mention was the cost of the therapy for one child, which could be $30,000 or more per year. With five million kids suffering from allergies and asthma in this country, this type of therapy is clearly not going to solve everyone's problems, but it is an option for severe, life-threatening asthma. You might wonder, "Why give immunoglobulins? I thought the whole problem with allergies was too much of an immune response." Well, that's true. But gamma globulin, in a very large intravenous dose (much larger than that used to prevent hepatitis), gives the immune system a potent jolt and lowers the response to allergens.

Modulating the nervous system plays an important role in asthma therapy. Prednisone, one of the most potent asthma drugs currently available, strengthens the adrenal glands, which help the body fight stress. The adrenals make cortisol, which tends to increase resistance and reduce inflammation. Stress over time forces the adrenals to produce an abundance of cortisol and gradually become exhausted. The defenses become frayed, and inflammatory conditions and allergies come to the fore.

It's long been known that stress can trigger or worsen an asthma attack. At the same time, asthma attacks themselves stress the nervous system, creating a kind of vicious circle of nervous system overload. Patients with asthma are frequently confronted with the feeling of near-asphyxiation. This engenders a primitive panic reaction, which makes efficient breathing difficult. The asthma attack becomes, in part, a basic conditioned response that becomes imprinted on the neurophysiology of the patient. It is, to a certain extent, a "behavior" that is sometimes difficult to unlearn. Asthma sufferers find themselves on a kind of metabolic roller coaster, with rapid alternations in tone of the autonomic nervous system. The nervous system is dominated alternately by the parasympathetic side and the sympathetic side. A chronic parasympathetic dominance can induce constricted breathing. To switch their autonomic nervous systems into the sympathetic mode, many people with asthma become addicted to stress, whether from life circumstances, coffee, sugar or adrenaline-like medication.

Truly holistic asthma management therefore involves attention to the regulation of the nervous system. This may include training in deep relaxation and relaxed abdominal breathing. Biofeedback techniques, with emphasis on breathing retraining, can help patients reimpose some measure of control on their runaway physiology. Control of asthma is predicated on restoration of the autonomic nervous system to a more stable, balanced state.

To sum up, victory in the struggle against asthma may not have to await spectacular breakthroughs in pharmacological management. Simple techniques are now at our disposal to help us reverse the dismal trend toward worsening asthma statistics.

Smoking

Years ago, songs, books, and movies depicted the voluptuous joys of smoking. "These Foolish Things," a romantic ballad of the thirties, presented smoking as a universally glamorous pastime. In the 1942 movie *Now Voyager*, Bette Davis and Paul Henreid savor their cigarettes with afterdinner drinks, in a classic scene that makes smoking an integral part of the game of romance. Today, most Americans are too guilt-ridden to smoke with delicious abandon. We are unable to escape the association of cigarettes with heart and lung disease, fetal growth retardation, and cancer. Tobacco companies no longer downplay the unavoidable evidence connecting cigarettes and cancer but have tried to disclaim the accusations that they manipulate the nicotine levels of cigarettes to sustain people's smoking habits.

Yet is smoking all bad? Besides the fact that it might kill you, seemingly not. There are actual health risks that are associated with stopping smoking. People who stop smoking have a slightly higher risk of developing ulcerative colitis. Many people gain weight after they stop smoking. Others develop gastrointestinal distress or constipation, and find they can't go to the bathroom without a cigarette. Why these odd effects? As an antiobesity agent, smoking can squelch appetite. It helps some people cope with stress and can act as a gastrointestinal tranquilizer. Nicotine has even been proposed as a "smart-drug" for Alzheimer's Disease. We do not know all the pharmacological effects of smoking, but there is more to them than a displaced need to suck the thumb.

Beyond all the discussions about whether nicotine is a drug, it clearly plays a role in the metabolism as a pharmaceutical agent, especially in the blood sugar cycle. When you eat a meal, the liver stocks and releases glycogen, a type of quick-release sugar that counteracts feelings of hunger. Three to five hours after eating, the liver stops releasing glycogen and you start to feel hungry. Smoking releases blood sugar from the liver. As a smoker, either you can choose to eat, supplying the blood sugar your body is craving, or you can smoke a cigarette. The cigarette does not contain sugar, but the nicotine triggers a release of stored sugar from the liver, thus satisfying the smoker's craving for food.

Certainly this kind of antihunger effect does not compensate for the serious side effects of smoking, including death by lung cancer or emphysema. But it does suggest why it is really difficult for some people to stop — smoking has become part of their daily metabolic process. This is why I encourage some kind of nicotine replacement as part of a smoking cessation program. This could be in the form of a patch, chewing gum, or aerosol spray. The idea is to gradually taper off, with smaller and smaller doses of nicotine, until the body has had time to adjust to living without this powerful pharmaceutical agent.

Smoking can also play an important role in a person's psychological equilibrium. The gesture-impulse of smoking should not be viewed as a moral failure but rather as an emergency method of holding back a flood of stressful emotions. For many people, the act of smoking is a conscious moment of relaxation — of just stopping for a moment and performing a physical ritual time-out that offers removal and relief from the stresses of the day. There are better ways of doing this, but smoking is convenient and was for many years socially acceptable. Nicotine also offers a kind of energy buzz that some people give themselves as a psychic reward after completing a mildly stressful task. Unfortunately, the relaxation break and the buzz offer only temporary relief; they permit the real health disaster to continue to build. I compare smokers to unscrupulous contractors who use inadequate materials to build a dam, knowing that the dam will eventually break. As a reformed smoker, I can admit that my own behavior became erratic under the tremendous pressure of living on the hospital wards during my medical training. When facing an ominous situation with a patient, I would sometimes find myself retreating to the bathroom for a surreptitious cigarette. I even found myself inventing stressful situations to provide myself with a pretext to satisfy my addiction. Without the cigarette, I would have had to stand my ground and face whatever I was dodging. But there's no dodging the serious health risks of smoking, no matter how powerful its psychological attractions.

How Smoking Degrades Health

Smoke degrades health in a remarkable variety of ways. First, cigarette smoke contains a whole array of chemical pollutants, including aldehydes, aeroleins, nicotine, nitrous oxide and dioxide, carbon monoxide, phenols, allergenic proteins, and carcinogenic tars. Several of these are immune depressants, and the immune system reacts to all of them.

Only in recent years did the public learn that nicotine was not the sole destructive element in tobacco. The *New York Times* published findings on tobacco research showing that cigarettes contain substances even more addictive than nicotine: aldehydes, which are equally dangerous and have neurotoxic effects. Unlike nicotine, which is the active principle of tobacco, aldehydes also appear in the body as byproducts of fermentation, caused by yeast or bacteria. Cheap, inferior wines are laced with aldehydes, for example.

Second, cigarette smoke cripples the natural protective function of the tissue that lines the respiratory tract from the nose to the lungs. Normally, tiny microscopic hairlike cilia filter the air to remove bacteria, particles of dust, and pollen and push them toward the gullet so they can pass into the digestive tract. Elements of cigarette smoke, especially nitrous oxide and dioxide, paralyze the cilia so that bacteria and dust remain in the lungs and cause infections. Passive smokers, especially children, suffer from this effect as well.

The immune system mounts a defense against the smoke particles that make their way into the lungs, sending white blood cells called macrophages to ingest the particles. The macrophages are soon overwhelmed by the massive quantities of "pollution." If you look through a microscope at macrophages from a smoker's lung tissue, they are bloated with coal-black carbon particles. Worse, they are seriously weakened and are unable to respond effectively to bacteria, their other principal target. Other white blood cells called natural killer cells are also weakened by the smoke particles. They are less able to recognize viruses and tumor cells, including cell mutations induced by carcinogenic tobacco tars, and they kill aberrant cells less effectively. In cancer patients, the weakening of the natural killer cells can encourage the cancer to metastasize, or spread throughout the body.

Another immune reaction causes damage to the lung tissue that eventually leads to emphysema — lung damage so severe that the lungs can no longer oxygenate the blood. The reaction begins when glycoproteins — a component of cigarette smoke — lodge in the deepest recesses of the lungs. The immune system detects these foreign proteins and sends hosts of white blood cells to attack them. This excess immune activity causes secretion of an enzyme that breaks down the walls of the lung tissue, and macrophages are then called in to gobble up the destroyed tissue. The macrophages prevent the enzyme activity from being turned off, and a cascade of tissue breakdown follows. The dead tissue collects in the lungs, creating an ideal medium for bacterial growth. The ravaged tissue that remains is less and less able to supply the body's needs for oxygen.

These same tobacco glycoproteins also cause an allergic reaction, inducing the body to produce more of the immunoglobulin E (IgE) antibody, an antibody specific to allergies. The IgE antibody can set off an immune overreaction, resulting in constant sneezing, wheezing, coughs, runny noses, rashes, and asthma attacks.

At the same time, cigarette smokers produce less of other types of antibodies, the ones that attack bacteria, and their T cells and B cells also react poorly. All of these multiple forms of imbalance gradually take their toll, causing serious damage to health over a long period of regular smoking. The good news is that except for emphysema, the body can bounce back to health in a relatively short time after smoking stops — in a matter of months. But when large areas of lung tissue have been destroyed, the effect is permanent.

How to Stop Smoking

I have many patients who say, "I can't understand why I smoke. It is so useless and self-destructive." They worry so much about their lack of self-control that their addiction to smoking begins to erode their self-esteem.

My first step in helping them is to reassure them that if they are wondering why they find it so difficult to stop, they are on the right track. Once they discover why they smoke, then and only then are they ready to stop smoking. In fact, I tell them, "Don't try to stop smoking just now. Let's find out what smoking does for you and first find another way to satisfy that need."

Once they understand the psychological and metabolic components of the smoking addiction, they enroll in my smoking cessation program. Usually I prescribe a nicotine patch, gum, or aerosol to replace the nicotine they're used to, so they can gradually taper off. I prescribe a diet with more protein than carbohydrate to break the body's craving for sweets, and suggest frequent, smaller meals throughout the day, to break the nicotine/ blood sugar habit. I suggest that they reduce their intake of caffeine, which depletes nicotine from the blood so quickly that the craving is perpetuated. Caffeine also tends to worsen hypoglycemia, causing wild shifts in blood sugar. With no caffeine in the system, the liver will release blood sugar more slowly and evenly. I also give them these antioxidants and vitamins:

- Antioxidants, to counteract the deleterious free radical effects of smoking. Dosages: vitamin C, 1000 milligrams per day; vitamin E, 800 International Units per day; mixed carotenoids, 25,000 International Units per day.
- Fish oil, to reduce susceptibility to emphysema and asthma. Dosage: two or three 1000-milligram capsules daily.
- Magnesium, to keep lungs healthy and spasm-free. Dosage: 400 to 600 milligrams elemental magnesium daily, in magnesium citrate, glycinate, or chelated form.
- Vitamin A (retinol), to provide additional cancer prevention. Dosage: 25,000 International Units per day (but no more than 5000 International Units daily in case of pregnancy)
- N-acetyl-cysteine (NAC), to act as a powerful antioxidant and specifically control mucus production. Dosage: 600 milligrams three times daily.

On the neurophysiology side, I often recommend acupuncture, which can help control addiction by releasing endorphins, which are natural neurotransmitters that block pain and induce euphoria. Some of my patients find that meditation techniques can help them stop and release the stresses that they formerly staved off with cigarettes. To help with motivation, I also suggest they write ten compelling reasons why they want to stop smoking; put a copy of the list in their wallet or purse, on the refrigerator door or office desk, or anywhere handy; and leave one copy with me and one with a significant other. This combination of psychological reconditioning and nutrient support has enabled many of my patients to overcome the addiction to smoking. Fortunately, many people are continuing to remove themselves from this major risk for respiratory illness.

A Look to the Future

The prognosis for respiratory health continues to look brighter as we project current trends into the twenty-first century. Lung cancer and emphysema rates will go down as smoking dies away as a social custom — we hope! With that culprit largely eliminated, we can expect to increase our awareness of the multiple causative factors in sinus and lung problems and to reduce the occupational and environmental hazards that can cause respiratory problems.

Certain sufferers of emphysema will benefit from the innovative lung reduction surgery now being pioneered. This technique actually removes areas of diseased lung tissue, which contain spaces that trap air in the lungs of patients with emphysema. Paradoxically, the reduction in lung volume by removal of diseased tissue actually increases endurance and reduces shortness of breath in properly selected patients, with a minimum of side effects. Unfortunately, this has also been a striking example of the lack of recognition of intelligent medicine by the government health care system and insurers, since Medicare recently decided to stop paying for this beneficial procedure.

We are beginning to identify faulty genes that can render us susceptible to allergies and asthma. In the future we may look to a genetic solution to some of these problems. We are also shifting from a drug-based approach to a green approach, or ecological approach, to treating allergies and asthma. As evidence emerges showing the crossovers between food and respiratory reactions, we will make advances through diet modification. We will continue to discover and improve on nutritional and other therapies that use the body's own metabolic processes, rather than powerful drugs, to correct respiratory problems.

CHAPTER FOURTEEN

Keeping Eyes Bright and Ears Sharp

Hearing and sight — most of us take them for granted during our adult life. But many have had the experience of seeing an older parent start to withdraw from life as hearing fails, and it becomes too difficult to enter into a family conversation or even talk one-to-one. Closer to home, you yourself may find that those little granny glasses perched at the end of your nose have started to become very useful, not for affecting the John Lennon look but for making it through the daily paper.

Significant changes in hearing and sight can occur with aging. Some are a minor nuisance, and some can threaten our enjoyment of simple daily pleasures or even our livelihood. Prevention is the key to warding off the more serious forms of decline. Like the skin, our eyes and ears flourish and function well with general good health habits. General systemic factors, from sugar metabolism to blood circulation, can significantly affect our hearing and our vision. Also, there are some specific nutrients that can support good hearing and vision. Environmental dangers include the long-term effects of ultraviolet radiation on vision and the long-term effects of environmental noise on hearing. Let's take a closer look at the factors that influence both these invaluable senses.

Hearing Loss—Is It Inevitable?

"Hey, can't you turn that down?" our parents used to yell at us. "I can't hear myself think." But we knew better — rock and roll was supposed to be loud. In fact, if there's one crucial emblem of American youth culture it's loud music, very loud music. Rock and roll in the sixties, disco and heavy metal in the seventies, rap and hip-hop in the eighties and nineties — no matter how the styles have changed, the common denominator is that they're supposed to be loud. You were not getting the full effect unless you could walk into the arena and feel the bass line thumping in your viscera. Better yet, you could push your way to the front, stand directly in front of those towering guitar amps, and get blown away by the power chords. One of the champions of loud and louder rock and roll was Pete Townshend of The

Who, who liked to climax his show with a screaming explosion of feedback and amplified cacophony as he and the other members of the band smashed their instruments to bits at full volume.

These days, one of Pete Townshend's favorite charities is H.E.A.R., Hearing Education and Awareness for Rockers, founded in San Francisco by former bass guitarist Kathy Peck, who suffered severe hearing loss in her early twenties after several years of playing amplified rock. Her mission is to alert people to the risks of high-decibel music and noise, and she actually recommends earplugs for rock and roll concertgoers. But rock and roll isn't the only threat to our hearing. In our modern industrialized environment, we're assaulted from every side by a cacophonous world of noise: urban traffic, highways, airplanes, office machines, lawn mowers, and so on. For entertainment, we strap on stereo headsets or settle into our seats in the digital-surround-sound movie theater, experiencing rocket blasts and explosions or the throbbing roar of a *Tyrannosaurus rex*.

Over time, these assaults take their toll. A study in the *New England Journal of Medicine* reported that approximately 4 percent of people under forty-five years of age and 29 percent of those sixty-five or older have a handicapping loss of hearing that interferes with social or job-related communications. It's been estimated that more than 28 million Americans have hearing impairment, and the prevalence of hearing loss increases dramatically with age. More than 36 percent of persons over the age of seventy have a handicapping hearing loss. Even more disturbing, many younger people are suffering hearing loss before their time. One study of students at the University of Tennessee found that 60 percent of entering freshman had hearing loss, and 14 percent of them had hearing similar to that of the average sixty-five-year-old. The most probable culprit is noise.

To some extent, hearing loss is another disease of civilization. One study of a Sudanese tribe living deep in the African bush found that people of any age in that community had better hearing than a comparable group of American farmers; and more significantly, the older people heard as well as the young. In addition, some diseases, many related to immune disorders like lupus, are known to cause hearing loss. But medical science classifies hearing loss with age as an "idiopathic" disorder; in other words, we don't know why, it just happens. While hearing loss is associated to some extent with the loss of neuroepithelial cells in the inner ear and with reduced blood circulation, this is only partly a "natural process." It is certainly precipitated or pushed along by cumulative noxious influences throughout life, including noise trauma, the toxicity of drugs and medications, and other environmental factors.

Noise

It's increasingly evident that loud sounds can harm hearing, including the loud sounds that more and more are part of our entertainment media, our workplaces, and our urbanized environment. Studies have shown measurable hearing loss in people exposed to high-intensity noise, even noise that's below OSHA safety thresholds. We should be concerned about cranking up the headphones while jogging, loud rock concerts, and even loud movies, which are increasingly mesmerizing audiences with megabass surround-sound and thrilling and perhaps literally deafening audio levels. And noise doesn't affect just hearing. Studies of noise in hospitals — P.A. systems, medical machinery, hallway conversations — have suggested that high noise levels may raise stress levels in patients and even retard healing. In our increasingly clamorous environment, noise pollution may be every bit as serious a problem in some urbanized areas as air pollution. High ambient noise levels can have real medical consequences, including anxiety disorders, insomnia, stress-related conditions, and syndromes of immune disregulation that we don't think of as being hearing-related, as well as actual hearing impairment.

We tend to get used to our noisy environments and don't realize how extreme they are until we spend a night in a country home or inn and find the silence "deafening." So it's important to be alert to the problem and to take preventive measures. A good rule of thumb for music levels is to keep them low enough to enable you to hear other sounds above the music. It's especially important to be careful with car stereos and Walkman-type headphones, which can unleash a lot of concentrated sound energy. When you can't avoid high sound levels, the solution is to use earplugs. These can be made of foam rubber or plastic, and they come with an EPA noise reduction rating on the label. Stuffing cotton or tissue in your ears is not effective.

Noise is measured in decibels, and anything 80 decibels or higher is potentially damaging, particularly over sustained exposure. The louder the sound, the less exposure is needed to cause damage. A lawn mower producing a 95-decibel sound level will cause hearing loss in 4 hours, while a rock concert or stereo headset producing 110 decibels can cause damage in half an hour. Sitting for 2 hours in a surround-sound movie theater listening to gun battles, explosions, rocket launchings, and dinosaur roars can be a risky experience. You may notice temporary hearing loss or ringing in the ears after such an exposure, or you may not, but repeated exposure over the years can be damaging. The highest noise reduction rating you can generally find from earplugs available in a drugstore is about 30 decibels, which is not really strong enough for 4 hours at a rock concert but is certainly better than nothing. A lower rating, say 15 decibels, can be used for running the lawn mower or going to see the latest Schwarzenegger extravaganza.

Drugs and Medications

Many drugs and medications are ototoxic — that is, they can cause hearing loss. They range from some common antibiotics to sophisticated designer drugs to . . . aspirin! Yes, aspirin and other so-called salicylates have been associated with hearing loss and ringing in the ears, especially with high dosages or long-term use. Studies have shown that aspirin combined with noise exposure has a synergistic effect: people who work in a noisy environment and also self-medicate with aspirin suffer greater hearing degradation than would be expected from simply adding the two factors.

Some diuretics can cause hearing loss, including Lasix, which is commonly used for older patients with congestive heart failure. The anticancer agents used in chemotherapy are frequently ototoxic — we are increasingly seeing loss of hearing sensitivity in younger and middle-aged people who are given chemotherapy, especially women with breast cancer. Some antibiotics can also cause hearing loss, especially those of the aminoglycoside family. These are powerful antibiotics used often in treatment of surgical patients, or elderly or immune-compromised individuals. Some susceptible individuals may even suffer hearing impairment with long courses of more common antibiotics, such as erythromycin or the penicillin derivative amoxicillin.

In fact, a recent study of ear infections in adults (otitis media, the infection of the inner ear that is common in children) found that adults who took antibiotics had a slightly lower rate of recovery in clinical tests than those who took no antibiotics, and those with a history of prophylactic or preventive antibiotic use also had a lower rate of recovery.[1] In light of this, the government has put out a position paper recommending conservative use of antibiotic treatment for children with ear infections, which usually get better without treatment. Unfortunately, individual pediatricians remain at the mercy of practice standards in their communities, in a medical/legal climate that pushes them into prescribing medication to prevent the very remote but real possibility of hearing loss and consequent liability. No one gets sued for prescribing antibiotics, even if their long-term effects may be adverse. We tend to aggressively treat kids with antibiotics for their ear ailments to ward off the specter of deafness. Yet, studies show that food allergies are more often the culprit of ear problems in kids, and the vast majority of otitis media infections will resolve themselves spontaneously, without antibiotics.

At the same time, the number of myringotomies — surgical procedures to open up the ear tubes — has skyrocketed, replacing tonsil surgery as the most common type of ear, nose, and throat surgery. Myringotomy is commonly prescribed for children, and involves inserting a tube to remove fluid from the blocked middle ear, thus relieving uncomfortable pressure on the inner ear. In our childhood everybody was getting tonsillectomies, which are now completely out of fashion, and now kids are getting myringotomies. Yet, these surgical procedures and aggressive antibiotic therapies may start to weaken the auditory system even in childhood. What's more, I think the phenomenon of ototoxic reactions should remind us to be cautious about the use of antibiotics in particular, and the use of other powerful drugs in general.

Environment and Allergies

Our environment assaults our ears in more ways than one. Air pollution can potentiate allergies, causing chronic inflammation of the Eustachian tubes, which may in turn predispose a person to hearing loss. Passive smoking can directly irritate the Eustachian tubes, leading to the same results.

Nutrition

There is some evidence of a nutritional component to hearing threshold ratings. The cochlea, which are the organs of the inner ear that translate sound vibrations into nerve impulses, have a high concentration of vitamin A, and special sensory receptor cells contain or depend upon vitamin A. Studies have shown that supplementation with vitamins A, D, and E improved hearing loss and, in some cases, tinnitus. Animal studies have shown that the combination of noise exposure, hypertension, and a high-fat diet produced devastating hearing loss. More research needs to be done in this area.

That Ringing in the Ears

While hearing loss is a real risk, more people — in the millions — are probably actively suffering from tinnitus, or ringing in the ears, than from their hearing loss. This is especially common in middle age. Singer Barbra Streisand is among the sufferers. "I hear noises all the time," she has been quoted as saying. "It's pretty horrible; I long for the silence."[2]

Many factors influence tinnitus. Circulatory impairment and blood viscosity may predispose a person to having the syndrome, along with rapid or extreme fluctuations in blood sugar. (People taking medication for high blood pressure often complain of tinnitus as a side effect of the drug.) Managing cholesterol levels and the types of fats and oils in the diet can sometimes have a positive effect. Other therapies that sometimes help are the use of niacin, and the use of *Ginkgo biloba* as a circulatory-enhancing agent. Even acupuncture can be helpful, which suggests a relationship to an imbalance of the autonomic nerves that control circulation in the inner ear. Sometimes an injection of a local anesthetic near the ear (called neural therapy in Germany) will cause tinnitus and dizziness to abate, possibly because it rebalances autonomic nerve activity.

There appear to be some nutritional components to tinnitus as well. One study of army personnel with chronic tinnitus and noise-induced hearing loss found significant deficiency of vitamin B_{12}. Supplementation to restore normal blood levels caused some improvement in some patients. Other studies have suggested the potential of zinc and of magnesium supplements to improve chronic tinnitus in those who suffer some deficiency. One interesting study set up a multifaceted dietary plan for people with confirmed hearing loss and tinnitus who hadn't been helped by medical therapy. These subjects followed a diet with such elements as reduced sodium, reduced saturated fats, reduced animal protein, elimination of refined sugars, and increased whole, raw foods such as vegetables, nuts, and seeds. Most showed improvement in hearing thresholds and tinnitus. The implication is that hearing improvement may depend on multiple health factors. Again, more research needs to be done in this area.

Treating Hearing Loss

Hearing aids are still the mainstay of treating hearing loss, but we now have smaller and more dependable aids, some fitting entirely within the external auditory canal, with programmable amplification circuits that can reduce distortion. In the future, we may look to greater use of totally implantable aids, the so-called cochlear implants, which are designed to reproduce the electrical output of the auditory apparatus and to stimulate the nervous system directly. Since hearing is many orders of magnitude less complex than vision, it's easier to tackle, with some sound fidelity, the engineering of an artificial receiver and implantable miniaturized system of directly stimulating the nervous system and brain.

This technology already exists, though it's now a fairly rare, expensive, and experimental practice. It is used in some children and younger people who have profound genetic deafness. No one has tried using this with older people, though that may come.* We could think of a cochlear implant as the prototypical artificial sense organ. Given the amazing developments in computer miniaturization, it's not pure fantasy to envision a time of replaceable sense organs, which could gather sound or light for direct processing by the nervous system and brain, with a degree of miniaturization and fidelity that could rival that of our marvelous eyes and ears.

---

* I should mention that the use of cochlear implants in children is somewhat controversial. Some advocates for the hearing-impaired argue that the actual result is a very rudimentary type of sound mimicry, which they believe will divert children from the task of learning sign language and alternative means of communication, and remove them from the deaf community.

Science fiction has also speculated about the possibility of regenerating organs, and this too now has a basis in fact. Researchers at Albert Einstein College have investigated a way of repairing cochlea injured by noise: by regrowing damaged ear cells. The idea is to use neuronal growth factors to selectively enhance growth or regeneration of neuronal receptors and transmitters of sound impulses.[3] In the meantime, though, the best ear medicine is still prevention — avoiding ear-damaging noise levels, using earplugs when necessary, and being extra careful with drugs and medications that can have an ototoxic effect.

Seeing Clearly

Even in the glasses of thine eyes
I see thy grieved heart.

WILLIAM SHAKESPEARE,
RICHARD II

For centuries, people have talked of the eyes as windows of the soul. What many don't realize, however, is that the eyes are windows into the body as well. Shakespeare's line could apply just as well to cardiovascular disease as to torments of the soul. Practically speaking, it's very hard to look into the body and determine at what rate the blood vessels are aging. An angiogram of the heart is pretty crude — it involves squirting dye into the coronary arteries and looking for constrictions in the serpentine flow patterns. If you see them, you have an indication of pretty advanced arteriosclerosis, but this takes years to develop. By the time you see results from an angiogram, you've lost years of opportunity for preventive therapy.

On the other hand, you can look directly into the eyes and see the very delicate little capillaries there. With high magnification and proper lighting, you can discern early patterns of narrowing or breakdown of blood vessels due to high blood pressure, diabetes, or atherosclerosis. This is one reason why the eye doctor blinds you by dilating your pupils and then shining a light in there — it's not only to find out about eye problems but to spot degenerative processes of other systems of the body. An eye doctor can observe retinal swelling from fatty deposits of cholesterol from the bloodstream and can identify other patterns that forecast diabetes.

Regular eye exams are crucial not only for detecting serious eye problems like glaucoma but also for getting early warning of a whole range of other serious diseases, including systemic diseases like diabetes and hypertension, which are often first detected by eye doctor. Everyone over forty should have an eye exam every year or two years. People with diabetes should certainly have an eye exam every year, though they fail to do this all too often.

As for vision itself, most people retain good vision into their elderly years. Of course, everyone experiences the natural process called presbyopia, which means that we get more farsighted as we age. (Not a bad metaphor!) If you gradually find yourself holding the newspaper farther away as you read it, it's probably time for some reading glasses or, if you already wear a prescription, bifocals (preferably those that don't have that line splitting them in the middle). Be assured that this is not a degenerative disease but a natural phase of aging. It is not a sign of nutritional deficiency, nor can it be reversed with vitamins or arduous eye exercises. It's caused by a slight hardening of the lens, plus a decrease in the stretch of the tiny ligaments that support it.

Nevertheless, older persons are at higher risk for several specific diseases of the eye. The major ones are cataracts, macular degeneration, glaucoma, and diabetic retinopathy. The good news is that these diseases are in large part preventable. As with hearing, the key is a good overall health plan, with a good diet and regular exercise — the same approach that maintains good cardiovascular health, immune health, and so on. Furthermore, there are some key nutritional supplements, especially the antioxidants, that can ward off degenerative diseases of the eyes.

Macular Degeneration — The Black Hole of Vision

Macular degeneration, a degenerative disease of the eye that afflicts many individuals over the age of sixty-five, is the most common cause of blindness in that age group.

The macula is a tiny 1-millimeter-wide area at the very center of the retina. Macular degeneration happens because of cumulative damage to the delicate cells of the macula. When this happens, you start to experience a blurring or a black spot at the very center of your field of vision — the area that's crucial when you read, watch a television program, or recognize faces. In the extreme stages of macular degeneration, you experience a large blurry "hole" right in the center of your field of vision and are able to see only peripherally — the opposite of "tunnel vision."

An ophthalmologist can often detect incipient stages of macular degeneration in people in their forties. It typically begins in one eye and then appears later in the other. The odds increase with age: only 1.6 percent of adults aged fifty-two to sixty-four have it, but 11 percent of people aged sixty-five to seventy-four do, and 28 percent of people aged seventy-five to eighty-five. It's more serious in people over seventy and accounts for many cases of legal blindness.

For medical science, this is yet another idiopathic ailment of the aging process — meaning that we haven't yet pinpointed the microprocesses that set it in motion. However, we do know that oxidants are clearly a factor, as in many other age-related degenerative processes. It's true that smokers who inhale have a two and a half times increased risk, probably because of the constant exposure to free radicals generated by the smoke. Also, people with cardiovascular disease, high blood pressure, and diabetes have a higher risk of damage to the tiny blood vessels of the eyes.

When I started my radio show several years back, people would call in about macular degeneration, and I just had to say, "I'm so sorry, we don't have an answer for this." Little could I have envisioned that within a few years nutritional science would have developed the leading therapy. In fact, nutritional approaches are the major way we can prevent or improve this condition, except for a laser therapy that can slow deterioration in certain cases, and a new experimental protocol with radiation therapy. The key has been the explosion of knowledge about the antioxidant nutrients.

Actually, the clue to the linkage between antioxidants and macular degeneration was stumbled across many years ago. There were studies even in the fifties that suggested that vitamin E and beta-carotene could have a positive effect, but this likelihood wasn't pursued. Then, in 1988, conventional ophthalmology was stunned by the publication of a study by Dr. David Newsome that demonstrated that zinc supplements could greatly retard the progress of macular degeneration.[4] We've since learned that carotenoids — especially lutein, which is found in spinach and other leafy vegetables — are also strongly implicated in prevention.* These are essential yellowish pigments that protect against the wavelengths of ultraviolet light that are particularly damaging to the macula.

In fact, it's true that the more ultraviolet rays of sunlight reach the retina, the greater the chance that a person will develop macular degeneration. Sailors and ski instructors have increased risk, and so do blue-eyed people, whose eyes transmit more light to the retina. It stands to reason that good sunglasses that block the ultraviolet and high-energy blue wavelengths should assist in prevention.

Many people used to subscribe to what I term the "Bugs Bunny theory" of good vision: "Rabbits have good vision because they eat carrots, and carrots contain vitamin A, so vitamin A must be good for the eyes." Well, we do need vitamin A for night vision, and if you don't have enough vitamin A you will get night blindness, so there was some truth in that. But now we have a more complex nutritional view. A whole array of nutrients that work synergistically to maintain eye health. The eye is one of the organs that is most

---

* Green leafy vegetables contain assorted phytochemicals, which include both carotenoids and bioflavonoids.

sensitive to oxidative damage, and it can serve as a real bellwether for oxidative changes in the body.

You can now go to a health food store and purchase "eye formulas" with catchy names like Ocudyne and Ocuvite, which contain a mix of supplements that protect against macular degeneration. These include various antioxidants — zinc, selenium, vitamin C, vitamin E, beta-carotene — plus the carotenoids, and specific bioflavenoids called proanthocyanidins. (Recent research suggests that multiple supplementation with antioxidants, working together synergistically, may be more effective than any individual supplement taken alone.) An eye formula may contain vitamin B_2 (riboflavin), which is the B vitamin that is most identified as an antioxidant. Another useful supplement is bilberry extract, which was used as a special vision-enhancing supplement for the RAF fighter pilots who flew night missions during World War II. British doctors found then that the proanthocyanidin pigments in bilberry preserves could improve night vision.

Since problems with blood circulation may be a factor, vasodilators have been proposed for treatment of macular degeneration. One might also consider chelation therapy as a means of enhancing microcirculation of the retina. Researchers are also now looking into macular implants to repair macular degeneration. There is research into immune-modulating and growth-modulating drugs that might prevent or repair damage to the retina. For now, we have the powerful preventive instruments of the antioxidants, especially zinc and lutein.

Cataracts Can Be Prevented

Antioxidants can also help prevent cataracts, which are cloudy formations in the lens of the eye. Many people first heard about cataracts when their grandma or granddad had them, and perhaps had surgery to take them out. They are more common in older people and are caused by a clumping of protein in the lens, causing opacity. As a result, the vision becomes hazy and blurred. Paradoxically, sensitivity to light increases because a cataract interferes with the ability of the pupil to properly regulate the amount of light falling on the retina.

Modern cataract surgery has become increasingly sophisticated, safe, and effective. It involves sucking out the cloudy material from the inside of the lens and replacing it with a clear artificial lens implant. Sometimes an ultrasonic probe is used to emulsify the cataract into tiny bits, which are then sucked out of the eye. This process is called phako-emulsification. The lens implants are made of clear plastic, which cannot interact with the immune system. Since the lens has been removed, the cataracts cannot grow back. Sometimes the membrane that covers the replacement lens can

CAN SURGERY CORRECT YOUR VISION?

Beyond the dazzling variety of vision-correcting eyeglasses, bifocals, contact lenses, soft lenses, and tinted lenses, there are now surgical techniques that claim to fix myopia or astigmatism permanently. The incisional technique, called radial keratotomy, has been used for a while. It has some problems, including some weakening of the cornea and undercorrection of the vision impairment, leading to residual nearsightedness. There is now a system of computer-guided laser surgery that purports to take the uncertainty out of the procedure. A high-precision excimer laser, which produces short pulses of light, is used to sculpt the cornea to a new specification as a lens that will compensate for distortion in the shape of the eye. It's a little like the adjustments to the Hubble satellite telescope that fixed the basic flaws in the telescope mirror.

This procedure, called RIC, has now been approved by the FDA, and it's pretty safe and effective. There remains some concern, though, because rarely it is unsuccessful and falls short of the mark. Even though it is often very successful, the question remains whether it is worth the downside risks. I think one would have to be very motivated to eschew glasses and contact lenses and undergo RIC. However, someone who works in a challenging environment or is a soccer player, an Antarctic scientist, an actor, or a TV newscaster might have a justification for taking this route. But for most of us, eyeglasses represent a thirteenth-century technology that still has a place in the twentieth century. They're safe, and they work.

grow cloudy after cataract surgery, but the cloudy portion can then be burned off with a laser in a doctor's office.

Although modern cataract surgery is one of our better procedures, it is possible to prevent most cataracts. The key to prevention is nearly the same set of factors that guard against macular degeneration. Cigarette smoking can promote cataracts, in addition to macular degeneration. So can excess sunlight exposure and ultraviolet radiation, so the same precautions apply. The antioxidants will provide a good deal of protection. An eye product you take to prevent macular degeneration, if it has a broad spectrum of antioxidants, will simultaneously protect against cataract formation.

Deficiency of glutathione, a more esoteric antioxidant, also plays a specific role in cataract formation. It is an amino acid component of the protective system of the lens, and low glutathione levels have been reported in eighteen different types of cataracts. For a while I ran elaborate nutritional profiles on all my patients. This grew prohibitively expensive, and insurance no longer covered it, but I found some interesting things from these profiles. In particular, a very high percentage of my patients who had deficiencies of glutathione peroxidase, which is a selenium-dependent and glutathione-dependent antioxidative enzyme, also had premature cataracts in their forties and fifties. The use of glutathione as a supplement is controversial because it is not clear how well it is absorbed orally. However, it is a premier antioxidant, and there is some evidence that it can be maintained in the body through supplementation with its amino acid precursor, N-acetyl-cysteine.

Diabetics tend to develop cataracts at an earlier age than others because diabetes accelerates free radical damage. High insulin levels are associated with free radical production and with lipid peroxidation, which is a measure of free radical activity in the blood. There is also a diabetes-specific type of cataract that is caused by the deposition of a sugar called sorbitol in the eye. In diabetic patients, both sorbitol and fructose can be deposited in the eyes, where they can cause nerve damage and lens damage. Researchers have long been looking for a pharmaceutical drug that could act as an aldose-reductase inhibitor and inhibit the conversion from glucose to sorbitol. In fact, there is one already: the bioflavonoid quercetin. Designer drugs have been tested, but they are not as effective as quercetin and have not been approved by the FDA. Quercetin, a natural agent, is the best we have at this time.

Some supposedly conservative doctors still maintain that the benefits of antioxidants have not been definitively proved, and they don't recommend taking these supplements. They have been further stirred up by the one or two limited studies of high-risk patients who weren't helped by beta-carotene alone, even as they continued to smoke. In light of the preponderance of evidence, however, I will point out that a lot is at stake, and oxidative processes have been shown to play a key role in cancer, eye disease, cardiovascular health, neurological health, and on and on. As more and more studies suggest strong benefits for antioxidants in maintaining long-term health for so many systems of the body, I think it's a more truly conservative position to take the supplements. See chapter 16 for more on the antioxidants and the betacarotene issue.

What if you're already developing cataracts? Should you opt for surgery or vitamins? My suggestion is this: try the nutrients for six months. If your vision continues to deteriorate, go ahead and consider the surgery. Cataracts are not reversible.

Still, before agreeing to cataract surgery, you should always get a second opinion to see whether other problems might be affecting vision. Formerly an eye surgeon would await the moment when cataracts were supposedly "ripe" — in other words, the point at which any disadvantage of surgery would be outweighed by the advantage of restoring sight. But now cataract surgery has become so effective, and relatively safe, that eye surgeons may tend to promote it. While ophthalmologists are in general responsible and ethical, in the past a deplorable minority have prematurely or incorrectly recommended lucrative eye surgery for unsuspecting elderly patients. Fortunately, these excesses are being curbed through increased governmental vigilance. The point is to treat eye surgery like any other surgery, i.e., seriously. However, the key is prevention, because we do have good ways of forestalling the development of cataracts.

Glaucoma — A Circulation Problem

Do the eyes have circulation? Actually, they do, though it's not blood that circulates but a clear fluid called the intraocular fluid, which carries important nutrients to the tissues of the eye. Sometimes the natural drainage of this fluid can become clogged, and the resulting buildup of pressure in the eye is called glaucoma. The excess pressure can cause internal damage to the structures of the eye, including damage to the optic nerve where it enters the eye. Only peripheral vision is affected at first, but rampant glaucoma can cause blindness. Early detection and prompt treatment can usually control it.

Glaucoma usually builds up slowly. It is more common with age and with certain risk factors like diabetes. Many people don't notice that their vision is deteriorating because the glaucoma comes on gradually and first attacks peripheral vision. Glaucoma appears to be yet another "disease of civilization." In rural indigenous societies there is no increase with age, while in Western industrialized society glaucoma affects only 2 percent of people over the age of forty but 7 percent of people over seventy. In the United States there is a higher risk for African Americans, paralleling their higher risk of hypertension. An ophthalmologist or optometrist can test for glaucoma with a goniometer, a device that blows a puff of air onto the eyeball to measure the intraocular pressure.

A long list of factors can raise the risks of glaucoma, and it's more often caused by an underlying metabolic disorder than by something that is happening only in the eyes. I see it often as a disease of insulin excess, one of the manifestations of the carbohydrate-driven degenerative process that we call Syndrome X. Many of my patients have shown reduction in their intraocular pressure after switching from high-sugar, high-carbohydrate diets to my leaner Salad and Salmon Diet. In fact, the best prevention measures against glaucoma are the same ones you'd follow to reduce the risk of high blood pressure and arteriosclerosis (see chapters 12 and 16).

Other risk factors are not what you'd expect. Some people are concerned about caffeine, but it's not been shown to directly influence intraocular pressure. Contact lenses don't appear to affect glaucoma. On the other hand, repeated bodily inversions, such as yoga headstands and shoulder stands, and hanging from horizontal bars, can exacerbate glaucoma. Smoking can increase the risks, and so can the "tight necktie syndrome," in which pinched blood vessels in the neck can raise fluid pressure in eyes. New evidence points to popular inhaled steroid asthma medications as a risk factor for glaucoma.

The conventional medical therapies for glaucoma include beta-blocker drops, drugs to reduce fluid production in the eye, and local diuretics or parasympathomimetics to increase the outflow of fluid from eye. Several of them are available in the form of eye drops that control intraocular pressure in different ways. Someone with glaucoma might use up to three different kinds of eye drops, depending on what works. Some of them may have noticeable side effects, especially the beta-blockers, which infrequently cause depression, dizziness, impotence, diarrhea, nausea, and breathing problems. The parasympathomimetic drugs sometimes cause confusion in the elderly. There is also a laser treatment that opens up the ocular drainage canals and thus reduces pressure.

One of most therapeutic herbal agents for glaucoma is marijuana. While the incidence of glaucoma is higher in African Americans, there is one interesting exception. The Rastafarians, a religious sect in Jamaica, have an extremely low incidence of glaucoma — much lower than the general population. This appears to be due to their constant inhaling of locally grown marijuana. In fact, Jamaican scientists have formulated a specific glaucoma treatment from the active ingredient in marijuana: tetra-hydra-cannabinol, or THC. A drop of THC applied directly to the eye will cause a drop in intraocular pressure for about 5 hours, which is as good as any other glaucoma eye drop used in the United States. In spite of recent state referenda supporting the medical use of marijuana, for obvious reasons I don't expect that this will obtain wide acceptance in this country. A more acceptable herb to use for glaucoma is *Coleus forskohlii*, originally used in Ayurvedic medicine. An appropriate dose is 50 milligrams of the standardized 18 percent extract three times daily, taken orally.

To sum up: the best preventive plan against glaucoma is to pursue overall good health; follow the guidelines for good cardiovascular health; eat a low-carbohydrate, low-fat diet; and exercise regularly to maintain good blood flow to the eyes.

Retinal Disorders: Are Floaters Always Innocent?

Some people in their middle years begin to see "floaters": spots of light or dark that seem to migrate across the field of vision, sometimes associated with flashes of light. They are usually innocent, but they should prompt a visit to the eye doctor, since they may betoken the beginnings of a drying up or coalescence of the vitreous, the jellylike fluid inside the eye. Floaters are more common in middle age and later, when the vitreous tends to change character. Some people confuse these with ocular migraines, which induce shimmering auras without the headache pain of normal migraines. In people who have floaters, however, changes of consistency in the vitreous may cause it to pull at or pull across the retina, with a slight traction effect. This can cause retinal detachment, which is often heralded by a shower of sparks or bright flashes and ultimately appears as if a black curtain or a black card has blocked off part of the field of vision. Retinal detachment requires immediate and urgent attention. If it's caught in time, modern laser surgery can often reattach or "weld" the retina. Retinal detachment is more frequent in older people and the nearsighted, but overall it's not that common, and only a small percentage of the population will experience it. However, innocent floaters may herald retinal detachment, so precautions should be taken.

If you are susceptible — and your eye doctor should be able to give you some indication of this — you should avoid high-impact sports and jarring physical activities, since a sudden impact, a blow to the head, or an accidental blow to the eye can cause the retina to detach. So can changes in pressure due to sudden shifts in posture during exercise.

Retinal specialists can advise you on your risk of retinal detachment. My wife is an example of someone in this high-risk group. She began to experience the floaters, went to a specialist, and was more than a little scared when he told her she didn't have retinal detachment but did have a predisposition for it. If you are in this higher-risk group, you'll want to temporarily avoid high-impact activities like tennis, jogging, and high-impact aerobics, and take up low-impact activities like swimming or rowing instead, until your eye doctor gives you the all-clear.

Vitamin A has been suggested as a protective factor against floaters, so your basic eye tonic will probably provide some protection. There is some evidence that bioflavonoids can support the integrity of the retina, and they are included in some of the eye tonics. The bottom line: see your eye doctor immediately if you start to experience floaters for the first time.

Diabetic retinopathy, another retinal disorder, was quite uncommon a few decades ago. However, since more people with diabetes are surviving and living longer, they are becoming susceptible to complications of this disease, which is a leading cause of new blindness in the United States in adults forty-one to sixty. People with diabetes should take special care to have an eye exam every year, though an alarming number of them fail to do so. It's an overlooked opportunity, since laser techniques can forestall vision loss if the problem is caught early enough.

In diabetes, there is a tendency, called microangiopathy; for blood vessels to proliferate. When it takes place in the eyes, the blood vessels on the retina can build up in small bulges that can hemorrhage and damage vision. This proliferative tendency can be reduced by using anti-angiogenesis factors that inhibit the growth of blood vessels. Shark cartilage happens to be a rich source of these factors. There is ongoing research into whether shark cartilage or a derivative will prove to be a useful therapy in proliferative diseases, like cancer. The bioflavonoids, such as pycnogenol, bilberry extract, and rutin, are helpful in preventing capillary leakage or hemorrhage, and so do chromium, magnesium, and the full complement of antioxidants.

Preventing Computer Eyestrain

Magical tool or bane of modern life — whatever your opinion on computers, they're here to stay. It's a fact that the long hours many people put in at their personal computers or data terminals can cause physical problems. We've looked at a few of these in chapter 7. Some of the first indications of computer health risks arose in connection with computer terminals or monitors, as researchers began to investigate whether the radiation they emitted could cause problems such as cancer or cataracts for people who sat 18 inches away from them all day long, day after day. A simple cause-and-effect relationship was never clearly established, but computer manufacturers have nonetheless responded to these concerns by producing low-radiation monitors and terminals. But other risks remain, especially of strained vision as well as neck and back problems caused by prolonged unnatural postures.

In one study, 14 percent of all people making appointments with optometrists reported having computer-related eyestrain. The reports of eyestrain and sore eyes go up significantly for clerical workers who use computer terminals for seven or more hours a day. They may have blurred vision, dizziness, soreness, itching, headaches, or problems with contact lenses. Stale office air and poor lighting can compound the problem.

One of the most common factors compounding computer eye strain is dry eye syndrome, which causes a feeling of burning eyes and fatigue. Computer use causes a fivefold decrease in eye-blink rate, as people intently look at the material on the screen. (The normal blink rate is twelve blinks per minute.) As a result, more of the tear liquid evaporates from the surface of the eyes, leaving a dry, gritty feeling. Normally, eye-blinks replenish the liquid that protects the surface of the eye.

People who spend long hours at the computer monitor may also experience an actual decrease in focusing ability, which appears to be temporary.

Here are some tips to help reduce computer eye-strain:

• Position your monitor or arrange your workspace to avoid glare on the surface of the screen. Use an antiglare filter if necessary. Avoid having bright office lights in your line of vision at the same time you are working at the computer.

• Make sure your eyeglass prescription is accurate. If you are using bifocals or trifocals, make sure your prescription has a wide element to include the entire computer screen. If you alternate between looking at reading materials and the screen, try to place the printed materials close to the screen, or at the same distance from your eyes. You may need to have bifocals or trifocals tailored to the distances at which you place your reading materials and the computer monitor. Especially if you're over forty, you may need a special eyeglass prescription tailored to the distance that you sit from the screen.

• If you're shopping for a monitor, get one with a flat, nonglare screen and with a good sharp resolution. The "dot pitch" rating, which is one measure of resolution, should be at least .28mm (smaller is sharper). The built-in flicker of computer monitors can also cause eyestrain, especially in combination with the flicker of fluorescent office lights. A monitor that's rated as noninterlaced will have less flicker. Look for a monitor that meets VESA standards for flicker-free operation and Swedish MPRII standards for low electromagnetic radiation emissions.

• Laptop computers have improved a lot since the first ones were introduced with dim, low-contrast screens. But even some of the newer models, including color models, still have relatively low contrast screens that will contribute to eyestrain. If you're going to spend long hours at a laptop, make a bright, high-contrast screen a priority.

• If your eyes start feeling dry and gritty, consciously blink them to keep the tear liquid flowing. Keep eye drops near your workplace.

• Look away from the screen every 10 or 15 minutes. Let your eyes take a break and roam around the room for a minute.

Hearing and Vision: The Holistic Approach

Hearing and vision provide perfect examples of the holistic approach to good health. The best nutritional and preventive measures to maintain good hearing and vision are exactly the ones that support good health for the body as a whole. What's good for your heart is good for your eyes and ears. This means a healthy diet, low in saturated fat and high in nutrients; regular exercise to help circulation; and regular supplements with antioxidants to stave of the systemwide degenerative effects of free radicals. As in

---

Dry Eye

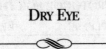

Dry eye is a common problem that particularly afflicts middle-aged women. While declining levels of estrogen near menopause may be implicated, hormone replacement therapy doesn't seem to do much good. Supplements of GLA oils and vitamin E help. A new and innovative medical approach currently in the testing phases involves the application of special estrogen drops directly to the eyes. Dry eyes may require higher doses of estrogen than are safely provided in the pills ordinarily used to treat menopause.

---

other bodily systems, with both vision and hearing we need to be aware of the potentially damaging effects of environmental excess, primarily noise in the case of hearing and overexposure to ultraviolet light in the case of vision.

A Nutrition Protocol for the Eyes

Nutrient	Daily supplement	Benefit	Food Source
The antioxidants			
Vitamin C	1000 milligrams	Help prevent	
Vitamin E	400 to 800 International Units	macular degeneration, cataracts, retinopathy	
Mixed carotenoids	15 to 40,000 International Units		Carrots, green leafy vegetables
Riboflavin (vitamin B$_2$)	50 milligrams		
Selenium	200 micrograms		
Zinc	50 milligrams		
N-acetyl-cysteine	600 to 1800 milligrams	Supports glutathione production (cataract protection)	Eggs

A NUTRITION PROTOCOL FOR THE EYES (cont'd)

NUTRIENT	DAILY SUPPLEMENT	BENEFIT	FOOD SOURCE
Bioflavonoids		Help prevent macular degeneration, cataracts, retinopathy	Blueberries, cherries, raspberries, red onions, buckwheat, many others
Quercetin	1000 to 5000 milligrams		
Rutin	500 milligrams		
Bilberry	160 milligrams		
Ginkgo biloba	50 milligrams		
Pycnogenol	50 milligrams		
Other eye nutrients			
Chromium	100 to 200 micrograms	Helps diabetic retinopathy, glaucoma	Brewer's yeast
Magnesium	400 milligrams	Helps diabetic retinopathy	Leafy greens, whole grains
Omega-3 oils	50 to 1000 milligrams	Helps glaucoma	Fish oil or flaxseed oil

CHAPTER FIFTEEN

Not Only Skin Deep:
Skin, Hair, and Nails

Nowhere does the general health (or lack thereof) of the body show so readily as it does in the appearance of our skin, hair, and nails. All of the considerable time, money, and efforts of the beauty industry are lavished on these three areas. The old adage "Beauty is only skin deep" may be true in some sense, but to maintain an attractive exterior you have to go deep inside. In fact, beauty is an inside job.

Hair and nails are actually derivatives of skin; both are made up of modified epidermal outer skin cells filled with hard keratin. The skin itself is constantly sloughing off the dead cells that make up the visible outer layer of skin. About once every 3 weeks the epidermis is totally replaced by cells that are produced in and have migrated from the deepest level of the skin, where cells are constantly dividing to provide fresh cells for the next level. What we take into the body nourishes the production of healthy skin, hair, and nail cells. In fact, only a few external applications can help these three areas.

The truth is that the maintenance of skin depends largely on nutrition. Along with nails and hair, skin is the fastest-growing and most superficial tissue of the human body. Abnormal growth patterns, defects in immunity due to infection by bacteria, viruses and fungi, and sensitivity to toxins and allergens are quickly and obviously manifested as skin problems. That's why it makes little sense to smear a cosmetic cream on the skin surface when the problem should be seen as a signal of a more profound imbalance in the body.

Some of the best things you can do to care for your skin are free or reasonably priced:

1. Don't smoke. This causes free radical damage to collagen, the structural material of skin, causing it to become less elastic. This is the origin of "smoker's wrinkles"—you can usually spot a smoker by them.

2. Apply a sunscreen, especially to your face, before venturing out on days when you'll get a lot of exposure to the sun (even in winter). One with a rating of SPF15 will extend your burn time by fifteen times, which should be adequate. If you're using other products, the sunscreen goes on first. Remember that a sunscreen does not start working until 30 minutes after it's been applied.
3. Make sure your diet contains plenty of fresh vegetables and fruits, which are highest in natural nutrients.
4. Supplement with a good antioxidant formula to cut down on free radical damage.
5. Drink plenty of pure well water or spring water. Avoid heavily chlorinated municipal drinking water.
6. Don't indulge in crash diets. Rapid weight loss or gain affects skin elasticity.
7. Get an oil change. Switch from saturated fats and hydrogenated oils to beneficial internal skin lubricants such as the natural linolenic and linoleic acids found in avocados, nuts, whole grains, and monounsaturated oils such as canola and olive oil.

Why Supplements Can Help

Food is the best source of the nutrients necessary for life. Your body best utilizes these nutrients when they are present in balance in foods. Food also provides the vitamins we need to build skin, hair, nails, and other tissues, as long as the vitamins and nutrients in the foods haven't been destroyed. You can add natural food supplements to your diet to help replace those lost. The nutrients that specifically affect skin, hair, and nails are vitamin A, vitamin C, vitamin E, vitamin B_6, biotin, silica, calcium, zinc, and the amino acid L-cysteine. Topical vitamin E has long been used to prevent scars. Research has shown that vitamin E can help prevent the formation of scars only if it's used when the scar is forming, because what it actually does is prevent the overgrowth of collagen that causes the scar.

Let's recall our supplement recipe used to treat challenged or at-risk epithelial tissue, which includes the skin, scalp, and nail-growing tissue as well as the lungs, mouth, and throat:

- Vitamin C: 1000 milligrams per day
- Vitamin E: 800 International Units per day
- Mixed carotenoids: 25,000 International Units per day
- Vitamin A retinol: 25,000 International Units per day (but no more than 5000 International Units daily in case of pregnancy)
- Selenium: 100 micrograms twice daily

- Zinc: 30 milligrams twice daily
- Folic acid: 10 milligrams twice daily
- Flaxseed oil: 1 tablespoon twice daily

To this we could add, for basic skin, hair, and nail health:

- Calcium: 1000 milligrams daily
- Vitamin B_6, 25 milligrams daily
- Biotin, 3 milligrams daily
- Silicon (as 2 percent orthosilicic acid) 6–20 drops per day (from Jarrow Formulas, Los Angeles, California)

Dietary sources of L-cysteine should be adequate — it's one of the sulfur-containing amino acids found in eggs, beans, and meats.

Cosmetics counters are laden with new products from cosmetics companies that claim to improve the skin by delivering vitamins to the skin by external application. We know that some vitamin E is absorbed by the skin. Vitamin C and zinc may affect collagen synthesis, but there's no proof yet that cosmetics containing them rejuvenate the skin. Because cosmetics aren't drugs and are not regulated by the FDA, they don't have to contain or deliver enough vitamins to make a difference. Cosmetics companies can just put in some vitamins and sell the product without substantiating their claims.

Avoiding Skin Problems

While getting a facial can make us feel pampered and, in fact, is good for cleansing the facial skin and keeping pores open so that the skin can "breathe," any harsh chemicals that might be used can actually cause skin reactions. It is much better for the health of your skin to think of an "inner facial" consisting of a change to a toxin-free natural foods diet; avoidance of constipation, which causes colon toxicity; and supplementation with essential fatty acids like flaxseed oil and/or primrose oil or borage oil. This can result in dramatic improvements in skin condition in 3 to 4 months. Be patient — it won't happen overnight. Remember that new skin is formed deep under the superficial layer and does not reach the surface until prior skin layers have been sloughed off. I promise you that if you make these changes, not only will your skin improve, but your general health and well-being will improve also. Do it every day without expecting results for just 90 days, and then you'll see a difference.

Stress, too, can cause skin problems (although in some instances doctors use stress as a catchall when they don't take the time to delve deeply enough to find a physical cause). Stress and anxiety do trigger the release of hormones and neurotransmitters that can sometimes promote inflammations, itching, and even acne. Stress may also deplete key nutrients. Try using meditation and biofeedback to reduce the stress; such techniques may partially rein in the inflammatory process.

On the other side of the stress question, we need to keep in mind that stress has become a popular notion embraced by the general public, and some people use this notion in their lives in a harmful way. In working with patients to reduce their stress, I often help them change their mind-set so that they don't get stuck in a cycle of self-reinforcement and self-fulfilling prophecies sustained by their belief systems. For instance, if you believe that stress will give you hives or make your hair fall out, you're setting yourself up for trouble. Our immune systems will actually respond to what we believe. There's a lot to be said for keeping a positive attitude, as has been objectively demonstrated.

I take a twofold approach in dealing with skin problems (and, in fact, in all my practice), which I think of as the mind/body approach. On the physical side there are specific protocols for the natural treatment of various skin problems like seborrheic dermatitis, acne, psoriasis, rosacea, eczema, and even precancerous skin lesions. They involve the use of herbs, nutritional supplements, and diet modification as well as tracking down hidden allergies to foods and environmental factors. I use all of these successfully in my practice.

Wrinkles

We've known for years that prolonged exposure to the sun can cause premature aging of the skin and excessive wrinkling. Now a team at the University of Utah has conducted a study that shows that the more you smoke and the longer you smoke the more wrinkles you get. In fact, according to the study, smokers have three times the rate of excessive skin wrinkling as those who don't smoke.

Smoking damages collagen, a fibrous protein found in the skin, which represents 30 percent of the total body protein. Damaged collagen appears to lead to faster skin wrinkling. Smoking coupled with sun exposure is double trouble; together, these two factors lead to even more severe wrinkling. So, for the best protection for your skin and to avoid excessive wrinkles, stay out of the sun and stop smoking.

It just makes sense to think about things you *can* do to save your skin because there are so many other things that you have little control over. Take "liver spots": even if you try to limit sun exposure now, you may get them anyway. By the age of eighteen most people have received 75 percent of their lifetime exposure to sun. If you are in your forties and you're trying to limit your sun exposure, you may still, depending on your genetic predisposition or the amount of sun you had as a child, end up with liver spots.

These have nothing to do with the liver except that they are liver-colored. Called "those horrid age spots" in ads for bleaching creams, which are only minimally effective, liver spots can be helped by the use of tretinoin cream (Retin-A) and other treatments. Retin-A is a synthetic vitamin A, administered nightly though a topical cream, which over 9 months or so can in some instances smooth fine wrinkles and lighten age spots. It is expensive, doesn't work for everyone, and has a subtle rather than a dramatic effect. Retin-A is obtained by prescription only and has a new name, Renova, in its newly approved use for wrinkle and spot treatment. Retin-A had originally been approved for acne, for which it wasn't very useful, and has been recycled for wrinkles. Retin-A can also be used to normalize the skin if you have dark discolorations or hyperpigmentation. Your dermatologist can help you determine whether it's right for you.

When you are using Retin-A, extreme care must be used to insure that the skin has minimal exposure to sunlight, since the Retin-A strips off a top, protective layer of skin, thus exposing the skin underneath to more ultraviolet radiation. Another drawback is that Retin-A has to be applied consistently for a long time before results are apparent.

A popular ingredient in nonprescription "rejuvenating" creams and masks is a compound of alpha hydroxy acids (AHAs) derived from fruit peels. They provide a gentle skin scrubbing effect, which is akin to that produced by Retin-A. Effects vary and are limited.

As the baby-boomer generation has gotten older, the market has been deluged with a plethora of cosmetic products that claim to retard and even reverse the aging process. The fact is that aging is a natural, inexorable process. Some of these products are useful and some are not. Use them if you want to (and if you can afford to) but don't rely on them.

Skin Cancer

A deep, dark tan was once thought to be healthy looking, but today there is overwhelming evidence that exposing the skin to the sun's rays and therefore to the sun's radiation is a health hazard. The American Academy of Dermatology reports that the incidence of melanoma, the most deadly skin cancer, increased by 1200 percent between 1930 and 1994. From those statistics it's easy to see that the increased use of sunscreens has not yet blunted this alarming rise in skin cancers. Sun overexposure and the demise of the ozone layer are clearly to blame, in part, but we still need more answers to explain the inexorable advance of melanoma.

Besides melanoma there are two other kinds of skin cancers. The most common type is basal cell carcinoma, which affects nearly 600,000 people annually. But the important fact is that it is 99 percent curable if detected and treated early. Watch for its usual appearance as slowly growing, raised, translucent nodules, which if not treated may crust, ulcerate and sometimes bleed. About one-third of these cancers are found on the nose. The face, neck, and hands are other common sites for basal cell carcinomas.

Squamous cell carcinoma, the second most common type of skin cancer, affects some 150,000 people annually, killing over 2000 of them, but it is 95 percent curable with early detection and treatment. They are usually raised, red or pink, scaly nodules or wart-like growths that ulcerate in the center. Typically they develop on the rim of the ears, the face, the lips and mouth, the hands, and other areas that are frequently exposed to the sun.

Malignant melanoma, the least common and most deadly of the skin cancers, may suddenly appear without warning or can develop from or near a mole. It is found most frequently on the upper back and on the legs, but it can appear anywhere on the body.

Your doctor or dermatologist should give your entire body a thorough inspection, noting the location and condition of any moles, warts, or other skin blemishes, and then the skin should be rechecked periodically to make sure that there are no significant changes. This is the one of the most important measures you can take to guard against skin cancer.

There's also a diet component to skin cancer. High levels of saturated fat in the diet have been associated with precancerous skin lesions called actinic keratosis; they are the precursors of basal cell carcinoma. Again, we see how important diet is to health.

Many people now realize that lying in the sun to get a tan leads to premature aging of the skin and even to more serious conditions like cancer, so they tend to protect themselves with sunscreens or clothing. It's wise to keep in mind that ultraviolet radiation has a cumulative effect on the body — every bit of it, whether real or artificial — so stay out of tanning parlors. Exposing yourself to extra UV radiation just for cosmetic purposes is taking an unnecessary risk. If you've been told that your tanning booth gives "safe" UVA, not UVB, don't risk it! UVB, with the shorter electromagnetic wavelength, was thought to be the primary culprit in skin cancer, but submitting to intense amounts of UVA in a tanning parlor is questionable. There is plenty of evidence that UVA rays contribute significantly to aging of the skin and to the risk of skin cancer. (UVB is stronger in higher altitudes, near the equator, and at midday; UVA is the "background" ultraviolet radiation and is relatively constant throughout the day.)

Also, don't rationalize your overdose of sun exposure by citing the argument that vitamin D (which is made in the skin in the presence of sunlight) can prevent colon cancer or osteoporosis. To produce vitamin D, the body only needs light, not a suntan. Normal activities all through the year will supply your skin with enough sunlight. Stay out of the sun from 10 A.M. to 3 P.M., during the summer months when the sun is strongest, and use your head when evaluating health risks.

Some studies have shown that people who experienced repeated sunburn as teenagers are more likely to have skin cancer as adults—and this means the baby boomers. No doubt we're losing our ozone layer and sunlight's potential to inflict damage may be greater than ever. Whatever the various causes, baby boomers are at high risk for skin cancer. Because of this, it's important to keep a watchful eye out for changes in skin coloration, or the appearance of any new moles, nodules, or wartlike growths, and have them looked at by a dermatologist. Skin cancers can be quite effectively treated in the early stages.

Psoriasis

Psoriasis, an inflammatory condition of the skin in which the skin's outer surface proliferates into a flaky crust, is a disfiguring and sometimes painful problem. It can also affect nails, giving them a pitted or funguslike appearance. It tends to cluster in families, but conventional medicine has not found a cause.

Doctors who use the orthodox treatment for psoriasis usually begin by prescribing topical steroid creams. If they don't work, "PUVA" is offered: the patient is given ultraviolet light treatment and a drug called psoralen, which intensifies the light's healing effects. This treatment can have side effects because, while partially alleviating the psoriasis, the high-intensity light may damage the skin and trigger other problems such as skin cancer.

We can employ intelligent medicine to treat psoriasis in several ways. First, we recognize that skin problems usually arise as the result of allergy or internal toxicity. The psoriasis sufferer may have candidiasis or food allergies. Therefore, treating the skin itself is not the solution. In the case of allergy, the diet has to be modified so that the offending foods are eliminated. In the case of *Candida* infection, antifungal therapy will remove the stimulus to uncontrolled skin proliferation (see chapters 9 and 10 for more on *Candida* infection).

Also, certain vitamins, minerals, and other supplements that reduce the inflammation of psoriasis should be taken. Omega-3 fish oils are especially helpful. When treated with vitamin A, vitamin D, shark cartilage extract, and antioxidant nutrients, psoriasis can be healed naturally. Fumaric acid, a natural substance, the use of which was pioneered in Swiss skin clinics, is an important adjunct to psoriasis care. Sunlight and seaweed are also often helpful. The coming of summer or a tropical getaway brings relief to many psoriasis sufferers. In some patients, skin applications of a specially prepared prescription vitamin D cream called Dovonex helps to alleviate scaling.

The cream provides vitamin D to the growing skin cells, mimicking the vitamin D–activating effects of sunlight. A new natural topical skin treatment promises to revolutionize the treatment of psoriasis. Popularly marketed as Skin-Cap spray or ointment, the active ingredient zinc pyrithione is effective for psoriasis as well as flaky eczema. A special shampoo form of Skin-Cap reverses stubborn scalp psoriasis as well as dandruff.

Acne

Although we think of acne as a teenager's problem, in fact many people are bothered with it in midlife and at various times throughout their lives. Chronic acne sufferers are often dosed with antibiotics. Unfortunately, these can cause chronic yeast infections accompanied by intestinal disturbances, sometimes leading to chronic vaginitis. Retin-A is still sometimes used for acne, though it isn't that helpful. Some patients are given Accutane, an oral form of Retin-A, which can give the skin a dry, unnatural look and can create liver abnormalities and elevated cholesterol levels.

Even as teenagers we knew that a chocolate bar on Saturday afternoon would sometimes produce "zits" before school on Monday morning. Yet when a dermatologist mentions nothing about our diet and starts prescribing, we suspend our disbelief. Well, your teenage self knew better! Dietary clean-up is the basis of natural therapy for acne.

Excess saturated fat and hydrogenated oils must be eliminated. Certain foods trigger acne in susceptible people. For some, it is sugar or chocolate; for others, dairy products. Still others react to iodine in shellfish or excess iodized salt. Some experience exacerbations with spicy foods. With a little experimentation and self-observation you can find out for yourself what foods trigger or exacerbate your acne. Then let your doctor know what you've observed; that can contribute to a better partnership with your doctor and perhaps shorten the time to a successful cure.

While cosmetic antiaging creams and ointments are generally ineffective, there are natural, noncosmetic creams and ointments that can help specific conditions, such as acne. Topical applications of azelaic acid, newly available by prescription, help many acne sufferers. For more difficult cases, a special prescription lotion prepared by mixing zinc and erythromycin does the trick. Other surface-active agents include tea-tree oil and specially prepared niacinamide gel. Acne rosacea, clusters of pustules on an inflamed base, responds well to Metrogel, a preparation of the parasite drug metronidazole in a gel form.

Intestinal toxicity due to chronic constipation, which often accompanies a poor diet, can force the skin to become an auxiliary eliminative organ. When your diet includes enough fresh and cooked vegetables and fruit, this problem will most likely disappear naturally. Therapy with acidophilus and natural fiber products with bentonite can promote colon cleansing.

Hormonal problems sometimes underlie acne. Surges of male androgenic hormones can cause the sebaceous glands to overproduce a greasy substance called sebum, which blocks pores. Reduction of animal protein in the diet and substitution with high-fiber grains, beans, and vegetables actually tames unruly hormones by facilitating their elimination from the body. In women, the application of topical progesterone cream from wild yams can ease premenstrual or menopausal acne. This can be found in health food stores under such brand names as Pro-Gest. More important, this same cream has been shown in studies to help keep bones strong, prevent osteoporosis later in life, and help keep wrinkles at bay. This is something that I think women will find very useful, as it has a wonderful effect on skin and even goes beyond that to provide gentle hormonal support.

As we discussed in the chapter on the endocrine system, stress can overstimulate the adrenals, which respond by an unbalanced production of androgenic hormones. Relaxation through biofeedback or meditation may alleviate stress-induced hormone overproduction.

Allergies to airborne chemicals can also trigger acne. For example, chloracne is a common form of skin eruption found in chemical workers exposed to chlorine. Skin testing can identify sensitivity to these chemicals.

Nutritional supplements that can reduce acne include primrose or borage oil, vitamin A, zinc, selenium, vitamin B_6, and chromium. Herbal blood cleansers like burdock, Oregon graperoot, dandelion, and goldenseal produce beneficial effects in many patients.

INTELLIGENT MEDICINE TIPS: ⎯⎯⎯⎯⎯⎯⎯⎯⎯⎯⎯⎯⎯⎯⎯⎯

For acne, try the following regimen:

> Vitamin A, 15 to 25,000 International Units daily, but restrict to no more than 5000 International Units in women contemplating pregnancy
> Vitamin B_6, 25 milligrams daily
> Zinc, 30 milligrams twice daily
> Selenium, 100 micrograms twice daily
> Chromium, 100 micrograms twice daily
> Borage oil, two to four capsules containing 240 to 300 milligrams GLA, daily

Eczema

The mainstay of conventional therapy for eczema, a form of allergic dermatitis, is the use of steroidal skin creams. Individuals with eczema often have other allergies such as asthma. This is the tipoff that this individual's eczema may also have an allergic component or may even be entirely caused by food or other allergies, as is often the case.

The radioallergosorbent (RAST) blood test or skin testing can often pin down the culprits. For those with complex allergies or serious eczema, a trial of an hypoallergenic protein powder called UltraClear often brings dramatic relief. This is available from nutritionally oriented physicians for supervised use. Suspect foods can then be eliminated and reintroduced one by one, and thus the offending foods can be identified.

Many patients with eczema also have *Candida* infections, which can be treated with diet modification and antifungal medication. As with other skin problems, restoration of normal gut ecology is essential.

Supplements that help eczema include primrose or borage oil, flaxseed oil, omega-3 fish oil, zinc, and vitamins A and E. I personally helped to formulate a topical preparation called Glycort, distributed by the Allergy Research Group (telephone 800-545-9960), which is derived from licorice and acts like a natural steroid application without the side effects of synthetic steroidal creams.

Eczema can cause severe inflammation of the skin. That's what had happened to Barry, who came to me with severe eczema: his face, arms, trunk and legs were lobster-red. He also had constant nasal congestion and wheezing, and his skin was so taut and inflamed that he had difficulty flexing his fingers and arms. He was scarred by years of scratching and overzealous application of steroid cream.

Since there was no normal skin available to skin test, I performed a blood test to discover the allergies that I knew Barry must have. The test results were positive to so many foods that I was stumped about what diet to recommend. He started with only vegetables, a few noncitrus fruits, and the hypoallergenic protein powder UltraClear. (Many traditional detoxification regimens for eczema highlight supposed allergic responses to citrus fruits. Other common food culprits include eggs, milk, wheat, tomatoes, and yeast.)

This diet, together with supplements of vitamins, minerals, and essential fatty acids, produced a reduction in Barry's inflammation in just 2 weeks. By then, a stool test had revealed a massive overgrowth of intestinal yeast. We prescribed antifungal medicine, and Barry's skin improved further. Eight weeks later, new healthy pink skin began to show beneath the flaking debris of Barry's old eczema: he was shedding the old skin like a snake. The bonus? He was 15 pounds lighter and very pleased with the new self that was emerging.

Gradually safe foods were reintroduced for Barry. He began to eat lamb, fish, and certain beans for his protein; amaranth, quinoa, and buckwheat became his grain staples; squash replaced French fries and potato chips in his diet; and healthy garden salads accompanied nearly every meal. Barry's congestion and wheezing also abated. He's a walking ad for alternative skin care and the added benefits and sense of well-being that a healthy diet can bring.

Seborrheic Dermatitis

This term refers to a flaky red rash that often affects the "T-zone": the region of the face around the eyebrows, on the forehead, and adjacent to the bridge of the nose. It is sometimes accompanied by bothersome dandruff of the scalp. Once it was treated exclusively with steroid creams, but even conventional dermatologists now recognize that seborrheic dermatitis is caused, at least in part, by a fungal infection of the skin. Topical Nizoral cream or, if natural remedies are preferred, tea-tree oil can alleviate the redness and flaking. A more fundamental approach to this unsightly problem looks toward the eradication of systemic *Candida* infection with diet modification and intestinal balancing. Oral vitamin B_6 and a topical skin application of vitamin B_6 cream are helpful, as well as oral supplementation with zinc and flaxseed oil (see chapters 9 and 10 for more on *Candida*).

I used these successfully with Arthur, who at forty-five had had seborrheic dermatitis almost all his life. His forehead and cheeks were perpetually dry, red, and inflamed. Skin applications of tea-tree oil helped only slightly at first, so skin testing for allergy to *Candida* and related skin fungi was undertaken. Red blotches appeared on his arm where the test substances were applied, confirming the suspected condition. A sugar-free, yeast-free diet and oral antifungal medication, along with generous supplements of vitamin B_6, flaxseed oil, and zinc, produced total remission in 3 months.

I've given these examples of specific problems to illustrate the power of natural approaches to skin problems, especially when conventional approaches fall short of total cure or create unwanted side effects. The interesting thing is that people who don't have skin problems but want to maintain their skin at its best into middle age and beyond can apply many of these same principles.

Healthy Hair

Healthy hair is a natural adjunct to a really healthy person. If you want to keep your hair healthy, you have to avoid the enemies of healthy hair: too much sun, vitamin deficiencies, illness or other stresses, certain drugs like sulfa drugs and birth control pills, and cosmetic assaults like perming or dyeing. There is also the issue of environmental contamination, as from chlorine.

Damage from the sun can be avoided by following the example of people in other cultures where there is harsh sun — they cover their heads to protect the hair and the hair follicles from ultraviolet damage. Products are readily available that protect the hair from solar damage, essentially "sunscreens" for the hair. Remember, not only can sun damage the hair, but also the heat from hair dryers is unquestionably associated with hair damage and hair loss.

Chlorine, used in swimming pools, is a bleach and it does have a damaging effect on hair. Not only does it affect the texture and color of the hair, but it can also weaken hair at the follicle. Sports magazines for swimmers usually have advertisements for products that are designed to protect the hair from chlorine damage.

If you have pets, it's easy to see how hair is affected by diet. Try feeding your dog or cat one of the nutritionally rich pet foods and watch how the animal soon develops a completely different coat: dryness disappears and the coat becomes thick and lustrous. The same thing happens in humans when sufficient nutrients are added to the diet.

Conversely, poor diet and especially crash dieting have the opposite effect on the hair, and hair loss may occur. The nutrients that are sometimes implicated in hair loss are the essential fatty acids, so I give flaxseed oil or the amino acid L-cysteine.

DOSAGES: Flaxseed oil, four to six 1000-milligram capsules or up to one tablespoon daily; L-cysteine, 500 milligrams three times daily, not with food.

What's so insidious about hair loss is that it can be latent. You go on a crash diet, then resume your normal eating habits, and later lose hair, so it's hard to establish antecedents. It's hard to recognize that the crash dieting or the illness (or whatever it was) was causing the hair loss.

Many people don't recognize the relationship of hair condition or hair loss to illness. Sometimes there is a latency period of months after an illness before the hair loss occurs. Hair is, in fact, one of the most vulnerable parts of the body. After chemotherapy, the hair loss occurs about 10 days later; what this really represents is free-radical damage and a profound interruption of nutrition to the rapidly growing hair follicle. Any nutritional deficiency or illness is liable to show up in the skin and nails and also the hair.

I'm not saying that all hair loss is a sign of disease or poor health; there is a programmatic loss of hair that occurs hormonally, particularly in men but also in women. As they age, most women will also experience some hair loss. It happens to some women in their forties as a prelude to menopause.

Whether you're a man or a woman, if you find that you're losing more hair than you suspect is normal, you should certainly see your doctor to investigate the cause. For instance, I often tell women who have had hair loss to try discontinuing birth control pills or hormone replacement therapy. While estrogen may rejuvenate hair and skin in some women — and logically speaking it should, because the hormones involved have an antiaging effect — for others there is a paradoxical side effect. Loss of scalp hair is listed as a side effect of estrogen in the *Physicians' Desk Reference*, though it is infrequent. Hypothyroidism can cause dry skin and thinning hair; thyroid medication can reverse this. Any kind of autoimmune disease, such as lupus, can cause hair loss.

Generally, a safe, conservative approach to hair care is the best way to keep hair healthy. Harsh treatments like dyeing, straightening, and perming should be avoided. I see African-American women with serious hair thinning problems who have been using hair relaxing products for 30 years or more. They say, "If this is from the hair relaxing products, why didn't I get it 30 years ago?" It's like anything else: a continued assault will produce more damage than an occasional insult, and there may be a cumulative effect on the hair and scalp.

Serious health concerns are now being raised about hair dyes, which have a high potential for causing skin irritations, allergies, and immune problems because they're in a category of chemicals that have been associated with carcinogenesis: the aromatic compounds or phenolated hydrocarbons with aromatic chains. Studies have shown that people who use them have a higher incidence of certain autoimmune diseases, and there is some evidence, still incomplete, linking them to certain cancers.

Finally, I should say that I don't believe in the "fertilizer theory" of hair growth. Many people start taking supplement after supplement in vain when they are basically dealing with a natural, genetically based hair-thinning or balding process. It's true that some hair loss or thinning is related to debilitating diseases, medication, hormonal changes or problems, or specific individual nutritional deficiencies. It can derive from any one in a series of weak links, or from broad-based deficiencies such as those caused by overzealous dieting or anorexia nervosa. The bottom line is to look at your general health picture and make sure you're getting sufficient nutrients across the board, as pointed out in chapter 16.

Healthy Nails

Nails that chip, peel, or break too easily are often a sign of age or poor health. Menopause and adrenopause can affect the nails because of hormonal deficiencies. Nails are a reflection of the body's health — so much so that a bout with illness can leave a trace as horizontal ridges in the surface of a nail, especially the thumbnail.

People who are perpetually in ill health or have chronic conditions will often have nails that are thin, split, and grooved with ridges. There are even characteristic patterns associated with certain diseases; for instance, people with kidney diseases have a spooning of the nails — nails that curl upward. People with gastrointestinal diseases like colitis have some of the worst nails I've seen: thin, split, and grooved. These patients often ask, "Can't I take supplements of gelatin to improve my nails?" You can put a lot of supplemental nutrients into the body, but unless the body is in generally good health, the nutrients won't be absorbed and utilized. First the underlying problems have to be discovered and corrected. Undetected hypothyroidism, for instance, can cause problems with nails — another of the body's signs that something fundamental is wrong.

On the other hand, if a person is in generally good health, it's quite likely that gelatin, the protein derived from the hooves of animals, will work to strengthen the nails. Calcium is also a factor in nail health, and vitamin C and zinc are growth factors just as they are in skin and hair. Biotin is a growth factor for nails also. It's part of vitamin B-complex, but for nail enhancement it's given in much higher doses. A recent study by Hoffman LaRoche indicated that 3 milligrams per day of biotin, which is quite high in relation to most people's usual dietary intake, could enhance nail growth and reverse symptoms of thinning, cracking, brittle nails. Biotin is the closest thing to a quick fix for nails.

Toenails that are thin or that split easily may signal a fungus growing around or under the toenails, circulatory problems, or poor nutrition. New, safer oral drugs are now available to treat fungal nails, but they work best in conjunction with a low-sugar *Candida* diet.

A Look to the Future

As in other body systems, it is likely that a combination of preventive strategies, nutritional supplementation specifically targeted to deficiencies, and high-tech solutions of the future will yield skin and hair whose biological age belie their chronological age. Meanwhile, it is the task of intelligent medicine to separate hype from reality and wishful thinking from plausible science. Hope must be balanced with a certain degree of graceful resignation, because ultimately the skin and hair mirror to some extent the passage of time. We need a little philosophy to leaven our medical research.

PART THREE

TAKING CHARGE
OF YOUR HEALTH

CHAPTER SIXTEEN

Eating for Health and Pleasure

We know today more than ever the importance of diet in maintaining good health. Everywhere we look, from television commercials to supermarket aisles, we see and hear claims of "Low-Calorie!", "Zero Cholesterol!", "High In Fiber!", "Fat-Free!", and even "*99% Fat-Free!*" Advertisements for weight-loss programs, liquid diets, and low-calorie desserts fill the pages of magazines and bombard us over the airwaves. Health food stores contain a veritable cornucopia of foods, diets, vitamins, and nutritional supplements.

Of all the healthy diets — high-protein, macrobiotic, food-combining, gluten-free, vegan, my own Salmon and Salad Diet — how do you decide which one is the right one for you? How does one separate fact from fiction? What supplements, if any, should you be taking?

When my patients consult me about their diets they often expect that I am going to "punish" them by taking away something that they love to eat, or they tell me how strenuous and serious are their own efforts to restrict everything that they consider "bad." It's time to chuck the moral issue of good food versus bad food and come to accept the fact that food is a complex issue for many of us. Perhaps separating the emotional and moral issues from the actual process of eating will enable us to derive not only ample nutrition but also a sense of pleasure from eating.

Pleasure is certainly one of the many gifts of an enjoyable meal. If you have unpleasant "baggage" associated with food or with mealtimes, now is the time to put that old "baggage" on the shelf and leave it there. Come to your next snack or meal with a new awareness of the pleasure you can derive from the look, smell, texture, taste, and even sound of food.

Once you've decided that food should pleasure you in all your senses, you will have started down a path that can lead to a happier, healthier you. Naturally, when shopping you will look for fruits and vegetables that are at their peak of freshness and that have a fresh, pleasing aroma. To please your eye, you will want variety of color and texture. The feel of a smooth food like pureed butternut squash will contrast with the feel and sound of something crunchy like radishes or green pepper in your salad. If you've been stuck in the habit of coming home and pulling something out of the freezer and popping it into the microwave, you can start to change that today by preparing just one more fresh meal per week.

Get into the habit of self-nurturing by cooking as many of your own meals as possible, or cooking with friends or family. If you have kids, let them learn to cook, too. As long as you start with good fresh ingredients and a simple recipe, and don't overcook, you can't really go wrong. Set your table and make it attractive, perhaps with flowers or your favorite place mats. Don't save these things for special occasions! Start making this a daily practice. You will develop your creative side, and you will derive many physical and emotional health benefits from it.

Food is associated with a sense of physical and emotional well-being from our first day of life and remains important throughout our lives. What I suggest is that you examine your attitudes toward food and self-nurturing and decide whether *you* think they serve you well. After all, whether or not we acknowledge it, we always act in accordance with our own belief systems, so time spent examining just what we do believe about food can give us needed information.

If you feel you want to make some changes, many paths are open to you, and you will need to spend some time choosing one. That may leave you wondering which path is right for you. I am going to share some of my personal experience and some of the things I've learned working with my patients. I think you'll have some good guidelines when you've completed this chapter.

Standard American Diet (SAD)

The diet that I (along with the rest of the baby-boomer generation) was raised on was probably the worst ever in terms of health. The epitome of middle-class eating was thought to be blemish-free, commercially produced white bread (some brands now have as many as fifty-two added chemicals!), plentiful cold cuts, and steak or a roast. The prosperous postwar boom had provided many Americans with processed food and as much meat as they wanted. Yes, there was a fledgling health food movement in the 1950s, but for the most part, the occasional "juice bar" in an urban center was populated mostly by beatniks and Russian exiles. The rest of America was growing fat, literally, on the postwar boom.

By the time I was in medical school, I knew that the American diet was contributing to the increase of disease in this country among people who ostensibly had a healthy lifestyle. At first I thought that meat was the culprit, so I experimented with macrobiotics and vegetarianism. But I've learned over the years that a macrobiotic or vegetarian diet may be right for some people and not right for others. I have come to believe that there is not one dietary path that is right for everyone. Believe me, this is not the easiest philosophy for me to hold. Everyone wants to know where you stand; the so-called diet doctors prescribe a diet that you must follow; they stand behind it — that's it — there's no other way! Well, perhaps there are many paths to dietary rectitude; so I've come to believe in a more pragmatic approach without holding to one ideology.

In fact, I don't think there's a place for morality or ideology in this arena; they don't mix with a scientific empirical approach. There's a science to optimizing people's health nutritionally, and its importance shouldn't be minimized. On the other hand, a good diet is not a panacea for everything.

Once the optimal diet approach for an individual is found and followed, it can help to optimize the health of many of the body's systems — the cardiovascular system, of course, but also the immune system and even the nervous system. A balanced nutrition plan pays off with better health, but it's not the only factor in health. I often find myself advising patients who are making valiant efforts to eat a certain proportion of this or that food group, or to never eat this or that, to just ease up on themselves.

Although there is not one diet for everyone, there are some general guidelines to follow in choosing what you will eat. In this chapter we'll give highlights of approaches that seem to work for many people, and we'll also deal with some common issues that give people concern. We'll also offer a diet approach that is heart-healthy and preventive of sugar diseases: the Salad and Salmon Diet. This is not a list of food groups and portions but a flexible diet plan that will accommodate many different tastes.

What to Eat?

The subject of proper diet is endlessly debated in nutrition circles. Controversy rages over many issues, such as the role (if any) of animal protein in the "ideal" diet. Such concerns sometimes move otherwise pacific vegetarians to fits of savage indignation.

Here are some guidelines that can help virtually anyone form the basis of a healthy eating style. Remember, of course, that each of us is unique in food preference and biological makeup. There is no single "ultimate approach" to diet selection. What we're looking for is a diet that promotes optimal personal health, not rigid adherence to one dietary philosophy.

Nutrient-Rich versus Calorie-Dense

An important basic principle in food selection is to prioritize foods that are rich in vitamins, minerals, fiber, and protein and packaged with minimal caloric accompaniment. An example of a nutrient-rich food is salmon. It's loaded with protein, vitamin A, vitamin D, selenium, and heart-healthy omega-3 oil. Another is broccoli, which is chock full of fiber, vitamin C, the carotenoids, calcium, and cancer-preventive indoles (more on these later). The calorie-dense antithesis of these foods might be a rich dessert pastry, packing a caloric wallop in terms of sugar and synthetic shortening but with little in the way of substantive nutritional value. A diet that emphasizes high-nutrient and low-calorie content is especially important as you age and your metabolism slows down.

Think vegetables! And think about fruits and other low-calorie, nutrient-rich foods. By eating lots of vegetables and fruits, you're less likely to fill up on fatty foods. Vegetables have fewer calories than meat or cheese, so you'll not only be getting needed nutrients but restricting your calorie intake, which has been shown in animal studies to sharply reduce the incidence of cancer, and even prolong life.[1]

Low-Fat Mania

These days, every major magazine is full of low-fat articles and recipes, many of them meatless for the sake of cholesterol and fat reduction. If you peruse the shelves of your local supermarket, you will also notice that nearly every item has a label boasting its absence of cholesterol, even foods like peanut butter and pita bread that never had cholesterol to begin with.

In fact, the collective cholesterol angst is so strong worldwide that the McDonald's fast-food chain recently announced a plan to begin selling an all-vegetable burger in the Netherlands, and that in the United States, grated carrots will top salads instead of cheese. (These moves also represent a cost-saving measure for the giant fast-food chain.) But I think we may be going overboard on the antifat business.

Some people apply fuzzy logic to their reasons for not eating fats. It goes something like this: "Fat is the calorie stuff that makes you fat and has something to do with heart disease, so eliminate fat and you'll stay slim forever and never die." Right? Wrong! Taken to its extreme, low-fat mania results in the exaltation of poor-quality high-calorie foods like "low-fat" desserts, cookies, breakfast pastries, and pasta items made with refined flour. Don't fall for the low-fat hype.

The Cholesterol Connection

Though Americans now take the cholesterol-heart disease connection for granted, many researchers are not so sure.

Here are a few of the reasons why:

1. An equal number of scientific studies refute the notion that high cholesterol is responsible for coronary heart disease as link the two. But as

the low-fat ideology gained adherents, studies disproving the cholesterol hypothesis were shunned by prominent medical journals, and therefore the public did not hear about them.

2. "Either way, you're gonna die." This argument can be summarized as follows: Even though the rate of fatal coronary disease is lowered in individuals with high cholesterol by lowering their cholesterol levels, their overall mortality rate is not lowered. The same people will die of other causes at nearly the same age. According to some studies, lowering cholesterol may ultimately extend life expectancy for low-risk individuals by only 3 days to 3 months. Eighteen days to 12 months of increased life expectancy can be seen in high-risk individuals.

3. Studies being conducted on women and cholesterol have different results than the highly publicized, public-mandate studies, which have been done only on men. In fact, Margo A. Danke, M.D., who is at the forefront of women's health research, states that "a cholesterol-lowering diet in women may paradoxically *increase* coronary heart disease risk rather than reduce it."

4. Many doctors, like Alan R. Gaby, M.D., believe that the whole cholesterol controversy is simply a way to mask the real underlying poisons in our diet, chiefly "large amounts of dietary sugar, refined flour, margarine, processed or heated vegetable oils, and food additives."

5. Men with very low levels of cholesterol (below 160 milliliters per deciliter of blood) have 32 percent higher rates of violent death like suicide and trauma, as well as death of cancer, respiratory and other diseases, and stroke.

6. The original research on cholesterol and coronary heart disease, which caused the outcry against cholesterol in the first place, was found to be flawed, marred by statistical misinterpretation.

Oil Change

That's right—get yourself an oil change. Some fats are healthy; others are not. Avoid margarine and hydrogenated fats used as shortening in cookies, breads, candies, and baked products. Cut down on butter and fried meats. Frying seals in fat and renders chemically unstable refined polyunsaturated vegetable oils rancid ("oxidized" is the formal biochemical term.) *Oxidized* cholesterol and fat may be the true culprits in heart disease.

When the fast-food giants advertise their "healthy" move from lard to polyunsaturated vegetable oil that is touted to have no cholesterol, remember that the vegetable oil is an unstable compound and oxidizes readily, especially with repeated heatings, producing free radicals that can cause all kinds of harm to the body. Like the move from butter to margarine, this switch doesn't deliver the health benefits it claims.

Some oil is necessary in the diet, but make an effort to get it from food sources like the omega-3 oils found in cold-water fish such as salmon, trout, tuna, and sardines or from vegetarian sources like walnuts and purslane. Also make use of heart-healthy monounsaturated olive and canola oils and even avocado oil. They help even out blood sugar levels and have newly proven benefits for people with diabetes, such as reduced resistance to insulin, lower blood pressure, and protection against arteriosclerosis.

Frying foods is not recommended, but if you insist on frying, peanut oil is probably your healthiest bet. For sautéing or stir-frying, when you want to use the oil as a condiment for added flavor, use a little sesame, walnut, or olive oil, or even corn or sunflower oil if a blander taste is desired.

Consider keeping all oils in the refrigerator, since once they are opened they begin to lose their freshness (or oxidize). Oxidation is caused by the polyunsaturated fat molecules reacting with air to produce a rancid taste. Most people prefer oils that don't change taste, even during frying, and those are the oils that are higher in monounsaturated fats.

Avoid the tropical oils like coconut oil and palm oil, and also cottonseed oil, which is often blended into processed foods and salad dressings. Since cotton is not classified as a food, cottonseed oil, a byproduct of cotton production, is grown with pesticides, fertilizers, and other chemicals that have been banned by the FDA for use on food crops.

RATING THE SUPERMARKET-AVAILABLE OILS

OIL	COMMENTS	STABILITY
Olive	Staple of the Mediterranean diet since ancient times; very versatile, flavor varies from mild to bold; excellent for salad dressing.	OK for cooking
Peanut	Flavor varies from bland to mildly peanutty taste; best oil for frying.	Good for cooking
Canola	Made from rapeseed, a member of the mustard family; good for salads and baking; bland taste.	OK for cooking
Sesame	Available from toasted or untoasted sesame seeds; toasted oil is pungent, so use sparingly for added flavor when sautéing or roasting.	OK for cooking
Sunflower	Taste is bland; use when you don't want oil to overpower food. Almost as inexpensive as vegetable oil; For frying use the oil labeled "high-oleic" from health food stores.	OK for cooking

RATING THE SUPERMARKET-AVAILABLE OILS *(cont'd)*

OIL	COMMENTS	STABILITY
Corn	Comes from the germ of the corn kernel; slightly sweet taste that some people like for salads; very slightly more expensive than sunflower oil.	Borderline for cooking
Safflower	Made from a thistle grown in India; popular for salads.	Poor for cooking
Vegetable	Usually made from a mixture of oils, especially from soy beans; it is often partly hydrogenated. This is the cheapest cooking oil, and its low resistance to oxidation makes it a very poor choice for any heating. It is bereft of the nutritional value of less processed oils.	Not for cooking

Vegetarianism — The Mantle of Virtue?

A carefully planned and executed vegetarian diet has many proven health benefits. But all too frequently, junk-food eaters assume the virtuous mantle of vegetarianism and gorge on all manner of nonnutritious sweets, chips, and fried foods that they pick up in health food stores. The unbalanced eating styles of many vegetarians leave them prey to deficiencies of critical nutrients like protein, iron, zinc, B vitamins, and essential fatty acids. The paucity of protein options fosters inordinate carbohydrate cravings.

I've seen patients who were vegetarian and ate absolutely no animal protein — in other words, had a diet almost totally bereft of cholesterol — who still had very high cholesterol levels. One patient, a strict vegetarian for religious reasons, had dangerously high cholesterol levels. I determined that he was consuming too much fruit, fruit juice, and starches. His problem was a susceptibility to high triglycerides, which translated to high cholesterol levels, which were causing cardiovascular damage. Because he was a committed vegetarian, I couldn't offer him starch-free foods like fish and chicken and eggs, but I was able to bring his cholesterol down by engineering his diet to be lower in starch, fruit, and refined sugar and higher in proteins from legumes like beans and tofu.

While a vegetarian diet may be a good cleanser for people who have spent most of their lives on a diet heavy in foods from commercially raised animals, continuing a totally vegetarian diet for too long can often backfire, especially for women. The bottom line: vegetarianism is a boon for some, a bane for others.

The Glycemic Index

As I frequently point out, sugar disease is the basis of much physical degeneration in the modern world. Not just sugar, but other simple or refined carbohydrates, can trigger insulin overproduction with consequent overweight, high blood pressure, high cholesterol, heart disease, and ultimately diabetes. Glycemic index is a measurement of the body's response to carbohydrates — how quickly the food is converted into blood sugar. Carbohydrate-free foods such as meat, fish, poultry, salad, eggs, oils, and butter have glycemic-indices of zero. Broccoli has a very small amount of carbohydrate and thus has a low glycemic index. As noted in chapter 6, the high glycemic index foods are products like bread, pasta, mashed potatoes, and dried fruit. The high glycemic index foods have a powerful roller-coaster effect on mood and energy as well as long-term effects on the endocrine system. (Look again at chapter 6 for more on the glycemic index.) They are not inherently unhealthy, and they provide the key to performance for athletes competing in, say, the Tour de France. But they are distinctly unhealthy for the normally active or slightly sedentary.

Prioritize low glycemic index carbohydrates like tofu, beans, brown rice, and kasha. These foods slowly release their stored sugar without precipitating insulin surges, unlike dried fruit and fruit juice, cold cereal, flavored yogurts, pasta, breads, and most "natural desserts."

Sitting down to eat a large plate of pasta, or eating other large portions of high glycemic index foods, can be especially risky. With a large portion, you are more likely to exceed the ability of your system to produce sufficient insulin. You're challenging the insulin response, which tends to induce high cholesterol levels and levels of fat-enhancing hormones.

Time of day is also important: a high-carbohydrate breakfast muffin or dish of cereal will set up an instability pattern for the day. This is why some people say about their diet, "As long as I don't start eating I'm fine." It's not that they're starting, it's what they're starting with. Consider an alternative low glycemic index breakfast, such as lentil soup or even an egg. You can moderate the effect of carbohydrates somewhat by eating them in combination with protein. In effect, eating beans or chicken with your rice "time-releases" the glucose absorption into the blood stream and reduces the steep insulin rise.

If you're interested, see Barry Sears's book *Enter the Zone*, which is listed in the Resource section, for more on the glycemic index. As we've said before, you don't need to worry too much about the details of glycemic index numbers or get into counting them the way people count calories.

The point is to be aware of high-carbohydrate, high-sugar foods, whether processed or natural (read those nutrition labels!), and limit them in the diet. Especially limit the amount in any one meal, to avoid overload demands for insulin.

When to Eat

This is almost as important a question as what to eat. A study of the eating habits of Japanese sumo wrestlers gives us a case study on how to put on massive amounts of weight. They eat relatively little during the day and start with a massive meal in the evening, followed by a rest. Then they have a big midnight snack and go immediately to bed. The combination of gorging and sleeping gives them the desired massively heavy physique. To maintain a more normal body shape, do the opposite. Have a hearty breakfast to forestall craving for junk food later in the day. Eat moderate-size scheduled meals punctuated with complex carbohydrate and protein snacks. For example, hummus on a rice cake, or chopped almonds and walnuts in a cup of plain yogurt, makes a good between-meal "nosh." Eat light if you're eating late to avoid the morning blahs. Don't "graze" on sugary foods (even too much fruit) after dinner when calories can't be worked off. If your lifestyle allows, consider making lunch your big meal of the day, and have a lighter supper in the evening. That way you'll consume most of your calories during the day while you're still active and will burn more of them.

Protein Alternatives

Most Americans are trying to cut down on their intake of the classic red meat protein sources of the past: steaks, hamburgers, chops, and stews, laden with saturated fat. Marine sources of protein are a desirable alternative for those who like them. It was once thought that seafoods like lobster and shrimp were laden with cholesterol, but in fact, these foods do not raise cholesterol levels in humans. Bivalves (clams, oysters) actually have been shown to lower cholesterol in human experiments.

Also consider eggs, which have been shown by many studies to be a reasonable protein source. The widespread notion that eggs boost cholesterol in people is the height of scientific absurdity. Only an insignificant minority of the population have this problem. But when the eggs are powdered, as may be the case in prepared foods, the cholesterol is oxidized, and this renders it more likely to induce atherosclerosis. Powdered eggs and products made with them should be avoided. Many prepared baked goods or wheat products that list eggs as an ingredient are likely to include powdered eggs — from cakes and noodles to (obviously) pancake mix.

Organic, free-range chicken, preferably baked or grilled, is also a good option for high-quality protein. Remember that how the chicken is prepared is as important as that it's chicken. Some people hear, "eat lean poultry" and say, "Oh, I'm at McDonald's so I'll have the chicken McNuggets or the chicken sandwich — it's better than red meat." But this doesn't cut it. Those nuggets and ground chicken patties are saturated with oil, which may be vegetable oil but is easily oxidized with heat and full of dangerous free radicals. (See more on oils, page 413.)

Vegetarians and the economy-minded can look to tofu, beans, lentils, split peas, and other legumes as excellent sources of protein that can also help them meet their fiber quotient. They are rich in phytochemicals, which have an anticancer effect, particularly against breast or prostate cancer. Individuals who are at higher risk for cancer of the breast, uterus, colon, or prostate do well on a vegetarian or semivegetarian diet.

Eight ounces of yogurt a day not only will provide some of your protein but, more importantly, will boost your body's immune system, help fight off disease, reduce hay fever and allergy symptoms, provide you with plenty of calcium, and, if you're a woman, fend off recurrent episodes of vaginitis. Women are especially susceptible to vaginitis after a course of antibiotics, and yogurt will help restore the balance.

One word of caution: if you want all the health benefits of yogurt, stay away from flavored and sweetened yogurts, and do make sure that the yogurt you buy actually *contains* active cultures and is not just made with active cultures. Yogurts that have been heat-treated after culturing contain no live cultures! Some of the national brands are nothing more than artificially colored, artificially sweetened, jam-flavored pretenders. Some even have chemicals added.[2] Frozen yogurt is a highly sweetened concoction of thickeners and flavorings that has little left of yogurt in it but the flavor.

For sugar-free flavorings, dust yogurt with cinnamon, sprinkle with toasted sesame seeds or chopped roasted almonds, or add vanilla flavor or orange, apple, or pear slices. Or add a little low-sodium onion mix and turn yogurt into a dip for raw celery, cauliflower, broccoli, or pepper spears.

Meat May Not Be All Bad

The worst kind of saturated fat is the kind in the red meat and the processed sandwich meat that's available in our supermarkets. That meat now contains more fat than it does protein. Many people are wisely reducing their intake of meat. The 1950s ideal dinner of steak and potatoes was a dietary aberration. As history always shows us, the pendulum has started to swing in the other direction. We are increasing our intake of plant foods and lowering our intake of animal foods. However, this doesn't mean we should cut out animal foods altogether. Some meat (yes, even red meat), minus the drugs and hormones pumped in by modern farming techniques, might not be so bad for some of us after all. The move back to moderate meat consumption has begun. Some people, of course, never abandoned it.

Take the case of one of my patients, Lynn, an environmentally aware, health-conscious woman in her late thirties. For years she was a strict vegetarian and lived mostly on beans, rice, fruits, and vegetables like most of her friends. However, Lynn came to me because her hair was very dry, her nails brittle, and her skin pale. She was sleepy much of the day and couldn't figure out why. Her blood tests reflected anemia and low iron and vitamin B_{12} levels.

My prescription came as a surprise to her: small quantities of meat, preferably red meat, every day, in addition to the basically healthy diet she already maintained.

Lynn complied and watched her symptoms reverse themselves within a matter of weeks. Lynn admits that she felt guilty at first, when her vegetarian friends saw her putting organic ground beef in her shopping cart at the health food store. Like many Americans, she still worried about cholesterol and fat. But so far her cholesterol levels have not risen appreciably, and her triglycerides are actually down.

Cholesterol and fat not withstanding, many children of the meat-loving fifties, like Lynn, may also reap a psychological benefit from eating a small amount of meat as a nutritionally justifiable "comfort food."

The important thing is that we are not talking about the commercially raised meat available in most supermarkets but about the organically fed animals that are given no antibiotics, hormones, or other drugs or chemicals. The newly available beefalo, bison, and wild game meats are a trend that I hope will spread. These meats are low-fat and hormone free; they have much more protein than domesticated meat and yet contain only one-sixth the amount of fat, a level that compares favorably with many beans and grains. This kind of organic meat is available in some supermarkets around the country and is supplied by mail order companies as well (see the Resource section). From them, you can order by mail everything from organic, free-range chicken to bison steaks and ostrich meat. This meat is higher in beneficial omega-3 oils and significantly lower in overall saturated fat. Of course, it's protein dense and naturally iron-rich.

We've got to remember that we're part of a food chain. Maybe we're enjoying the benefits of eating lean chicken rather than processed meat, but we could gain even more by paying attention to what our chicken eats. To rephrase the old adage: "You are what you eat eats." This is the basis for the "free-range," "range-fed," "organic" poultry, egg, and dairy trend. For example, chickens fed natural feed laced with marine oils lay eggs rich in heart-protective EPA (eicosapentaenoic acid); meat from bison grazed on traditional prairie grasses instead of corn is leaner and lower in cholesterol, and possesses a more heart-healthy fatty acid composition. Well-exercised "organic" barnyard chickens yield less fatty meat, free of antibiotic and hormone residues. "Natural" animal products are making a comeback.

Fiber: It Works for Moths

As George Burns once quipped, "Fiber can't be all bad. Have you ever seen a fat moth?" British physician Colin Burkitt is the godfather of fiber. He based his entire career on demonstrating that many modern diseases are fiber-deficiency conditions. They run the gamut from coronary artery disease to diverticulosis and colon cancer. Many foods containing fiber have now been demonstrated to be very effective in preventing these diseases.

Fiber is not simple; it has multifaceted functions in the body. The good news that it doesn't have to be gritty or hard and chewy. There are two types of fiber: the soft, soluble kind that acts as a sponge and the insoluble gritty kind like cellulose that speeds the intestinal transit of food. Certain types of fiber act to lower excess amounts of hormones, particularly female hormones.

Generally, fiber is consumed in inadequate amounts in this country. The average American eats 5 to 15 grams of fiber a day, but a more optimal amount would be 25 to 35 grams. It isn't hard to increase your fiber intake; you can get lots of fiber from broccoli or from applesauce. It's a very good idea to protect yourself by increasing your fiber intake in simple, sensible ways.

Some diet enthusiasts heroically stuff themselves with granola, fruit, salad, beans, nuts, and healthy cruciferous vegetables. As a result, flatulence has made major inroads among the health-conscious. (Products like Beano, found in health food stores and pharmacies, can help with this side effect.) Thus, emphasize fiber, but in moderation, each according to his or her capacity. Don't be a fiber fanatic.

Keep It Fresh and Organic

When selecting fruits, vegetables, and prepared foods like baby foods, insist on organic products. They are free of toxic residues that may render even the healthiest foods harmful or even deadly. Insist on freshness, too. Fresh foods are tastier because the nutrients they contain have not been degraded. With the current organic produce explosion, more fresh options are available year-round.

Raw versus Cooked versus Frozen

Carrying on an interminable debate, "raw-fooders" insist that subtle nutrient qualities are damaged by cooking, while the "cookers" reply that careful food preparation renders food more easily assimilated. The answer: choose both, selecting a mixture of raw and lightly steamed food items. Give *boiled* veggies a wide berth — unless consumed in their broth in soup dishes, they are leached, lifeless remnants of their former selves. Frozen vegetables without additives or preservatives may be better than wilted fresh vegetables, but they are a bit of an unknown because of potential handling problems. Repeated cycles of thawing and refreezing damage nutrients and flavor. Freezing your own fresh vegetables may be an alternative.

Phyto-Pharmaceuticals

Science is gradually discovering categories of food components that go beyond simple vitamins and minerals in their ability to prevent disease. Most people have familiarized themselves with the "alphabet vitamins" and the commonly known minerals, but there are probably hundreds of nutrient components, many of which we are just discovering. This represents a new wave in nutrition discovery, teeming with new and unfamiliar names that we don't yet need to commit to memory. Examples are the cancer-fighting indoles present in the cabbage family vegetables like Brussels sprouts and kale; natural phyto-estrogens in soybeans and other legumes, which prevent breast cancer in women and prostate cancer in men; and polyphenols found in berries and green tea, which may combat heart disease as well as cancer. Carotenoids, which rev up the detoxification pathways that prevent cancers, are found in most fruits and vegetables, including parsley, carrots, citrus fruits, broccoli, cabbage, cucumbers, squash, yams, tomatoes, eggplant, peppers, soy products, and berries. Emphasize all these foods, and stay tuned for new research developments.

Natural versus Synthetic

Our food is laced with far too many chemicals, the safety of which has not been tested over time. As a matter of fact, we as a population are being ruthlessly subjected to what amounts to wholesale scientific experimentation. Newly patented "designer chemicals" are permeating our diet as never before. We're absorbing multiple food additives that no humans have ever consumed before this century. The long-term effects of artificial sweeteners, hydrogenated oils, and artificial food colorings, flavorings, and preservatives are unknown. I recommend that you avoid them all.

Avoid At All Costs

- Nitrate-laced smoked and processed meats. (Nitrates are linked to a higher incidence of gastrointestinal cancers.)

- Foods fried in lard or hydrogenated vegetable oil. (Most fast-food eateries use one or the other. These are linked to cardiovascular disease.)
- Domestic *raw* clams and oysters. (There is a risk of hepatitis or viral gastroenteritis.)
- Frozen "Diet Cuisine." (These are often heavily additive-laden. Make your own portions from fresh ingredients free of chemicals.
- Supermarket breakfast cereals in boxes featuring cartoon character illustrations. (These are synonymous with high sugar and artificial ingredient content.)

Not So Natural

Avoid overdependence on the following foods: corn, wheat, baker's yeast, milk, potatoes, tomatoes. But they're natural, you say? Think about it. These highly utilized food sources are all relatively modern introductions — the result of agricultural domestication in recent centuries. (Some believe our bodies evolved hundreds of millenia ago to subsist on paleolithic foods: meat, fish, eggs, fowl, roots, berries, and vegetation — the so-called caveman diet.) Many individuals have food allergy or intolerance to one or several of the above. If in doubt, eliminate, rotate, or seek professional allergy testing.

Unhealthy "Health" Food

All that emanates from the health food stores is sacrosanct — or that's what you'd been led to believe. Although the health food industry holds itself to higher standards than the commercial food industry as a whole, beware of misleading items. Carob candy, for example, if used injudiciously, renders you as obese as the richest European chocolates. Soy margarine is no less sinister than common commercial brands. "Vegetable protein hydrolysates" in certain meat substitutes are a clever euphemism for MSG. In other words, don't suspend your wariness just because you're shopping in a health food store.

Food Combining

The notion that food groups must be invariably consumed alone is sheer pseudoscientific bunk left over from the nineteenth century and recently revived. There's no evidence to show that human digestion accommodates proteins one way and carbohydrates another. Many protein-carbohydrate mixtures exist in nature (nuts, beans, and seeds, for example.)

But for some, especially those with delicate digestions, a few food combining tips apply. Avoid mixing sugar, fruit, or fruit juice with starches, as in traditional American breakfasts like a toasted bagel with jelly and juice, pancakes with maple syrup, or cereal topped with generous helpings of fruit and sugar. The resulting fermented mix in the gastrointestinal tract fosters flatulence and bloating.

The Spice of Life

Because of the availability of products from all over the world in our supermarkets, and because we can get fruits or vegetables that may not be in season here, Americans tend to think that we eat a varied diet. In fact, the American diet is extremely monotonous. Think over what you've eaten during the last four days, and it's almost certain that you've had wheat and dairy products daily, and probably eggs, corn, tomatoes, potatoes, and citrus fruits. Those are the most common allergenic foods, and it is known that repetition of a food can render you susceptible to food allergy. So make an effort to get variety in your diet — not just wheat and corn, but other grains such as rye, buckwheat, spelt, amaranth, and quinoa. A wide variety of foods will provide you with more of the unique, healthful, disease-fighting nutrients that food alone can supply.

Beware of Perfectionism

Don't get caught up in dietary perfectionism. Perfectionism is self-abuse of the highest order. As in the Victorian era, the flip side of rectitude can be debauchery and unbridled hedonism. Learn to be steadfast but not rigid, and allow flexibility. The exception is when addiction to substances like sugar, caffeine, or alcohol makes total abstinence a preferable strategy. Learn to cheat playfully, without guilt or heavy self-recrimination. If you like, you can balance minor dietary lapses with a day of light eating or increased exercise.

The Salad and Salmon Diet

This is a diet I frequently talk about on my radio show, "Health Talk," and that I prescribe often for my patients. This diet is extremely healthful and is beneficial for weight loss, for cholesterol and blood pressure reduction, and for control of diabetes. It will also help minimize allergies in some patients. It's enjoyable, easy to follow, and centers on delectable "spa cuisine."

I present this in the spirit of dietary flexibility and individuality. This is not a controlled diet like the conventional diets for losing weight, but a new way of thinking about what you eat. Rather than mincing out portions, the

Salad and Salmon Diet focuses on healthful ingredients that you can mostly enjoy with abandon, while restricting or banishing troublesome "diet-busters" like sweets, flour products, pasta, fatty meats, processed foods, and superfluous deserts.

The Salad and Salmon Diet is also not a new way of grouping foods. In grade school, we were instructed that it was important to eat from each of the major groups: the meat group, the dairy group, and so on. You'll remember that a few years ago we were given the new word—throw out those other groups and start with a new pyramid of groups, with complex carbohydrates as the broad base and dairy and meat closer to the narrow apex. But this is an oversimplified way of looking at foods. Instead of looking at food products like meat, dairy, or bread, we should be thinking about food components like protein, carbohydrates and fat. Instead of grouping foods, we should be think about how food is prepared. "Eat your vegetables" isn't a holy writ—there's a gulf of difference between a big heap of mashed potatoes or french fries and a few boiled new potatoes in a salad, or between Mom's stewed-to-pieces green beans with ham hock and lightly sautéed green beans in a stir-fry with chicken breast, or even raw with a dip.

There are only three key groups in the Salad and Salmon Diet: the foods to emphasize, the foods to enjoy in limited moderation, and the foods to avoid.

Emphasize Healthful Protein

Sources include

- Fish (especially fresh salmon, trout, tuna, and mackerel) which are good also for their content of omega-3 oils.

You can eat any reasonable quantity, every day if you like, preferably cooked by broiling, poaching, baking, stir-fry or grilling. If you like, cook with a small quantity of olive oil. Experiment with the creative use of herbal marinades made with garlic, thyme, or Cajun spices. Beer makes a good marinade for fish. Try sautéing fish in wine; the alcohol will evaporate and the fragrance of wine will be sealed in. Avoid breaded fish, since the fat retention and starch content add unnecessary calories. Sushi can be an excellent way to eat mackerel, salmon, and tuna in their healthiest un-cooked form. American-style sushi restaurants are opening all across the nation.

Beware mayonnaise-laden tuna, shrimp, or lobster salad. If you do make it at home, use sparing amounts of low-calorie mayonnaise. Better yet, make your own version with a little olive oil, some chopped scallions and celery, and some minced hard-boiled egg white.

Canned tuna, salmon, sardines, and mackerel are popular and okay for convenience, but look for water-packed varieties or those made with natural olive oil. Avoid smoked fish in which the beneficial essential fatty acids have been damaged by the smoking process; salt or other preservatives are usually added. Properly done, freezing does little to deplete the nutritional benefits of fish and hence is acceptable, especially where it's difficult to find fresh fish.

Farm-raised fish like catfish or "domesticated" trout and salmon may seem like the fish equivalent of organic meats, but actually they may concentrate more pollutants in their flesh than free-swimming ocean varieties. This is because acid rain and runoff from adjacent soils may pollute the artificial ponds in which they are raised. They are also given antibiotics and are fed unnatural feeds such as grains, which may affect their nutrient composition.

Pay attention to local advisories on the PCB content of fish, especially from fresh-water and coastal sources. Swordfish in particular is a popular variety, but excessive consumption may transmit too much mercury. This is true of tuna to a lesser extent, but up to three portions weekly of either should be okay. A recent study in Japan, a country that consumes a lot of tuna, showed a direct correlation between mercury levels in hair analysis and frequency of tuna consumption. Some states even warn pregnant women from consuming more than a certain amount of fish from suspect waters. The key idea is to diversify your fish menu — don't eat all of one kind or from one source.

- Shellfish, shrimp, lobster.

Try these with a simple garnish of olive oil and lightly seared garlic in lieu of traditional butter sauces. Raw shellfish can be chancy because of the risk of bacterial contamination and of hepatitis and other viral diseases. Cooking is better unless you know the source is safe. Hot sauce on raw shellfish can actually partially protect you from bacterial contamination, as can a glass of wine. Despite their cholesterol content, shrimp and shellfish do not increase your blood cholesterol levels.

- Skinless breast of chicken or turkey; beefalo, or game meat.

For meats, use the same methods of broiling, baking, stir-frying, or grilling that you use for fish. Try marinades using rosemary, sage, or garlic, perhaps with a little vinegar. Beefalo and game meat are tough, so tenderize with a mallet or marinades. I support the concept of using meat as a condiment or side dish or as one element among many in a stir fry. Asians and Latin Americans often use small amounts of meat to add flavor or an accent to dishes that are primarily vegetarian.

Be cautioned that delicatessens and supermarkets sell turkey loaves that look the same as turkey breast but are not. Insist on breast of turkey cut from a real bird, or you may be getting the poultry equivalent of bologna when you order turkey slices for your chef's salad. Turkey burgers are great, but make sure they are prepared fresh from lean turkey breast rather than from a grind that incorporates fatty skin and mystery parts.

- Tofu, beans, lentils, split peas, other legumes.

A recent survey showed tofu to be America's most-despised food, but many have learned to enjoy creative products such as tofu hot dogs, soy burgers, and even tofu bacon and cheeses. Firm tofu is probably most popular as a meat substitute in a stir-fry.

Beans are a good source of protein at any meal, even for breakfast, when a nutritious bowl of lentil or split pea soup is a preferable alternative to sugar-laden granola with milk and fruit. Eat as much as you like — it's hard to overdose on beans. Use canned kidney beans, black beans, or chick peas as a garnish for your chef's salad. Dehydrated bean soups make a good snack.

- Eight ounces of plain low-fat yogurt, as described earlier in this chapter, flavored with ginger, cinnamon, or fresh spices instead of stewed fruits and sugar.
- Optional: Eggs (poached, hard-boiled, or scrambled) three times a week. Omelettes are a wonderful opportunity to stretch the nutritive value of eggs, as you can include other less calorie-dense foods. Avoid using cheese, but try sautéing greens, onions, green peppers, tomatoes, or spinach until they wilt, using one of your tablespoons of olive or canola oil (see below).

Emphasize fresh vegetables and greens

Sources include

- Green leafy vegetables, salads, sprouts.

Eat daily, as much as you want, but use light olive oil with lemon juice, garlic, or vinegar as dressing. Avoid the highly processed bottled dressings, which are chock-full of sugar, additives, and hydrogenated oils. Try tahini dressing made from sesame paste for a Middle Eastern flavor. Blend with tofu in the blender for a creamy dressing. Sprouts are another good protein source, in addition to containing valuable vegetable nutrients.

Avocados, while relatively high in calories, have minimal carbohydrate content and don't induce carbo cravings. Half an avocado daily can be an enjoyable snack.

- Cabbage-family vegetables, including broccoli, cauliflower, and Brussels sprouts.

These are best cooked lightly. Forget the soggy, overcooked, heavily buttered or creamed styles of our youth. Try them lightly sautéed, stir-fried, steamed, or uncooked with a yogurt dip. A little shredded purple cabbage is a surprisingly sprightly addition to a salad or a stir-fry.

Emphasize healthful drinks

- Drink eight glasses of mineral or spring water per day, flavored with a dash of lemon or a squeeze of lime, if you like. Carbonated seltzer water is fine. Make use of flavorful herbal teas for taste — warm in winter, iced in summer.
- Fresh vegetable juice, such as carrot or beet juice made with a juicer.
- Consider healthful green drinks. These are powder mixes of freeze-dried high-chlorophyll plants, like barley greens, spirulina, and blue-green algae. ProGreens, from Nutricology, is one such product. These are a good source of phyto-nutrients, concentrated plant nutrients for immune support and cancer prevention.

Enjoy in healthful moderation

- Four ounces of whole grains per day, such as brown rice, millet, bulgur wheat, buckwheat, quinoa, amaranth, barley, rolled oats.

Here we have to limit the quantity, because these are carbohydrate sources, and we should limit the form to whole grains rather than breads and pasta to keep the glycemic index low.

There are several fiber-rich grains in kernel form that cook up like variants on rice. They make good side dishes, topped with a little light olive oil and fresh spices rather than butter. You can also mix them with vegetables, fish, poultry, or beans in casseroles. Many delicious traditional dishes are based on whole or cracked grains, such as the Middle Eastern tabouli, made from bulgur wheat, or the Eastern European kasha, made from buckwheat.

Rolled oats are all right for an occasional quick breakfast, but with routine use you might use up all your carbohydrates at breakfast, limiting your options later in the day. Remember, starting the day with starchy food tends to kindle carbo craving. Eating a poached egg or two with a small portion of rolled oats will slow the delivery of the carbohydrate calories.

- Two rice cakes per day as an alternative to bread. Garnish with hummus, bean paté, a slice of turkey or chicken breast, a little light tuna or shrimp salad, or a dollop of low-fat yogurt flavored with dip mix.
- Olive, canola, or flaxseed oil. These are the "good oils," but try to limit your intake to two tablespoons a day.
- Sesame seeds, pumpkin seeds, sunflower seeds, walnuts, hazelnuts, and almonds make a good snack food. Use them unsalted, raw, or roasted — 2 ounces a day.
- One apple, pear, or orange or half a grapefruit per day; fruit intake should be limited.

Eat no more than once or twice per week

- Corn, potatoes, sweet potatoes, winter squash, carrots, and beets because of their high carbohydrate content.
- Other fruits, jams, jellies, fruit juice, and dried fruit because of their high sugar content.

Avoid

- Commercially raised beef, veal, pork, lamb, organ meats, luncheon meats, sausages.
- Alcoholic beverages, sweet sodas.
- White rice and all flour products: breads, muffins, cookies, noodles, pasta, cakes, crackers, matzoh, breakfast cereals (except Wheatena, oatmeal, or oat bran).
- Margarine, butter, lards, other oils.
- All nuts other than those mentioned above, nut butters.
- All other dairy products, frozen or flavored yogurt, soy-based or rice-based frozen deserts.
- Salt, soy sauce.
- Ketchup, mayonnaise, commercial salad dressing (these have high oil, sodium, and sugar content and are often laden with preservatives, colorings, and artificial ingredients.)
- Breaded or fried foods.
- Refined or unrefined sugar, artificial sweeteners, honey, barley malt, maple syrup, rice syrup, and other natural sweeteners.

Are Supplements Necessary?

There are still huge unknowns in nutrition. We know that everything we need to thrive upon is in food, but we don't know how to completely reproduce the whole package of vitamins, minerals, nutrients, and trace elements that we must have to remain healthy. Don't be fooled into believing the ads that say an instant breakfast or a diet shake provides everything you could get from a balanced meal. It doesn't and it can't.

There are hundreds of thousands of nutrient components in a stalk of broccoli, but we don't yet know what they all are or how they interact with each other and within our bodies. Since food is the best source of the nutrients we need, and the only source of some nutrients, and our bodies can best assimilate and utilize them when they are present in food, our first concern should be making sure that we are getting as much as possible from the food we eat.

To do that we need a sensible diet plan that we enjoy and that works for us. Then we should make sure that our food comes from as clean and chemical-free an environment as possible and that it's fresh, so that the nutrient content has not been destroyed or lost.

Today, fresh foods are often transported for several days across the country, so the nutrients are naturally reduced because of exposure to oxygen. To counteract this, you can find yourself a good health food store that sells (1) fruits and vegetables either organically grown or grown with a minimum of chemical fertilizers and pesticides and that have *not* been irradiated to prolong their shelf life, (2) meat and dairy products obtained from animals raised without hormones or other growth-promoting drugs, and (3) grain products that are not bleached or bromated. Also, you can add natural food supplements to your diet to help replace those lost.

The processing of food to "improve" taste and extend shelf life is a major cause of nutrient deficiency. When brown rice is processed by grinding, bleaching, and other processes to form white rice, 80 percent of many trace minerals like magnesium, manganese, copper, and zinc are lost.[3]

An equivalent loss occurs when whole wheat berries are reduced to bleached white wheat flour, one of the mainstays of the standard American diet.

Nutrients can be lost in other ways. Various cooking techniques like microwaving can oxidize nutrients in foods, resulting in lower nutrient content. So can some types of preservation, like canning fruits and vegetables.

Nutrients are lost from the soil by repeated growing of crops, and they are not being replenished. Selenium, for example, is depleted in much of our soil, and the growers don't want to spend the money to supplement it because it's not required for plant growth — but it is required for human growth.

Nutrients are lost as well when crops are harvested before they have naturally ripened. The produce, picked when it is still green, is then force-ripened with chemicals, like ethylene gas. That's one of the reasons the tomato you buy in the winter, out of season, tastes like cardboard and bears little resemblance to the succulent summer vegetable you grow in your garden. The gassing also reduces nutrients, as do EDTA and other chemicals added to foods; EDTA, used to preserve the green color of frozen broccoli, lowers vitamin B_6 in the vegetable. Vitamin B_6 is now recognized as one of the nutrients that protect against heart disease.

By now, if you are getting the idea that the food we eat today does not reach our stomachs with all its health-giving nutrients intact, you're right. In order to remain healthy, most of us need some supplementation of the lost nutrients. An individual's needs for any nutrient can vary widely, however. The U.S. Recommended Daily Allowance (RDA) can be only the vaguest of guidelines.

The RDA was adopted over fifty years ago to determine what levels were needed to ward off diseases like scurvy and rickets. Current research shows that people have widely varying nutritional requirements. Also, the RDAs are kept low for political reasons. The government uses them as the standard for all sorts of government-provided or government-assisted food programs like Women, Infants and Children (WIC) programs, prenatal nutrition programs, meals for the elderly, veterans' programs, and school lunches. If the RDAs are low, the food will cost less. Every time they are raised, the food industry has to supply expensive food additives to meet the RDAs and to provide impressive labels for food packages.

What Dr. Roger Williams, one of the pioneers of nutritional medicine, calls biochemical individuality is important in determining what supplements are needed and in what amounts. This is the notion that people can vary greatly from any norm; some will have weak and some robust pathways for synthesizing various enzymes. An individual's nutritional needs are also influenced by varying factors like environmental pollution and stressors, chemical exposure, physical exercise, stress, and age. But this hasn't been acknowledged by the National Academy of Sciences, which sets the RDAs. For most nutrients, they recommend practically the same RDAs whether you are young or old. Accordingly, when you consider supplements, it's best to forget the RDAs and consult a nutrition specialist, since each individual's needs are unique.

Since the RDAs certainly do not represent current scientific thinking, I usually advise shoring up your nutrient intake with well-designed multi-vitamins or combinations of nutrients like antioxidant formulas or osteo-porosis formulas that specifically target your individual risks. Even though individuals have varying needs for nutrients and supplements, there are a few general recommendations that can be made for adults in midlife. Let's look at the supplements that will provide a good base on which to build individual prescriptions.

Antioxidants

Antioxidants are important to those approaching fifty and beyond because certain diseases of aging, like heart disease and cancer, are caused in part by damage from free radicals. Free radicals create a degenerative pattern within the body; antioxidants (sometimes called free radical quenchers) reduce free radical damage and can slow or prevent some degenerative diseases, including cancer and heart disease. Reducing free radical damage with nutrients like vitamin C, vitamin E, and the carotenoids may slow or even prevent certain degenerative diseases. Vitamins C and E may also help prevent cataracts, and vitamin E may slow the progression of Parkinson's disease.[4] Other nutrients, such as zinc and selenium, are precursor elements that the body uses to manufacture its own antioxidants.

While one or two of the recent major studies designed to verify the benefits of beta-carotene in heart disease prevention and cancer risk reduction seemed to have disappointing results, the results may not be all that they seem. These studies were bold nutrition experiments based on the often-noted association between high dietary intake of beta-carotene-rich foods and reduction in cardiovascular disease and cancer risk. The problem may be that the effectiveness of a single nutrient like beta-carotene may be compromised when it is isolated from the wide spectrum of plant nutrients associated with it in foods. We know that beta-carotene belongs to a family of nutrients called the carotenoids, which include lycopene, which reduces the incidence of prostate cancer, and lutein, a pigment that confers protection against macular degeneration (see chapter 14). It may be, too, that the trials evaluating synthetic beta-carotene as a solo nutrient were just too short or tackled excessively high-risk populations like long-term smokers.

The suggestion from the ongoing research is that the antioxidant hypothesis, far from being dead, remains promising. Current research suggests that a combination of nutrients working together synergistically may be much more effective than isolated antioxidants and may eventually be found to confer protection against cardiovascular disease, cancer, and a variety of degenerative conditions. The present recommendation is not to look at isolated beta-carotene as the effective supplement but at a carotenoid mix. Additionally, startling evidence is at hand showing decisive benefits from another antioxidant, vitamin E, even when it is used as an isolated supplement. Recent studies have shown that vitamin E in supplements can reduce heart disease recurrence in patients who have already suffered a heart attack by as much as 75 percent.

Some scientists have also questioned the value of common recommendations for vitamin C supplementation. A recent government-sponsored study by Dr. Mark Levine and others, published in the proceedings of the National Academy of Sciences, cautioned against excess vitamin C consumption at the same time it suggested an upward modification of the RDA of vitamin C by more than threefold, from 60 to 200 milligrams. This study suggested that while optimal preventive benefit could be achieved with much higher doses of vitamin C than are now recommended, the body could only use a limited amount, and megadosing potentially increased the hazard of kidney stones. As for toxicity, many scientists challenge the test-tube observation that vitamin C produces oxalic acid, which leads to kidney stones — it just doesn't work that way in the body. Since by various estimates one-fifth of Americans are dosing with vitamin C at levels of 1000 milligrams or more daily, wouldn't it stand to reason that we would see an epidemic of kidney stones or other substantial side effects? Yet, we haven't seen this. In my personal experience of treating thousands of patients with high doses of vitamin C, sometimes intravenously at doses of up to 75,000 milligrams per day, I have not seen one case of kidney stones developing. As for the needed amount, many studies suggest that challenging disease states like cancer or diabetes, or demanding life circumstances like aging or exposure to the pollution of cigarette smoke, engender a need for higher amounts of vitamin C. Evidence continues to indicate that higher doses than the new proposed RDA can prove therapeutic to the immune system, the circulatory system, and the respiratory system in particular, with special benefits for asthma sufferers. Surgeons continue to value vitamin C in substantial doses for assisting in wound repair, as they have for many decades.

Other Key Nutrients

Besides the antioxidants, there are other key nutrients that it might be wise to include in any supplementation program. Zinc has proved helpful in forestalling prostate disease, but most important, it supports the function of the thymus gland, which is the mainstay of immune-system longevity. Particularly for women, some bone builders are needed: calcium, magnesium, vitamin D, and the B vitamins. Also, the essential fatty acids (EFAs) tend to be lacking in the American diet, particularly the omega-3 and omega-6 oils, which can be supplemented with fish oils (omega-3) and borage oil (omega-6).

Both the omega-3 and omega-6 oils form prostaglandins, which control all cellular metabolic functions. They are extremely important, and our

ANTIOXIDANTS: WHAT EXACTLY ARE THEY?

The body's antioxidant system includes enzymes, scavengers, vitamins, and minerals such as selenium, manganese, and zinc. Antioxidants are able to generate safe chemical reactions or deactivate unsafe reactions within the body.

But *antioxidant* implies something that fights oxygen. Isn't oxygen something we need to survive? Yes, but ironically, oxygen is toxic under certain conditions.

Chemical compounds are composed of two or more atoms joined by chemical bonds. These bonds are formed by electrons, which are electrically charged. Oxygen has paired electrons, but sometimes in unstable formations, so they can participate in chemical reactions that produce compounds called free radicals. Free radicals grab electrons from other stable compounds, creating a degenerative pattern within the body. Substances that have reacted with oxygen are said to have been oxidized.

Free radicals can be created in the body by radiation, environmental pollutants such as herbicides, air pollution, ozone, and tobacco smoke. They can be consumed in rancid fats. At the same, they can be created by normal biological processes, including normal oxygen metabolism, reactions involving metals like iron, and the formation of hormonelike substances, prostaglandins.

Antioxidants fight this process, which damages the body's immune system and increases a person's susceptibility to colds, infections, and disease. Free radicals are also implicated in long-term degenerative disease processes such as heart disease.

ability to synthesize these nutrients may be impaired due to vitamin/mineral deficiencies, excess transfats, sugar, or alcohol.

While it's best to derive as many nutrients as possible directly from your diet, most people benefit from supplements, since vitamin-rich foods are not always what make up our daily diet. The table shows some good sources for the key nutrients, and my own recommendations for a daily supplement that will benefit most people in midlife and premenopausal women.

KEY NUTRIENTS: FOOD SOURCES AND RECOMMENDED SUPPLEMENTS

NUTRIENT	FOOD SOURCES	RDA	RECOMMENDED
Mixed carotenoids	carrots, cantaloupe, spinach, squash	*	25,000 I.U.
Vitamin A	as above	5000 I.U.	8000 I.U.
Vitamin C	citrus fruits, strawberries, green leafy vegetables, peppers, potatoes, tomatoes	60 mg.	500–1000 mg.
Vitamin E	nuts, whole grains, (like oatmeal, wheat germ, brown rice), oils	8 I.U.	200–400 I.U.
Selenium	salmon, dairy products, seaweed, whole grains, garlic, liver, shellfish	*	200 mcg.
Zinc	pumpkin seeds, oysters, spirulina	15 mg.	25–50 mg.
Calcium	dark green leaves: salad greens, bok choy, broccoli, collards, yogurt, nuts, and seeds (including tahini, made from sesame seeds), seaweed, whole grains, dried beans, sweet potatoes	800–1200 mg.	1000 mg. (1500 mg. for pregnant women or those over 50)
Magnesium	organic grains, vegetables	400 mg.	500 mg.
Folic acid	leafy green vegetables, most fruits, liver	180 mcg. (women) 200 mcg. (men)	400–800 mcg.

Key Nutrients: Food Sources and Recommended Supplements
(cont'd)

Nutrient	Food Sources	RDA	Recommended
Vitamin B_6	vegetables, brown rice, nuts, fish	1.6 mg. (women	25 mg.
		2.0 mg. (men)	25 mg.
Vitamin B_{12}	meat, eggs, milk, seaweed, soybean, tempeh	2.0 mcg.	25 mg.
Vitamin D†	fish oils, dairy	200 I.U.	800 I.U.
EFAs			
Omega-3	fish oils	None	1000–3000 mg.
Omega-6	borage oil, flaxseed oil, black currant seed oil	None	1000–3000 mg.

I.U., International Units; mg., milligrams; mcg., micrograms.

* Need for this in human nutrition has been established, but no RDA has been set.

† The active form of vitamin D is a hormone and is closely regulated by the body. While commercial supplementation (in foods like milk and dairy products) represents one source of this important vitamin, it is also manufactured by the skin in the presence of sunlight.

Some Guidelines on Taking Supplements

- If you decide to take antioxidants, remember that there are many other antioxidants in vegetables and fruits that you won't be able to get in a pill; eat at least five servings of these antioxidant rich foods per day.
- Don't rely on your multivitamin to provide you with sufficient antioxidants, even if the label says "contains the full antioxidant group." These often skimp on quantity. You'll want to take a separate antioxidant formula or separate pills for each antioxidant.
- When you buy a vitamin E supplement it is best to get the natural form, since it is more active. Read the label carefully; you want d-alpha-tocopherol.
- Experiments have shown that it's beneficial to take calcium supplements before retiring for the evening; they are better absorbed while you're sleeping. Calcium is also absorbed well with meals, so hedge your bets.
- Men and women don't have the same supplement requirements. Until

after menopause, women may need iron supplements, but men don't. Excess iron stored in the body can cause health problems.[5]

- If you're a premenopausal woman and you are taking an iron supplement; try taking it with a vitamin C supplement or a food source, which will help the absorption.
- If you're not used to taking supplements, there may be some mild side effects. Iron and calcium carbonate, for instance, can cause constipation until your body adjusts to the higher levels. Magnesium and vitamin C, on the other hand, can cause diarrhea or GI bloating. So you may want to build up your intake gradually.

Some care must be exercised in adding vitamin and mineral supplements to the diet. Many manufactured foods, sometimes because they have little nutritional value in themselves, add vitamin and mineral supplements to the food before it's packaged. For example, food manufacturers fortify flour, bread, and cereals with iron. They have unfortunately overlooked the fact that *too much* iron is associated with risks of its own. Since it is nearly impossible to keep an accurate count throughout the day of what supplements you've ingested from commercially prepared foods, this is another reason to avoid these foods altogether. Taking a vitamin and mineral supplement on top of heavily fortified foods could give you an excess of certain nutrients, like iron or vitamin D, which could be harmful.[6] Remember that the body has to carefully maintain a balance of nutrients for health, so supplementation should ideally be done under the supervision of a doctor or nutritionist.

In choosing which supplement brands to buy, I think it's best to select from a large reputable company. There have been some great assay wars in which companies have attacked their competitors for not containing the amounts of vitamins that are listed on the bottle. But those are now behind us, and the vitamin industry is subject to scrutiny from informed consumers and consumer groups. You may pay a little more for the products of a large reputable company, but they'll be up to the highest standards.

If you're still confused about the difference in brands, ask to speak with a clerk who knows the products. Vitamin and health food stores, especially, often have someone who is very knowledgeable about vitamin and supplement products. Don't be afraid to ask questions. Remember that the only dumb question is the one you *don't* ask.

Longevity

Would you like to live longer? Do you want to boost your immune function? Do you want strong, healthy bones throughout your life?

Who wouldn't answer yes to all of these questions? Well, the simple truth is that the foods you eat can make a huge difference in the quality and length of your life. For instance, if you boost your fiber intake you may help prevent many diseases that could shorten your life. Low-fiber diets are linked with a high death rate from all kinds of diseases. Immune suppression is linked to a deficiency of many trace minerals, especially zinc. Finally, some studies have shown that diets that emphasize meat may weaken bones.

There's no doubt that nutrition plays a powerful role in human aging. Alas, there is no single longevity food or nutrient. Rather, there's a whole range of varied nutrients that can work together to bring about a longer life span.

Longevity Picks

These are foods that either have been proved to fight disease or play important roles in maintaining good health and vigor.

VEGETABLES

Vegetables, and to a lesser extent fruits, epitomize the nutrient-dense concept, which means high levels of nutrients and low levels of "antinutrients" like fats and refined carbohydrates. In 1982, a National Academy of Sciences study first echoed your mother's old admonition to "eat your greens" but with a new twist: you'll lower your cancer risk. That call was echoed by the 1988 Surgeon General's *Report on Diet and Nutrition*, the first effort to define a rational longevity program based on disease prevention through dietary means. Many vegetables are high in mixed carotenoids, which show demonstrable protective effects against many cancers, including those of the lung, stomach, esophagus, and colon. The vitamin C in fruits and vegetables may mitigate against cancer (red peppers are especially high in vitamin C), and the fiber content of fruits and vegetables acts to lower cholesterol.

Fruits and vegetables also contain boron, the trace mineral most recently acknowledged as an important nutrient. Boron has been found to prevent calcium loss from bones, which may explain why women from countries where milk products are not available but who do eat large amounts of vegetables do not suffer a high rate of osteoporosis.

FISH

Drive around a fishing area, and you will see bumper stickers that say "Eat fish — live longer." Fish are an excellent source of the antiaging minerals magnesium, selenium, and copper, and they provide a low-fat source of protein. A new impetus for fish consumption came with the discovery that Greenland Eskimos had few heart attacks while they subsisted on a diet far from what Nathan Pritikin would have approved of — mainly fatty fish and blubber, with practically no vegetables. It was discovered that a component of fish oil known as EPA (eicosapentaenoic acid) works against fatty buildup and hardening of the arteries. Its richest sources are mackerel, trout, salmon, tuna, sardines, and herring. Studies have also shown that EPA is helpful in treating rheumatoid arthritis and in protecting against breast cancer.

WHOLE GRAINS

Most industrialized countries have shifted from whole grains to refined, a shift that has been paralleled by an increase in degenerative diseases. Whole grains are excellent sources of B vitamins as well as magnesium, boron, and fiber. The advantage of fiber from a longevity standpoint is that fiber blocks the absorption of cholesterol from food and may even help the body eliminate cholesterol already in the system. Fiber speeds the transit of material through the intestines, which keeps cancer-causing irritants from accumulating.

BEANS

Beans are an excellent source of soft soluble fiber, which may be even more beneficial than coarse bran fiber in lowering cholesterol levels and raising levels of beneficial HDL cholesterol, according to experiments by James Anderson, M.D., at the University of Kentucky. Beans have a low glycemic index, which means that they produce no sugar "high" but rather a steady release of caloric value, making them an excellent antidiabetic food.

ONIONS AND GARLIC

Onions and garlic boost beneficial HDL cholesterol, kill bacteria, regulate blood sugar, thin the blood, and have been found to block cancer in animals. The antihypertensive effects of garlic have been well documented in China, where garlic is used as a medicine. The immune activity of natural killer cells has been found to be enhanced by 140 percent in people who eat raw garlic. (If raw garlic turns you off, garlic concentrates in pill form work just as well.) The National Cancer Institute is currently studying the anticancer effects of the sulfur-containing compounds found in onions and garlic. It is best to eat garlic raw, as cooking neutralizes some of its cardiovascular benefits. On the other hand, nutrition researcher Dr. Jules

Constant has found that the blood-thinning effects of onions are not impaired by cooking.

WATER

An important nutrition verity is that lots of water is necessary. Some experts consider six to eight glasses per day to be optimal. But not just any water: some elements in tap water can threaten longevity. One study traces cancer incidence to the trend toward increasing levels of organic chemicals in drinking water between 1957 and 1972. Chlorine, added to water to kill bacteria, has been linked to increased cancer susceptibility as well. In addition, a striking concordance has been noted between water softness (a trend accelerated by the use of water softeners) and cardiovascular mortality. Pure spring water, if it's from an unpolluted source, has a high content of beneficial minerals such as magnesium, which supports longevity.

OLIVE OIL

Olive oil is a source of monounsaturated fats, which are also present in peanut oil and canola oil. People living in the Mediterranean basin who consume large quantities of olive oil have a surprisingly low rate of cardiovascular disease. One interesting study has shown that the addition of olive oil to complex carbohydrate diets, which are already cardioprotective, actually enhanced their cholesterol-lowering effects.

Promising Contenders

SHELLFISH

Once maligned as major sources of cholesterol, shellfish actually produce only a negligible rise — or even a fall — in serum cholesterol when eaten. They are extremely rich sources of zinc.

BREWER'S YEAST

A source of B vitamins and chromium, brewer's yeast acts as a blood sugar regulator and is a rich source of selenium, which is helpful in preventing cardiovascular disease and cancer. One caution: People with yeast allergies or *Candida* infections should avoid it.

LOW-FAT YOGURT

Nobel Prize winner Eli Metchnikoff touted live-culture yogurt as a miracle longevity food as far back as the early 1900s. Studies continue to support its immune-potentiating effect. Yogurt contains natural antibiotics that resist infection; the friendly bacteria it introduces into the colon help degrade cancer-causing bile acids. Yogurt also provides absorbable calcium for people with lactose intolerance, conferring resistance against osteoporosis.

Weight Loss and Diets

I have a strong recommendation for people who have been struggling to keep their weight down: Don't diet! Expunge the four-letter D-word from your vocabulary. Select a healthy eating plan instead, one that is realistic for you, and adhere to it more or less. Focus on health, energy, and vibrancy, not poundage or inches. Repeated binge-dieting actually increases the risk of obesity. The body has a primitive mechanism that responds to caloric restriction by increasing the tendency to store calories as fat. This is a useful response that enables humans to get through famines and lean times, but it works against the whole idea of losing weight by going on periodic low-calorie diets. This kind of dieting is precisely what you should do if you want to build up your body's fat-retention capabilities. Further, repetitive cycles of starvation and the body's effort to overcome the effects of starvation, which is the binge, begin to powerfully distort the body's production of insulin. The high levels of insulin drive the blood sugar down and cause profound hypoglycemia, which in turn causes inordinate hunger. This is the futile see-saw that repeat dieters put themselves on unknowingly. Get off the diet merry-go-round before it's too late!

My message to you, if you've been on the diet see-saw, is to make sure that the eating plan you follow is constructed for health, not for weight loss. Because of all the advances of modern medicine — the so-called miracle drugs and cures — lots of people lose sight of the fact that we are still bound by the limitations of nature in many areas. Understanding how our bodies metabolize food can make us more able to accept our limitations and not attach moral tags to events that have physiologic causes.

Remember, too, that changes take place in our bodies with age. Our metabolism slows down, but we don't usually reduce our food intake, and we become somewhat less active. All these things add up to perhaps a few more pounds. In fact, if you are a woman, it's possibly beneficial to have an "extra" 10 pounds of body weight after forty to see you through menopause. Studies show clearly that thin women have more trouble with hot flashes and other menopausal symptoms. That's because fat cells produce some

---

THINGS YOU CAN DO TO LOSE WEIGHT GRADUALLY

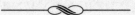

1. Build your diet around vegetables, some fruits, and low-fat proteins.
2. Never skip meals, especially breakfast. Never starve yourself.
3. Opt for a breakfast that's composed of foods with a low glycemic index, like split peas, lentils, vegetables, or low-fat proteins, and smaller amounts of whole grains. They release sugars gradually into the blood instead of flooding it right after eating.
4. Eat smaller, more frequent meals—at least three meals during the day and two between-meal snacks.
5. Never eat a meal just before napping or going to bed at night.
6. Eat most of your calories in the first part of the day. Make your evening meal your lightest meal.
7. Exercise to burn fat. Moderately paced exercise sustained for at least 20 minutes is best.

---

estrogen, so having a few extra pounds will help even out the hormonal fluctuations of menopause. Further, a slight increase in weight can help safeguard against osteoporosis, due to the protective effects of estrogen.

A Look to the Future

As researchers continue to discover beneficial, significant nutrients, many of us may feel somewhat overwhelmed trying to keep up with all the foods that we should and shouldn't eat. But all you really need to know are the basics: if it's fresh and unpolluted and has no additives, chemicals, or synthetic ingredients, it probably contains what you need to thrive—whether or not we know the names and functions of all the nutrients it contains or the details of how they work in our bodies.

Use your common sense and follow the guidelines we've discussed about eating—and for heaven's sake, enjoy it!

A recent cartoon in *The New York Times* spoofed the culinary excesses of the recent past. In it a slender, muscular, yuppie-type man is depicted dining at a trendy restaurant—the Café Austerité—where the specials board reads: "Mesquite-Grilled Seaweed." The message is clear. It just may be that the extreme dietary Calvinism of the seventies and eighties is giving way to a more common sense approach.

CHAPTER SEVENTEEN

External Medicine:
Coping with a Toxic Environment

Baby boomers have a lot of advantages in terms of improved nutritional awareness and freedom from some of the major infectious diseases that took a toll in prior generations. Still, one crucial health factor may be undermining your best efforts: you're living in the twentieth century, in a world that is more and more toxic.

Environmental toxicity is the new scourge. We have added 60,000 artificial chemicals to our world in the past half century. Over 150 million tons of toxic waste are dumped into our nation's oceans and rivers every year. Everyone has heard about the effects of environmental pollutants on animal populations—seals and porpoises washing up dead from the sea, waterbirds and songbirds declining because of pesticides and agricultural runoff. What is making ocean life die? Scientists speculate that water pollution has weakened the sea creatures, allowing viruses to take hold and utterly destroy the immune systems of the animals. They then succumb to myriad diseases. Dead dolphins have been found to harbor up to fifty times the danger levels of toxic PCBs. We've also seen the ill effects on animals born in polluted environments—shells of birds' eggs so thin they're easily crushed, crocodiles with poorly developed reproductive organs.

But we're now at a new stage in environmental pollution where we can see significant health changes in the human population itself. Four people every day, on the average, are killed by exposure to hazardous substances in this country. Birth defects kill over eight thousand infants a year. Cancer kills nearly half a million Americans annually, and scientists suspect that an important cause is environmental contamination. Before toxic poisoning shows up as cancer or birth defects, it can announce its presence through vague symptoms of fatigue and malaise that are difficult to fit into a diagnostic box and give a name to. If you wake up exhausted or suffer from headaches, allergies, depression, and chronic respiratory problems, you may have absorbed toxins from the air and water around you.

Let's consider some of the latest warning signs of toxic overload.

The Estrogenized Environment

The toxic sea is within us. It appears that very tiny amounts of pollutants like dioxins and PCBs have an estrogenizing effect on tissue — that is, they have an effect similar to that produced by an excess of the natural hormone estrogen. In a very real sense, we can say that our whole environment is becoming estrogenized. This may be one factor that is contributing to the soaring rate of breast cancer and higher rate of other reproductive cancers in women. It's harder to say how the various systems of our body may be responding to such pollutants, and they may well be affected in ways that we haven't yet identified.

Cancer on the Rise

We are seeing a huge increase in cancer rates, which many researchers believe to be largely caused by environmental toxicity. Researcher Dr. Samuel Epstein contends that as many as 90 percent of all cancers are environmental, resulting from increased cell mutation or decreased immune system vigilance, and not necessarily due to dietary causes. Pollutants can enter the body through many pathways: in the food we eat, in the air we breath, or via direct absorption through the skin. Not always, but occasionally, we find a "smoking gun" that links pollution to cancer. Uranium miners in the Southwest have five times the normal rate of lung cancer. We are seeing in breast cancer biopsy specimens and pathology reports that women have increasingly higher levels of pesticides in their breast tissue.

A New Laboratory of Pollution

The end of the Cold War and the opening up of Eastern Europe and the former Soviet Union have provided a chilling spectacle of the horrors of unchecked industrial pollution. In some cities of Eastern Europe, the majority of children are constantly sick with asthma, respiratory ailments, and childhood leukemia caused by the clouds of coal dust and soot in the atmosphere. In parts of the Ukraine surrounding Chernobyl we're getting a chilling lesson in the increase in cancer rates that nuclear pollution can cause. Water supplies polluted with oil and chemicals are making whole towns and cities sick. The rivers in Eastern Europe are virtual chemical dumps, and pollution in the great inland seas of the former Soviet Union is decimating traditional fisheries. Life expectancies in some areas are no greater than fifty-five. This is really a model for us of the risks of unbridled industrial expansion without environmental controls.

The Twentieth-Century Disease

The diagnosis of multiple chemical sensitivity (MCS) is becoming main-streamed, and research centers have been set up at major teaching institu-tions to study it. MCS has also been called the twentieth-century illness, universal reactor syndrome, and environmental illness. The syndrome has a wide range of symptoms: fatigue, flulike symptoms, mental confusion, and all kinds of skin, urinary, joint, and muscle problems. The chemicals that can provoke this disorder are almost limitless, from the formaldehyde in new clothing to pesticide residues, passive cigarette smoke, lacquers, plas-tics, and more. In many cases, people can trace the onset of their illness and sensitivity to a single and overwhelming exposure to a chemical. There is now a whole school of medicine, environmental medicine, that is develop-ing methods to diagnose and treat this problem.

What's to be done? While many commendable efforts are being made to prevent pollution and clean up the environment, other forces are actively resisting those efforts. The best we can do at this time is to be aware of some of the worst environmental offenders and take prudent evasive action. In this chapter we'll look at some of the common sources of environmental toxins and discuss ways to keep them out of your daily life, especially out of your home and workplace.

Chemical Sensitivities

If you are reading this book in your home or office, chemical solvents and gases are escaping at this very moment from the carpets, glues, and insula-tion around you. Factors like these have led to the "sick building syndrome," in which scores of workers have found themselves stricken by multiple health problems on starting to work in a new building or after new carpets have been installed in their offices. In the street you breathe in the chemi-cal exhaust of automobiles. Plastics and synthetic fibers release vapors into your lungs. Modern agricultural methods have exposed you to steadily rising levels of pesticides and herbicides in your meats and produce. These chemicals persist in the soil for years. Your drinking water may be a reservoir for the toxic runoff of waste that has been dumped, both legally and illegally. It may also contain high levels of chlorine, which is intended to kill dangerous bacteria — but the chlorine itself poses a health risk. Your fruits and vegetables contain residues of pesticides, and according to a report issued by the National Academy of Sciences in 1987, pesticides in our food may cause a million additional cases of cancer in the course of our lifetimes.

An alarming footnote comes from a 1995 study of 252 Denver children diagnosed with cancer. There was a strong association found between the use of insecticides (for yard treatment) and soft tissue sarcomas, and between the use of ordinary household pest strips and leukemias. The authors concluded that "some types of home pesticides may be associated with some types of childhood cancer," but urged more studies to clarify which exposures, if any, are truly carcinogenic.[1]

Though toxic chemicals are not healthful for anybody, each person's body tolerates toxins in varying degrees. Some individuals can work directly with a chemical and seem to suffer no ill effects (though the effects may occur twenty or thirty years down the line, with a suppressed immune system that leads to diseases like cancer). Others may become so sensitized or overloaded that they will suffer when exposed to levels so tiny that they are barely detectable even by the most modern technology. Sensitive people appear to reach a "total load," or saturation point, earlier than others. They are the ones who suffer from MCS.

Unfortunately, this prominent cause of illness and fatigue has gone largely unrecognized by modern medicine. People with chemical sensitivities are believed by many physicians to be suffering from a purely psychosomatic disorder, and their fatigue and strange reactions to be signs of deep depression. It's hard for doctors to believe that such a wide range of extremely low levels of chemicals could cause so many different symptoms. Yet, the Department of Housing and Urban Development recognized MCS as a genuine disability in 1990, and there are bills in the U.S. Congress and in some state legislatures to acknowledge MCS as a health consequence of indoor pollution.

Doctors will often tell people with MCS, "this is in your head," and there may be some truth to this, but not in the usual sense. These are people who have been hammered by allergic reactions that are quite real. Dr. Iris Bell, a leading CFS researcher, has studied the neurophysiology of these people and speculates that they have brain abnormalities in the hypothalamus and the limbic system caused by some form of trauma. The trauma could be an environmental insult, or an illness, or a physical trauma that puts the brain into a susceptible state. We now know that the brain is very closely linked with the immune system; several neurotransmitters that operate in the brain also trigger immune reactions. It appears that these susceptible people can have a kindling reaction: anything that their immune system sees as a strong external stimulus can kindle an allergic reaction. So, starting with a few limited allergies, someone can develop a wildfire spreading of the immune reaction and become allergic to almost anything that the body perceives as foreign. There may be a brain abnormality involved, but a neurochemical one rather than a mental delusion, a byproduct of depression, or an effort to gain attention or sympathy. (See the Resource section for information and support groups dealing with MCS.)

While the medical profession is gradually giving more credence to MCS, particularly in the wake of recognition of Gulf War Syndrome, and undertaking more research into diagnosis and cure, I think this really represents the tip of the iceberg. People who suffer from MCS are like the canaries in the coal mine: they show a clear-cut and obvious response to a toxic environment that is affecting us all, though perhaps with more subtle and long-term effects.

We may never really know how much chemical exposure we can handle, or which toxin may finally overload our system and initiate a decline in liver function or a progression toward cancer. What we *can* do is begin to carefully scrutinize our lifestyles and environment for toxic exposure, and try to reduce the risks as much as possible on all fronts at once. We can also take steps to actively support our own natural detoxification pathways, especially through the liver, and to reduce the load we're placing on those pathways. We may also wish to undertake an active program of periodic detoxification as a long-term approach to health maintenance.

Guarding Against the Toxic Avengers

A recent low-budget movie starred a creature called the "Toxic Avenger." He was a seven-foot green monster that killed people by crushing them in his toxic embrace. While it made for a funny movie, the real toxic avengers are much more insidious. While they may not be completely invisible, they are often so deeply embedded in our modern lifestyles and culture that we are not really aware of them. The first order of business is to start paying attention to the sources of chemicals and toxins that we tend to take for granted as safe.

Although your first impulse may be to hide out in your home, the way primitive people hid in caves to protect themselves from the elements, that may not be a wise idea. Your home could actually be making you sick! The latest battle against pollution has moved indoors to homes and offices, where the average American spends 22 hours every day. More than 90 percent of American homes use pesticides, and the Environmental Protection Agency's 1990 study of four thousand homes in Florida and Massachusetts found "common" household pesticides at higher levels indoors than outdoors, simply because a closed house tends to keep toxins circulating, whereas they disperse in the open air. As many as sixteen million Americans may be sensitive to pesticides. Even when a pesticide is targeted for removal because it is toxic or carcinogenic, it often takes years to pull it off the market.

Similarly, offices and "tight" buildings (the new highly insulated ones, without adequate air circulation) can pose a pollution hazard. For instance, in 1980 a new high school was opened in Oakland, California, and students and teachers reported difficulty breathing. The problems was eventually traced to the library and storage rooms, in which books were shelved on particleboard. The particleboard was releasing formaldehyde into the school's inadequate ventilation system.

Indoor pollution levels can be up to a hundred times higher than those outdoors. Researchers at the Environmental Protection Agency have suggested that indoor pollution may be responsible for over ten thousand deaths each year. The World Health Organization has concluded that up to 30 percent of new or remodeled buildings are plagued by indoor pollution. In the state of California alone, seven hundred "sick" buildings are reported each year.

One of the most common indoor pollutants is formaldehyde gas, which is released from countless materials: imitation woods, particleboard, synthetic curtains, and carpeting. Constant exposure to formaldehyde can cause serious and even irreversible health problems, from extreme tiredness to acute rashes to dry, burning throat and nose, sinus infections, cramps, spasms, urethritis and vaginitis, headaches, and memory loss.

Formaldehyde. Radon. Asbestos. Mothballs. Dust. Poor ventilation. How can you determine whether your home is "sick"? There are actually "doctors" who "cure" homes — individuals who specialize in ridding homes of their toxins. They'll come to your home with air-quality monitors, gas and radon detectors, and analytic tools for testing formaldehyde levels, electromagnetic fields, and more. Environmental testing services utilize gadgetry reminiscent of the movie *Ghostbusters* in their effort to sniff out hidden toxins. The analogy is apt — they "bust" the ghostly toxins that can cause illness. (See the Resource section for references to some of these services.)

If you believe you may be suffering from exposure, what can you do? Direct testing of blood levels won't help much. I've tested many patients for toxic levels of chemicals and pesticides, but only one — a man who worked with lacquers — showed extremely high blood levels of a toxic substance. His levels of the chemical toluene were sixty times the allowable "safe" levels. He was indeed suffering multiple symptoms, including severe fatigue and malaise.

Most patients show "normal" blood levels, but I believe that toxicity may occur at levels far below the official detection limit. Another possibility is that toxins are sequestered in the fat — but to do a biopsy you need a large-bore needle and a significant amount of fat, and I don't perform that test lightly because it is uncomfortable.

However, there are certain chemical markers of overexposure. For instance, if the urine contains hippuric acid, it's likely there is a problem with formaldehyde. That's because hippuric acid is a byproduct of formaldehyde breakdown. I sometimes test for that. I also test the urine for mercaptopuric acid, a byproduct of vigorous detoxification. Similarly, levels of another acid, glucaric acid, show whether the liver is working overtime to metabolize toxins.

For patients who are sensitive to sulfites, which are present in wines and are sprayed on some fresh vegetables to preserve them, the urine can be tested for sulfites. Individuals who have a problem with sulfur metabolism are thought to be more susceptible to Parkinson's and allergic diseases. The mineral molybdenum can strengthen the pathway that eliminates sulfites.

I also test for antibodies to chemicals. Toxins not only are poisonous but can engender a genuine allergic response, in which the blood carries antibodies that can be measured.

How to "Cure" Your Personal Environment

If your house is "sick," or if it's making you sick, how can you clean and cure it? How can you improve your personal environment to reduce the level of toxins? First, look for sources of chemical pollution. Countless chemical substances in your home can cause toxic reactions. The sidebar on page 423 lists some of the common ones as well as the symptoms caused by overexposure. Then, think about sources of potential toxins in your life — the air you breathe, the water you drink, the food you eat — and consider ways to reduce toxic substances in each of these areas.

AIR

It may be that nature has the best filter for indoor pollution: bring the outdoors inside. W. C. Wolverton, a former researcher at NASA, claims that common houseplants are able to absorb harmful gases and chemical compounds. A two-year study found that plants like English ivy and golden pothos removed significant amounts of benzene, formaldehyde, and other toxic gases in enclosed chambers.

Air filters can also help. Fiberglass air filters are the most commonly available. However, according to physician Joseph D. Sacca, the fiberglass particles (which can cause severe irritation) shed easily, invisibly coating surfaces in the home. To clean air, it's safer to buy filters with activated carbon granules to remove chemicals and gases. Negative ionization machines, often combined with air filters, can help by attracting and removing dust particles from the air. They put a charge on particles, which can then be sucked up more readily by air filters.

INDOOR POLLUTION: COMMON CAUSES AND SYMPTOMS

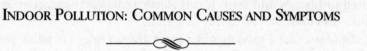

Acetic acid is present in certain fabrics and plastics and as a solvent for gums and resins. It causes irritation of the eyes, skin, nose, and throat.

Acetone is a solvent for oils. It is colorless and sweet-smelling and irritates the eyes, nose, and throat. It's also the basic ingredient of nail polish remover, which should be used only in a well-ventilated area, not a small, enclosed bathroom.

Ammonia is a colorless gas that has a pungent smell. It causes irritation of the eyes, nose, and throat as well as chest pains.

Arsenic is used to manufacture pesticides, paints, wood preservatives, and bronze alloys. It causes organ damage and death.

Benzene is a colorless liquid that removes grease and is used in the manufacture of varnishes, lacquers, linoleum, dyes, synthetic leather, and rubber. It's a known carcinogen and damages bone marrow.

Cadmium is a heavy metal used in many electrical and mechanical appliances, batteries, rubber and plastic, insecticides, photography materials, and semiconductors. It is a cumulative poison, which can build up in the body over many years and cause permanent kidney disease, sometimes high blood pressure, and sometimes increased calcium excretion that can worsen osteoporosis.

Carbon dioxide is a colorless, odorless gas used in fire extinguishers and other chemical processes. Overexposure causes headache, dizziness, elevated blood pressure, and increased heart rate.

Carbon monoxide is a colorless, odorless, poisonous gas in the exhaust of engines, furnaces, and fireplaces. It causes headaches, nausea, weakness, confusion, and sometimes coma and death.

Chlorine is a poisonous gas used in bleaching and disinfecting. It irritates the nose, throat, and lungs. It is also added to many municipal water supplies to kill bacteria; drinking large amounts of chlorinated water has been associated with increased cancer rates.

Formaldehyde is a colorless, pungent gas used to manufacture particle board, plywood, foam insulation, paper towels, grocery bags, household cleaners, and the backs of carpets. It can cause allergic reactions and fatigue.

Hydrocyanic acid is a liquid that smells like bitter almonds and is used in plastics and dyes. It can cause weakness, headaches, confusion, and difficulty breathing.

Lead is a metal used to solder pipes and is present in paint, pottery, china, and machinery. It is toxic to many organs in the body and can poison the brain, nervous system, and blood.

Mercury is a metal used in drugs, fungicides, electrical apparatus, and dental amalgam, and it was recently banned from use in paints. It damages the brain, kidneys, and central nervous system, causing a wide range of symptoms.

Nitrogen dioxide is a poisonous gas released by gas stoves and furnaces and kerosene heaters. It irritates the eyes, nose, and throat and impairs the lungs.

Paradichlorobenzene is a chemical used in mothballs and is a known carcinogen.

Perchloroethylene is used as a dry-cleaning fluid and solvent. It can injure the liver; cause nausea, dizziness, and fatigue; and irritate the eyes, nose, and throat.

Radon is a naturally occurring, colorless, odorless gas commonly found in areas where rocks and soil contain granite, shale, or phosphate. It is the second leading cause of lung cancer, and harmful levels have been found in many homes.

Toluene is a liquid obtained from coal tar and is used as a solvent. It causes weakness, confusion, dizziness, headaches, nervousness, and rashes.

Trichloroethylene is a liquid solvent used in dry cleaning, printing inks, paints, lacquers, and other products. It can cause headaches and fatigue.

WATER

If your water has detectable levels of pesticides or lead, you can buy water filters that will remove toxic chemicals. Many are available on the market; some are easily installed on your countertop, while others are installed beneath the sink. Carefully review their claims to be sure that they filter out lead, copper, bacteria, algae, and chlorine.

Shower filters are also available; in fact, shower water may be more harmful to you than tap water. Standing under the pelting force of a hot shower for 15 minutes opens your pores, allowing your entire body to absorb chemical-laden water, particularly chlorine. In the body, chlorine can be metabolized into even more toxic chemicals. See the Resource section for sources for shower and water filters, and for water-purification units for your pool, or for country wells, that don't use toxic chlorine. These new filters use silver and copper in a technique spawned by NASA space-age technology to clean water without corrosive chemicals.

FOOD

One way to avoid the risks of chemical overload is to buy organic foods whenever possible. One of the biggest sources of chemicals in your body is supermarket foods. Food adulteration, food coloring, and chemical food preservatives are extremely common. Over the course of a year, the average American consumes several pounds of these additives. There are also the inadvertent toxins in our food supply, such as pesticides in fish that result from toxic dumping in the oceans, lakes, and rivers.

Though organic foods are often more expensive than normal supermarket fare, the price you pay is well worth the health benefits you will reap. Demand for these products continues to increase, and prices for organic foods are beginning to fall.

INTELLIGENT MEDICINE TIP:

For an informative guide to pesticide residues in common fruits and vegetables, take a look at *Pesticide Alert*, by Laurie Mott and Karen Snyder (Sierra Club Books). According to the EPA, sixty different chemicals are used on green beans, seventy on cantaloupes and bell peppers, and over a hundred on apples. These amounts are typical for many fruits and vegetables.

PESTICIDES

Many people make an annual ritual of calling the exterminator and "bombing" their homes, spraying behind all the counters, and laying out mouse trays. This is something to reconsider, since studies have shown that pesticide levels inside the home can climb well above recommended levels and linger for a long period of time. What if your home is overrun by ants, cockroaches, fleas, flies, termites, or spiders? You don't want to share your bed with bugs, but killing the little critters with toxic chemicals can burden your own system as well. Here are some ways to control pests without poisoning yourself:

Ants: Sprinkle powdered red chili pepper, dried peppermint, or borax where ants enter. Plant mint around the outside of the house to drive them away.

Cockroaches: Mix baking soda, boric acid, and powdered sugar, and spread around the infested areas. You can also mix oatmeal with plaster of Paris. Either mixture will kill roaches. Put bay leaves in infested cabinets, as they will repel roaches.

Fleas: Feed your pet brewer's yeast tablets or powder — it contains B vitamins that cause natural odors that fleas abhor.

Flies: Buy or make sticky flypaper made of a mixture of boiled sugar, corn syrup, and water. Hang cloves, or put citrus oil in the room to repel flies.

All pests: Use an ultrasonic pest repeller to back up your campaign.

Medical Pollutants

Toxins come not only from the things around us but also from things we put inside of us. We have a greater awareness now of the potential toxicity of all kinds of implants and medical devices that are inserted in the body, from silicone breast implants to mercury compound fillings in the teeth.

I think of all the people who have artificial joints, artificial heart valves, artificial jaw replacements, silicone chin construction, breast implants, even artificial penis prostheses (there are thousands of men with these). We're putting a lot of artificial things in our bodies, and over time we're learning that not all of them are benign.

You may think, "I know I don't have any of these things in my body," but what about your teeth? Millions of Americans have fillings in their teeth that are made up of a compound containing mercury, a highly poisonous metal that has immune-suppressive effects. This kind of mercury toxicity is a real problem, and I see it in my practice quite often. Though not everyone with mercury in the mouth should have it yanked out, there are many patients who, even after medical and nutritional work, simply don't get well. They suffer a variety of bewildering symptoms that are typically related to mercury poisoning, ranging from depression, tiredness, and irritability to bleeding gums, swollen neck glands, burning sensations, diarrhea, irregular heartbeat, headaches, and muscle tremors. Mercury has been shown to depress the immune system.

The American Dental Association protests that mercury is stable when mixed with other metals such as silver, tin, and zinc in a filling. But mercury fillings have never been tested for safety by the FDA, and dentists themselves keep scrap amalgam in an airtight jar. The EPA has banned mercury from indoor latex paint because of the dangers of mercury poisoning, yet the vapor level in a patient's mouth after chewing during a typical meal is sometimes as much as ninety times higher than the vapor level in a newly painted room. Progressive dentists are therefore offering composite fillings as a safer alternative — and the white composite looks better than the old silver fillings as well!

Removing all your fillings is a drastic measure that can itself expose to you high levels of mercury. Vapors can be released into the bloodstream, and mercury fragments can even be swallowed. Patient and dentist must take special precautions, so it's best to work with a dentist who is experienced with this procedure and who will use a chelating agent to remove from the bloodstream any additional mercury that is absorbed during the procedure. An alternative is simply to replace old fillings with composite ones as they break.

Special Risks: Lead Poisoning

Lead may be among the most pervasive of environmental poisons, lacing our soil, water, crystal, and pottery. We have removed two major sources of lead poisoning from the environment by phasing out leaded gasoline and leaded paint. Even so, the National Academy of Sciences estimates that 600,000 tons of lead is dumped into the atmosphere each year. Nevertheless, experts contend that the biggest danger of lead poisoning continues to be old lead paint, which is still peeling from the walls of millions of American homes. Most houses and apartments built before 1950 contain lead paint, and until 1977, many brands of paint were laced with lead.

In children, lead poisoning causes pallor, retching, listlessness, and learning disabilities. The Centers for Disease Control have kept lowering the safe blood levels of lead for children to just a few *micrograms* per deciliter of blood. But lead is poisonous to adults as well — a lead level of as little as 25 micrograms per deciliter of blood can begin slowing red blood cell production, leading to anemia. Some historians credit the high level of dementia and illness among the ancient Romans to their sophisticated plumbing systems, which used lead pipes.

Lead is ubiquitous in our modern, polluted world. The soil in your yard may contain lead, mostly from old paint that has peeled off the outside of your house. In New York City, playgrounds under major bridges were found to be brimming with lead, from years of peeling bridge paint and auto exhaust fumes. Water is a common source of lead, mainly because of the lead soldering that joins pipes together. China, porcelain, and painted pottery often contain lead in their glazes. When correctly fired, the lead is supposed to be sealed in, but the glaze can begin to leach lead after being exposed to scouring soaps or the acids in fruit juices, wines, vinegars, and coffee. The FDA estimates that 14 percent of imported dishes exceed safe lead limits. And one study of brandy stored in lead crystal for over five years discovered that levels of lead soared to over 20,000 micrograms of lead per liter (the safe level in water is 50 micrograms). Lead-soldered food cans, once a menace, have now been outlawed.

Here is what you can do to protect yourself from lead poisoning. First, test your home with a do-it-yourself lead-testing kit (see the Resource section for references). These tests are easy to use and will let you know whether there are dangerous levels of lead paint in your home. Or look in your local Yellow Pages under "Environmental Organizations" or "Lead Paint Detection." To test your water, call the water safety hotline of the Environmental Protection Agency (800-426-4791). Lead contamination is most serious in areas with soft water, which tends to corrode pipes. Studies have shown that most lead is released the first time you turn on the tap in the early morning, or after it has not been used for six hours. Letting the tap run for three minutes to flush out the residue in the pipes will sharply reduce lead levels. Always use cold water for cooking and drinking. Hot tap water leaches more lead out of pipes.

To protect yourself from lead in the environment, you can "buffer" your body with other nutrients. Lead blocks calcium metabolism, and calcium is necessary for everything from strong bones to a healthy heart. More than 90 percent of lead is stored in bone. Calcium prevents its deposit in bones and teeth, but vitamin D appears to enhance lead absorption. Low-protein diets increase lead absorption, as does a high-fat diet. Even mild lead poisoning can interfere with iron metabolism. Other nutrients, such as magnesium, copper, chromium, vitamin C, and B vitamins all help protect against the effects of lead by blocking its effects on enzymes.

Several kinds of tests are available to check lead levels in your body. A simple and accurate method of determining toxic levels of lead in your system is hair analysis. While not 100 percent reliable, it provides a convenient, inexpensive screening test for toxicity. By itself, it's insufficient evidence for a program of therapy, but if the result is positive for lead, use other screening tests. There are blood tests and chelation tests that can pick up lead toxicity in people who have stored high levels of lead in their bones, even though the blood levels appear safe. Chelation therapy (see chapter 12, page 323) can then be used to remove lead from the body. I've seen patients with mysterious low-level, chronic fatigue feel rejuvenated after a series of chelation treatments. The spring is back in their walk, the energy back in their lives. Circulation is improved, and the body no longer has to work overtime to carry its load of toxic metals. To be safe, chelation therapy must be performed by an experienced practitioner, with careful monitoring during the procedure. See the Resource section for references.

The Liver: Our Natural Detoxifier

Perhaps the most important measure of toxicity in any form is the health of the liver. The liver is one of the most complex and remarkable organs in your body, and it's unquestionably the key to all detoxification.

Your remarkable liver weighs about four pounds, and it plays a hugely important role in digestion, metabolism, and detoxification. Chemicals, drugs, alcohol, solvents, pesticides, formaldehyde, and herbicides — all are detoxified by the liver. The liver's load is staggering, and its ability to detoxify varies tremendously from person to person. Some of us are exquisitely sensitive to drugs, caffeine, and alcohol, and others are like Rasputin — the diabolical Russian pseudo-cleric who was stabbed, poisoned, and shot, and wouldn't die.

Detoxification, like any activity of the metabolism, requires energy. That's why people who are toxic tend to get tired. Dr. Jeffrey Bland has looked at patients complaining of chronic fatigue and found that the vast majority had one or more forms of failure of the liver to rapidly and properly remove toxins from the blood. Research is bearing out the possibility that people who suffer from chronic fatigue, malaise, arthritis, and some other systemic complaints may be suffering from a systemwide breakdown caused by toxic overload. The body appears to be overwhelmed by toxins that are either externally absorbed or internally generated. (Even the hormones we generate, such as estrogen in women, have to pass through the liver in order to be eliminated from the body.) External toxins typically include food additives, chemicals, and environmental pollutants.

The liver can itself become damaged by an excess of the toxins it is supposed to process and remove from the body. These can sometimes be let into the body through a weakened GI system, as in the leaky gut syndrome, or through GI dysbiosis, in which a proliferation of the wrong kind of intestinal bacteria generates toxins. Even too much fat, protein, or carbohydrate in the diet can act as toxins that overwhelm the body's ability to break them down. Add to this daily doses of common over-the-counter medications like Tylenol, which severely strains liver function by depleting the critical antioxidant glutathione, and you have a recipe for disaster. Recent studies show that patients who take high doses of Tylenol, particularly with alcohol, are more prone to liver disease, while other anti-inflammatories like Advil seem to lead to higher levels of kidney disease. Since these are the two main detoxifying organs, this can become a vicious circle. People who suffer low-grade symptoms like headaches and joint pains, because of excess toxicity, then start to take some of these drugs regularly. The drugs put an increasing strain on the body's detoxification pathways and injure the very organs that are responsible for detoxification.

The good news: The liver is an astonishing organ with a tremendous capacity to regenerate. Even when a large portion of the liver is removed as the result of injury, it can recover in a matter of months. People can survive on a tenth of their liver, because it will carry on the entire liver's work.

The bad news: I see so many people with abnormal liver function that it is shocking. The liver enzymes that become elevated in abnormal tests indicate significant damage. Those tests often miss sluggish, torpid liver function. Studies have shown that mild liver dysfunction related to many drugs and chemicals, doesn't always show up on tests. I find that the most sensitive way to test for liver function is with a challenge. Caffeine, aspirin, and Tylenol are metabolized through major detoxification pathways in the liver. After giving a patient a challenge dose of these substances, you can see how quickly they are broken down and eliminated from the body by measuring urine levels. If levels don't decline quickly, it means the liver is not functioning as effectively as it should.

One sign of liver toxicity is light-colored stools. They indicate that the liver isn't producing enough bile, which suggests that it may not be functioning well.

To sum up, allergies, fatigue, chemical sensitivities, general malaise, and premenstrual syndrome can all be linked to a sluggish liver that isn't detoxifying substances vigorously enough. Once we have made a diagnosis of impaired liver function, we can then begin treating it through providing nutrients and unburdening the liver.

Detoxification and the Liver

The French have coined the phrase *crise de foie* — "crisis of the liver" — to refer to that sluggish, tired, and irritable feeling that can come on after a stretch of enjoying fine French cuisine and fine French wines to excess. They well recognize the potential burdens of toxicity and the crucial role that the liver plays in relation to it. Their answer to the crisis of the liver? That it's time to "take a cure" or "take the waters." They'll go to a spa, eat light cuisine, drink mineral water, have a mud bath or deep massage, or lengthy steam bath. This is a great European healing tradition of detoxification, which may even date back to our primate ancestry. The great apes engage in rituals of clay-eating, which seems to absorb intestinal toxins and acts as a means of cleaning out the system. A modern version might be the type of intestinal cleanser that you can get at a health food store, which contains psyllium, a fiber, and bentonite, a clay.

Detoxification is an old practice. In fact, traditions of fasting and dietary simplification are universal, cropping up in the rituals and practices of indigenous peoples around the world. Many of the world's great religions have traditional cleansing periods of fasting and simplification: the Lenten fast in Christianity, holiday fasts in Judaism, Ramadan in Islam. The diet of Zen Buddhist monks is a classically simple vegetarian diet featuring rice, vegetables, and bean curd. These traditions have a spiritual focus, of course, but there may be profound health benefits from a practice of regular and cyclical detoxification through fasting or a simplified diet.

Oddly, mainstream medical practice has largely ignored both the concept of detoxification and the therapeutic potential of this kind of cure. The time-tested methods of detoxification I recommend to my patients are simple and effective. They also require dedication and time, and initiate a slow, steady process of self-healing. This is probably why most medical doctors don't recommend them. Many doctors don't even seem to believe that toxins can build up in the body and cause disease. Yet, the medical profession has its own high-tech methods of detoxification. Dialysis, for instance is a form of detoxification for patients whose kidneys function too poorly to filter blood-borne waste products. Gastrointestinal specialists prescribe intravenous feeding to provide "bowel rest" for patients with Crohn's disease or ulcerative colitis.

Because of the somewhat daunting environmental onslaught, there's a new scientifically based focus on detoxification as espoused by nutritionally oriented physicians. Detoxification is really the new form of medicine for our generation. Practitioners look for factors of toxicity as an underlying cause of disease and use ancient, traditional methods of detoxification as well as modern technologically sophisticated methods like chelation therapy, which employs an array of different chemicals to remove poisonous heavy metals from the body. Nevertheless, the basis for a good detoxification program is a good diet and nutrition.

Diet is key in protecting and cleansing the liver. Saturated fat tends to build up in the liver, clogging it and decreasing bile secretion. Accordingly, it's best to steer away from animal fat and hydrogenated fat, and instead to emphasize monounsaturated oils like olive oil and omega-3 oils like those in fish and flaxseed. Lecithin, which contains choline and inositol (sometimes considered B vitamins), helps protect against fat buildup in the liver.

A diet that is generally low in animal protein and fat can also help rest the liver. That's because the byproduct of protein metabolism is ammonia, which must be detoxified by the liver. Protein can be obtained partially from vegetable sources, like beans and grains. Beans are also important because they contain sulfur substances that boost liver function, including methionine, an amino acid. Beet leaves and beet juice help liver regeneration because of their high content of betaine, a critical catalyst in the methylation pathway of detoxification. Caffeine and drugs should be avoided, even over-the-counter remedies like Tylenol and antihistamines.

For more on diet and detoxification, see chapter 9 on the gastrointestinal tract for an approach to fasting and for my "detoxifying feast."

Vitamin C aids the liver's conversion of toxins into harmless metabolites. One study, for example, demonstrated that college students who took vitamin C could process alcohol out of their blood much more quickly than students who didn't. It's interesting that alcohol is a model of a simple hydrocarbon, related to the many hydrocarbons that pervade our environment in the form of cleaning chemicals and petroleum products and byproducts. So vitamin C should aid in processing these environmental pollutants as well.

Other nutrients and vitamins that help the liver detoxify include N-acetyl-cysteine, an amino-acid precursor to glutathione. It's used in cases of Tylenol toxicity in hospitals, as when children swallow the contents of a bottle. Tylenol poisoning is one of the most severe kinds; it can destroy the liver in a matter of hours.

Another amino acid, taurine, helps the liver conjugate and remove many toxic residues, via the bile. Pantothenic acid (vitamin B_5) helps detoxify formaldehyde.

Niacin, which is helpful for lipid metabolism, can promote the release of toxins stored in fat. However, this type of therapy should be done only under a doctor's supervision, since doses over 500 milligrams can damage the liver.

Dr. Jeffrey Bland advocates a product called UltraClear, a scientifically based formula that he uses in conjunction with a very simple diet of fruits and vegetables. It provides a basic supply of necessary nutrients: basic proteins, carbohydrates, beneficial oils, and a rich source of vitamins that aid the liver in recovering function. This approach often helps people who are trying to get off the toxicity merry-go-round. (See the Resource section for references.)

You can also supplement your diet with herbs that are known to cleanse and protect the liver. The two most important are these:

Dandelion (also known as *Taraxacum officinale*). You may know dandelion as a common weed, but herbalists know it as an important cure-all. Its official name comes from the Greek *taraxos* (disorder) and *akos* (remedy). Dandelion has long been used as a liver remedy as well as a general blood purifier. It is extremely high in vitamins, minerals, and beta-carotene (dandelion has 14,000 International Units of vitamin A per 100 grams, compared with 11,000 International Units for carrots). Studies show that dandelion increases the flow of bile and relieves liver congestion.

Milk thistle (Silybum marianum). This common plant contains powerful liver-protecting substances, and its extract is stocked by the National Poison Control Center as an emergency treatment for ingestion of poisonous mushrooms (particularly the death angel mushroom). Studies have shown that it can prevent and correct liver damage. It increases the liver's level of an important antioxidant, glutathione, by up to 35 percent, and this is an important aid to detoxification. That may be why some experiments have shown that with the addition of milk thistle to the diet, the liver was protected from damage by toxic chemicals. Milk thistle has also been shown to help liver cells regenerate.

Other Detoxification Strategies

When you need to detoxify, take a tip from the European spa tradition — the nineteenth-century sanatorium approach to degenerative illness. Take some time off from work if you can, and get plenty of sunshine, exercise, and fresh air. Building up a good sweat through exercise can cycle toxins out of the body. Saunas and steam baths can also help you detoxify — something the Finns have known for centuries. The heat makes toxic substances literally ooze out of your skin as you perspire, and a shower afterwards washes them all away. Saunas must be accompanied by rehydration. In general, hydrating your system by drinking a lot of pure water can help cleanse your system.

The interest in this approach is evidenced by the popularity of American luxury spas in the Southwest and California, which offer massages, meditation, hiking, yoga, saunas, and a vegetarian or light diet. Of course, you don't have to go to an expensive spa to enjoy the benefits of these practices.

Using diet and sanatorium methods to detoxify is a simple and effective approach, which can initiate a slow, steady process of self-healing. Best of all, if you can incorporate some of these methods into your lifestyle on a regular basis, you'll make real strides toward reducing the effects of our toxic environment over the long term.

CHAPTER EIGHTEEN

Doctors and Medicine: How to Cope

For many, the medical system seems to have gone hopelessly awry—complicated, expensive, and without answers for many real problems. Gone are the days of the family practitioner who delivered babies, treated childhood diseases and adult complaints, and even listened to our anxieties and life problems. This kind of doctor is becoming a rarity. Instead we live in a world of specialists. We may have an internist who is at the front line of most complaints but who immediately refers us to a specialist, or several specialists, depending on the nature of our problem. In this era of managed care and HMOs, you no longer have a relationship with a doctor or even several doctors but a contract with a medical service provider whose staff may change frequently.

Because of the enormous costs of modern high-tech medicine, it is increasingly difficult to go to the ideal doctor. But in this changing new world of health care, intelligent medicine offers us a way to cope.

Dealing with Changes in the Medical System

Americans are increasingly going to have to settle for physicians who are simply competent, satisfactory, and relatively courteous and who communicate at a basic level. Unfortunately, there may well be less opportunity to undertake programs of prevention or to go to doctors for a basic understanding of the overall direction and prognosis of personal health. In the standardized medical system, people will find it difficult to get help in dealing with conditions that are stubborn, persistent, chronic, or obscure.

On the other hand, there are a growing number of physicians like myself who work with patients on an elective basis, sometimes to optimize health, sometimes to provide alternatives to standard perfunctory care or standard treatments, sometimes to help patients with refractory problems that aren't always helped by conventional medical care. They may practice under the name of holistic physicians, alternative physicians, nutritionally oriented physicians, or environmental physicians. As the crisis in health care deepens, we're going to see a greater number of Americans opting for this kind of care, even if it's not always covered by health insurance. This is part of the new world of intelligent medicine. In fact, studies have shown that many middle-income Americans are willing to pay for quality in service if it's important to them, including alternative health care.

The most rational approach — the intelligent medicine approach — is to use the system as well as you can and then reach outside it for special needs. If you find that you're not getting the depth of care you need, or the level of communication, then you may have to go outside your usual health care network.

In general, there are three kinds of reasons to go to a holistic physician. First, you may feel you're in pretty good health but want to optimize your health and performance and to identify patterns and pitfalls that may create problems for you later on. Second, you may have been diagnosed as having a clearly identifiable disease — like ulcerative colitis, rheumatoid arthritis, lupus — that is not well treated by conventional medicine. In cases like this, the conventional therapies may help somewhat without addressing the underlying problems. Third, your symptoms may fall between the diagnostic cracks, and your doctors aren't offering you any therapy because you don't have a clearly defined illness.

Later in this chapter, I'll offer some tips on how you might work with a holistic doctor. But whatever kind of doctor you are seeing, whether it's a rushed internist in an HMO or a physician in private practice, there are some basic guidelines you can follow to get the best care possible. I give you fair warning, though: this may require a fundamental shift in your attitudes toward doctors and the medical profession as you start to apply the intelligent medicine approach.

Take Charge of Your Medical Care

In American society, the doctor has often played the role of miracle-worker, problem-solver, dispenser of sage advice, trusted family counselor, compassionate care-giver. Medicine is one of the few professions that has consistently commanded a high degree of respect, at least until recently. If you were fortunate enough to grow up under the care of a trusted family doctor, you've probably unconsciously absorbed some of these attitudes. Certainly, many physicians have tried to live up to this ideal image.

The corollary of this attitude is that we've been led to expect to be passive objects of a doctor's care. "Doctor knows best," so take your medicine and don't ask questions. People think they're going to put themselves in the doctor's hands and throw themselves on his mercy. Patients come to me and say, "Doc, you're my last hope; here's my story." And I certainly do my best. But on the larger scale, this just doesn't cut it anymore. With the immense economic and social strains on our medical system, the great increase in technological complexity, and the increased mobility of our society, we can't afford this kind of attitude. We are going to have to become active participants in short-term *and* long-term health care. We're going to have to help our doctors, and help ourselves by being alert to possible health risks. Let's look at some key steps you can take to help your doctors by taking responsibility for your own long-term health care.

OPEN YOUR OWN HEALTH FILE

This is just as important as keeping track of your checking account and bills, which most people do for tax reasons or just to protect themselves. Health issues can be much more complex, with much more at stake.

You should keep a "repair and maintenance" file for yourself, just as you would for your car. Keep a health journal or set of notes, and make an entry every time you visit a doctor or a specialist or have tests done. Note down the date, the doctor's name and contact information, your symptoms or the nature of your complaint, the diagnosis, and the treatment recommended. (New software is available to help you do this on your home computer.)

This is not as much effort as it seems, and it can prove very useful later on. It's an especially important strategy if you're in the standard medical system or in an HMO. You may be seeing different specialists who don't talk to each other. A clinic may lose or misfile test results.

Sometimes, too, chronic or complex problems develop very gradually, and it's important to have the chronological information. Just as important, your health journal will give you an instant reference in case you need to contact any specialists or doctors in the future, or get copies of test results, or tell a new doctor about your medical history. There's a lot more mobility in contemporary America, and you or your doctor may move. If you are moving to a new city or changing health care providers, arrange for transfer of your medical records. Don't wait for a medical emergency to happen.

GET COPIES OF YOUR OWN TESTS, X-RAYS, MRIS, AND SO ON

Get into the habit of asking for a copy of any test that's done, and ask that X-rays or other images be given to you, or copies made for you. If you're developing a health problem, it's extremely important for your current doctor to see whether there's been some kind of progression or decline, and over what period of time it's taken place. Looking at one X-ray that shows some arthritis or bone damage in the present is much less useful than being able to compare today's picture with an X-ray taken earlier. I've seen confusion arise when there's a new finding, only a comparison will tell whether there is a serious problem, and it's difficult to trace previous results. Mammograms are a case in point. The comparative view is essential, and your present doctors really need to see the whole picture. This can be a problem if you've seen six different specialists and they've all ordered separate pictures. If you're getting sequential studies like X-rays or bone densitometry studies, try to get them done at the same institution, which will help your doctors make comparative evaluations.

Better yet, ask for your own copies and file them. Believe it or not, clinics do misfile and lose X-rays and MRIs. Usually patients are not given copies of these images, but you have a legal right to have copies of your entire set of records and images, including X-rays and MRIs, though a lab may ask you to pay for reproduction costs.

MAINTAIN A MEDICATIONS LIST

If you are taking multiple medications, keep a simple list of what they are, and the dosages, so you can convey this to any doctor you see. Most will ask, or should ask, so it's good to be prepared. Don't bring in a shopping bag with all your pills — just a list. Include any over-the-counter medications, since they may be affecting your health or interacting with prescription medications.

Help Your Doctors

The reality is that good doctors these days see a lot of patients and are often under considerable time pressure. They may be teaching or performing surgery, or making hospital rounds in addition to their office time. So the best thing you can do to ensure good care and attention when you see a new doctor, or see your regular doctor about a new complaint, is to be organized. You want to be able to give the doctor all the relevant information about your case as directly and efficiently as possible. Here are some guidelines to follow when seeing a new doctor, or seeing your regular doctor about a new complaint.

1. If you've seen other doctors about the problem, explain the previous diagnosis and course of treatment.

This will get your session off to the most efficient start. Even if your doctor may come up with a new and different diagnosis, this will provide a useful point of reference. It means the obvious tests have been done, and your doctor doesn't have to start from scratch. If you've seen several specialists, have a contact list available in case your current doctor wants to talk to any of them.

2. Offer any recent test results you may have copies of, and provide information about any current medications.

Here's where your personal health file comes in handy and where you can offer your list of medications. Bring actual printouts of test results, especially your most recent blood test. This will help your doctor get a much more useful picture of your condition right away, and arrive at a deeper diagnosis at your first visit, before doing new tests and waiting for results. This can save a lot of time and some expense. Just bring the most recent tests, not every test you've ever had.

3. Then start by describing your current symptoms, and name all of them, not just the "chief complaint."

If you follow your natural instinct, you'll probably tend to organize your story chronologically. Sometimes the way medical problems unfold in time really does make an interesting story. But your doctor has a completely different agenda. He or she wants first of all to know, "What are you suffering from *right now?*" What are your current symptoms, and their nuances? Some people do take great pleasure in unfolding the history of the problem, and how it started and developed along the way. But this makes the doctor wait for the punch line, without the crucial information, wondering why you're in the office today.

So the best approach is to first describe your current symptoms or diagnoses. This will probably lead to some question-and-answer exchanges and to the next logical questions, "When did the problem begin? How long have you been suffering from this?"

4. Be vivid and detailed in your descriptions of symptoms.

When describing your symptoms, be organized. Think about your how long you've had them, and try to describe them vividly, with all the details. Diagnostically speaking, the clues are in the details. Don't just say, "I've got a horrible headache, or a bad migraine headache." That's not enough. Say, "It feels like a hot poker is stabbing above my left eye." Say what time of day the symptom is strongest, what seems to bring it on, what if anything makes it feel better. Mention any connection to any aspect of your daily life, such as whether it's better at work or at home, at certain times of day, or during certain seasons. These facts might give a clue to environmental or stress-related influences. To avoid leaving anything out, you may want to list your symptoms on paper along with any factors that affect them.

5. Then give a quick chronology of when the symptoms started and when they escalated or new symptoms appeared.

Give a bare-bones chronology, with just the approximate dates for the start of each symptom or development, following a clear and concise time line. You might want to note this down on paper. But don't just hand the paper to the doctor; put it into your own words. It's important to have a dialog with the doctor and give him or her the opportunity to ask important questions.

6. If you're seeing several specialists, make sure each one knows who else is seeing you and what therapies or medications they are prescribing. (This is crucial if you're receiving different medications from different specialists, as we'll see in the section on drugs and medicine.)

Better yet, encourage your doctors to talk to each other. Unless they are part of a real clinical team they may be operating in complete isolation from one another. This is not uncommon. I usually ask my patients who else they are seeing, and I like to pick up the phone and touch base with a physician who is managing some other aspect of my patient's care. In about a minute of focused conversation we often discover something useful about how we should interact to help the patient. We might discern that we're working at cross-purposes, and be able to strike a better balance.

Choosing a Doctor: A Fresh Perspective

You may already have a good, long-standing relationship with a skilled physician in private practice whom you know and trust. If you're signed up with an HMO, you may have been assigned to a doctor or may be seeing different specialists. Whatever your situation, you may at some time feel the need to consult another physician. You might face the possibility of surgery or need to deal with a chronic health problem that seems difficult to treat. Or you may simply have questions about your long-term health that don't get answered with your current medical care. If you're one of these situations, it may help to get a fresh perspective on the problem.

The Second Opinion — and the Third

If you're considering surgery, should you get a second opinion? Of course. But the real issue is whether you should get a second opinion on other kinds of treatment, such as extended courses of medication, and whether you should get a *third* opinion if you're looking at major surgery. The second opinion is already an institutionalized medical practice. It's even subsidized by insurance plans. It's called for any time you're about to undergo a serious procedure: something serious, irreversible, consequential to your life. Unfortunately, people think about this for a surgical procedure but not for courses of drugs or medication. But they should. Taking a cholesterol-lowering medication, or an antihypertensive medication, can have a serious impact on your physiology and even state of mind. There are alternatives to these kinds of treatment and to many other "standard" medical treatments that may be much safer or more beneficial for you in the long run.

The standard second opinion for surgery is mostly for the benefit of doctors and insurance companies, to ward against the risk of malpractice or gross negligence, or to control costs. It doesn't really provide you with a true alternative perspective. The government has a real check-and-balance system. But in the second opinion system, a physician from a hospital across town will be commenting on the work of a physician in his own speciality. These physicians usually play by the same ground rules and often have to pass on each other's work. As a result, the second opinion is generally going to be a cordial opinion, a confirmation of the first doctor's findings. Only rarely will a specialist offer a conflicting view in a second opinion. The second opinion is usually a rubber stamp; it's not a matter of "Let's take a little different view of the problem."

I'm suggesting the value of a third opinion, in which you seek out the perspective of a doctor who is critical of standard medical procedures and has no vested interest in them — that is, doesn't derive income from doing them. A "third opinion doctor" who is not making a living from doing surgery, for example, won't suffer any political consequences in the professional community for offering a truly alternative opinion. If such a doctor is not keeping up with a huge case load by quickly prescribing the standard medications and going on to the next patient, he or she won't suffer by suggesting that a patient doesn't need a drug regimen, if there's an alternative approach and it's safe for the patient.

How to Get a Good Third Opinion

You can often get a recommendation or reference to a holistic or nutritionally oriented physician through friends or colleagues, just as you would to any doctor. You can write to one of the organizations listed in the Resource section and ask for a list of members in your area. There are also resources you can explore on the Internet. You may want to look up someone who has written an article or a book. Just remember that the ability to write an interesting or even important article or book doesn't in itself mean that someone is a good clinical practitioner. (I don't mind saying this, though I've written quite a few books and articles myself!)

For third-opinion purposes, don't get hung up on checking a medical pedigree: whether the physician is board-certified or is affiliated with the best hospital. Some of the best physicians around don't have the maximum credentials. (Of course, if you're looking for someone to perform a particular kind of surgery, then the surgeon should be board-certified and have had all the standard training, which a physician will receive only in a rigorous medical setting.) For holistic doctors or nutritionally oriented doctors, on the other hand, you really have to go with their reputation and standing.

Though you may have heard of a therapy that you think might help you, such as chelation therapy, you should leave it up to the physician to decide whether this is the appropriate treatment for you. A responsible physician who practices chelation therapy should be prepared to tell you that this isn't right for you or that conventional medical treatment would be more appropriate in your case.

There's a bit of a gray area if you think you might be helped by a chiropractor or an acupuncturist. A responsible chiropractor should be able to tell you if he or she doesn't have a therapy for you, just as a surgeon might tell you that you don't really need surgery. But be warned: this is not easy for self-serving practitioners, since they're aware from the outset that they will profit by providing the specific treatment a patient might ask for. That's why a true alternative opinion is useful. The bottom line: See at least one professional who does not have a vested interest in a particular procedure.

A Non-Western Alternative: Traditional Chinese Medicine

One of the alternatives that many Americans are turning to these days is traditional Chinese medicine, a practice often abbreviated as TCM. I have a real interest in this myself, and find it fascinating to explore the alternate views of illness and health that TCM offers, and compare them with our own medical tradition. Female disorders of a non-life-threatening nature are often good candidates for treatment by TCM, including PMS, painful or irregular menstruation, and certain menopausal symptoms. TCM is often useful in dealing with common medical problems that are poorly dealt with in the West, such as asthma and emphysema, which can be improved by acupuncture and traditional Chinese herbs. With many painful conditions, TCM can offer less toxic alternative therapies that can reduce reliance on harmful drugs.

You may encounter TCM in several ways. One group of practitioners includes physicians who have emigrated from China, the majority of whom are not licensed to practice medicine in the United States. While a few have gone through the rigorous additional training requirements to earn a medical degree here, many have not. They may be extremely adept in the use of herbs and acupuncture, though the degree to which they can communicate effectively with you varies. This may lead to some doubt about whether your complaints are being properly heard or whether the doctor is imparting the most effective treatment.

Traditionalists assert that only Chinese-trained veteran physicians are capable of mastering the intricacies of herbal combinations, acupuncture, and such esoteric skills as pulse diagnosis. They argue that effective treatment depends less on communicating with patients than with reading the subtle bodily signs of illness. Indeed, one of my mentors in TCM was a physician who barely could communicate in English but nonetheless possessed superb powers of observation, insight, and diagnostic skill.

Alternatively, the new availability of excellent training programs in TCM in the United States has given rise to a new type of Western practitioner possessing a modern scientific orientation as well as TCM skills. These practitioners, while less experienced than their Chinese counterparts, are often better able to communicate with patients. Some are M.D.s, while others are credentialed certified acupuncturists and/or herbalists. The issue of credentialing is confusing because it may be that a back-alley Chinatown herbalist possesses skills far superior to those of a board-certified American-trained M.D. with a certificate from a short training course in TCM. See the Resource section for more on certification.

Another issue is the way TCM is making its way into the self-care marketplace. Herbs like ginseng and ephedra, long mainstays of TCM formulas, are being marketed and popularized in over-the-counter pills, teas, and tinctures. While this allows the benefits of TCM to be mainstreamed, sometimes people are swayed by the Western notion that if a little bit is good, a lot is better. Some people are taking high doses of therapeutic agents out of the context of their traditional use. For example, some individuals may use ginseng, which is good for "energy," when TCM practitioners would find it contraindicated because of its potential for exhausting an already overtaxed system. Similarly, such diagnostic subtleties are trampled upon when Western thrill-seekers use ephedra-laced products like Herbal Ecstasy to get high rather than for its mild decongestant properties. It's been safely used for centuries in China, but there it is administered by experienced practitioners. If you think TCM may have something to offer you, take the same pains in checking references that you would in choosing any other medical practitioner, and don't self-medicate.

How to Approach an Alternative Physician

When you go for an initial consultation, expect to pay for the time as you would with a lawyer or other professional. After all, you're getting the benefit of the physician's knowledge and time and expertise, even if you're not embarking on a course of treatment. Consider your first visit to be exploratory.

Say to the doctor, "This is an initial consultation. I'd like to tell you about my problem and hear your suggestions, and then let's both make a judgment about whether you can help me." It shouldn't just be assumed that any given doctor can help any given patient. On the basis of your consultation, you can then decide whether you want to pursue the doctor's recommendations, or not.

A good physician should be prepared to say, "Look, I can't help you; this really isn't my area of expertise, but call so and so." Or even, "I'm sorry, but we just don't have a good medical answer for this problem." Maimonides, the great physician and teacher of the Middle Ages, told his medical students, "Thou should teach thy lips to say 'I don't know.' " This is one area where I sometimes fault some of my holistic colleagues, because even more so than mainstream doctors, some of them always have an answer. There's too much assuredness that the problem has got to be an allergy, or a food intolerance, or some other catchall category. Optimism is good, and it's worth taking the trouble to track down a solution, but there really are cases in which there is no solution. Part of the physician's job is to validate the patient's experience and to say, "Yes you do have this problem; it's not psychosomatic, but we don't have a very good answer for it right now." Sometimes the road to relief starts with accepting a situation, and adjusting one's lifestyle to deal with it.

Testing, One-Two-Three: The Physical Exam

Here's one typical scenario that a major health insurer underwrites: a yearly exam, with an EKG, and inspection of the prostate, and an elaborate blood test. The blood test is done at the time of the physical, and the results come back to the doctor a few days or a week later. But the doctor rarely suggests a followup visit to discuss those results. These blood tests are in fact being done simply to rule out very gross departures from the norm, rather than to detect more subtle problems. Having been screened for major problems, you will know that you're not going to die of cancer in six months, but you won't have the slightest additional bit of information about your health. Some additional information will go to the doctor, but probably none of it will be passed on to you. Maybe you'll get a letter in the mail saying that your test results were basically normal, and to have a healthy year!

As a physician, I don't subscribe to any one-size-fits-all testing guidelines. I want to know my patients well, and therefore I individualize the diagnostic workups. With a new patient, I'd be more likely to do a "routine" EKG, especially for an older patient who hasn't had one. Once I know my patient and his or her habits and lifestyle, I may feel that the patient can go longer between EKGs. If someone at fifty or fifty-five has an excellent lipid profile, is exercising regularly, and is following a good program of diet and nutritional supplements, I might feel comfortable having that person go for three to five years between EKGs, though some might consider this controversial.

Should you have a yearly exam at all? Yes, but you shouldn't have to settle for the old-fashioned standard physical. If you want to get more useful information from your physical, consider the following:

What to Ask Your Doctor

1. Ask to have a copy of the results of your blood test and other tests.

2. Make a second appointment with the doctor, when the test results are in, to discuss them. I normally see patients for a second visit and give them a lengthy analysis of the test results, with time for questions, answers, and specific recommendations. This is for well people too. An annual physical should be in two parts. First there is the initial information gathering: the time for you to express your concerns and for the physician to perform tests that are optimally directed toward specific concerns of the patient or doctor. Second comes the followup.

3. Consider a periodic secondary checkup with a specialist or doctor who is familiar with some of the more sophisticated and cutting-edge tests. While conventional physicians may provide excellent service in screening for serious health problems and preventing major disasters, they just may not have the time, expertise, or interest to pursue more advanced evaluations. However, you may have to spend out of your own pocket to get these additional medical services, since they may not be covered by standard health insurance.

THE WAY IT OUGHT TO BE

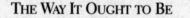

In an ideal medical system, the interaction between doctors and patients should be opened up to address issues that often don't come up in the standard office visit. Here are some questions that should be a regular part of the dialog between doctor and patient. Try discussing some of these things with your doctor.

Questions patients should ask their doctors:

- What do you see as my major health liabilities in the future?
- Though I'm well now, what should I be doing to prevent disease?
- Are there alternatives to the drugs you've prescribed for me?

Questions doctors should ask their patients in any checkup:

- In what ways would you like to optimize your health?
- Are you unnecessarily exposing yourself to harmful chemicals in your food, water, workplace, or home?
- Are you taking nutritional supplements?
- How do you relax?

Which Tests Are Necessary?

You expect to have *some* tests done when you go in for your yearly checkup, but which ones are really necessary? In my view, conventional practice suffers from overtesting in several areas — testing that gives us no therapeutically useful information or that may lead us further and further down a path toward unnecessary surgery or medication. Doctors always look for the "normal" response to a test — and there is such a variation between individual physiologies that in many cases "normal" doesn't mean very much.

At the same time that many tests are overprescribed, there are some quite useful, inexpensive tests that aren't done often enough. Let's look at some examples of each. Here are some questions I've had patients ask:

- Do I need an electrocardiogram (EKG) every time I see the doctor?

The EKG used to be a routine part of an annual physical for men and women over forty, and this is still a good idea. It's not an expensive test, but it's one that has on occasion been overprescribed, especially for elderly patients who might see two or three doctors, each of whom does another EKG.

- I'm concerned about my heart health. Should I have an annual stress test?

Another commonly overused test is the stress test, in which you walk a treadmill while your heart rate and blood pressure are continuously monitored. This should only be done when there is a strong suspicion of cardiovascular disease, based on risk factors or symptoms. Someone who has very high blood pressure and diabetes, and who smokes, would be a good candidate for a stress test. So would a mature person who has been fairly sedentary and wants to enter on a serious exercise program or go on a two-week white-water rafting expedition. It's also used for elderly persons who are undergoing surgery, in order to be sure that their hearts are strong enough to carry them through. But now, too many healthy thirty-five- or forty-year-olds go in for an annual checkup and hear the doctor heartily inform them, "We're going check out your heart with a stress test." This is really pointless. What's worse, it does result in a lot of false-positive results, which can undermine people's self-confidence and turn them into "cardiac cripples," afraid to exercise or even to get excited for fear of inducing a heart attack.

- Is it important for me to get a sigmoidoscopy?

Sigmoidoscopy, a visual inspection of the colon, is a test for rectal cancer that is medically useful but often needlessly prescribed. By the age of fifty everyone should probably have one sigmoidoscopy, or a barium enema, or colonoscopy to screen for colon cancer, and thereafter about every three to five years.

The simplest test for rectal cancer is the Hemoccult for blood in the stool, but it seems to give a few false negative results and a lot of false positive results, making it not a good diagnostic. There clearly are cases where sigmoidoscopy is called for — with a patient over the age of fifty who has polyps, or with a younger patient who has a family history of colon cancer. This is good medical practice. However, many physicians seem to have seized on this test zealously, applying it annually even when there's no real indication of polyps or other colon problems. Studies have shown that it takes at least five to ten years for an ordinary polyp to go from the minimal size detectable in a sigmoidoscopy to a cancerous stage, when it might reveal telltale signs of blood. Accordingly, it might make sense with some individuals to do a sigmoidoscopy every three to five years, which would provide plenty of time to catch any problems. On an annual basis — as an "insurance policy" — this is really overkill.

- Should I be tested for prostate cancer?

Most doctors perform a digital test on men over forty during the annual exam, feeling the prostate manually to check for problems. This is a good, quick, easy test. There is a current vogue, though, for the prostate-specific antigen (PSA) test, which really illustrates the downside of testing. When it came out, it was supposed to be a great boon to mankind. Typically given to men of fifty and over, it provides a fairly accurate early warning that prostate cancer will develop. The fact is that this is a relatively common and fatal cancer for this age group. When it was introduced, the PSA test was hailed as a major weapon in the battle against prostate cancer, but studies have shown that its use has virtually no impact on longevity or outcome.

Unfortunately, we don't have a very good treatment for prostate cancer. The test itself has done nothing to help us cure this illness. Worse, it has increased the misery of this disease by letting a lot of men worry for years in advance that they might be doomed, victims of a cancer that no one or nothing can halt. Eventually, some in this group will succumb to prostate cancer, or sometimes, after years of needless fearful anticipation, they will die of other natural causes. Either way, the PSA test has done little to improve anyone's quality of life.

It's made a lot of older men undergo therapies that are now thought to be superfluous and that have induced complications that worsen the quality of remaining life without producing any benefits. The standard care for early prostate cancer is now our old friend "watchful waiting." Radiation and surgery seem to be useless until the cancer has already taken hold, and they don't even work in every case. So the early warning gives us no edge. Ironically, the only group that does seem to benefit somewhat from an early warning is younger men, and they're rarely given the test because prostate cancer is so infrequent in this age group. This is a fairly expensive test, which does provide accurate diagnostic information but at this time has real medical value only in tracking the stages of an existing cancer.

An intelligent medicine approach might resolve this connundrum. If an elevated PSA level were to prompt a biopsy revealing cancer in an otherwise healthy seventy-two-year-old, given that the benefits of surgery or radiation are as yet unsubstantiated, this might suggest an enhanced form of watchful waiting. This could take the form of PSA monitoring, while the patient modifies his diet to a semivegetarian plan, relying heavily on natural sources of those healthy isoflavones and lycopene, such as soy, beans, and tomatoes, that have been shown to block prostate cancer. (We've mentioned these compounds, both phytonutrients, in chapter 16.) Also available are phytonutrient concentrates, which along with immune-enhancing vitamins might improve the outcome for such a patient.

- I still get my period. Do I need a mammogram?

Another test that's the subject of a lot of recent controversy is the annual mammogram for women who are in their forties or fifties. There is a consensus that women after the age of fifty, and after menopause, should have an annual mammogram. Typically, routine screening mammograms are recommended only for postmenopausal women. Before that time, and before menopause, it's up for grabs. Some doctors and medical organizations say it should definitely be part of an annual checkup for women over forty; others are saying, "Don't bother." Of course, if a woman has lumps in her breasts or a family history of breast cancer, the mammogram is definitely called for well before menopause. Unfortunately, part of the problem with mammograms is that mammograms in premenopausal women are very hard to read. In a recent study of how radiologists read mammograms, the specialists agreed on the need for a biopsy in 7 percent of a group of women, *but they didn't agree on which breast should undergo the biopsy!* Some said it was the right breast; some said the left. Women who are going through this should bear in mind that the current test is not perfect.

However, a new test uses a radioactively traceable injection of technetium-99 that will "light up" in areas of suspected malignancy. The hope is that this will provide a much less equivocal test result and reduce by half the need for biopsies. Also, the introduction of high density imaging (HDI) with ultrasound paves the way for avoiding about 40 percent of the breast biopsies now performed. I'm very sympathetic with women who have had two or three false-positive results from mammograms and had their breasts cut up for biopsies. It's understandable why they would want to give up on the mammograms, which is why this question should probably be decided on a case-by-case basis and not as a population-wide recommendation.

From all this you might think I'm on an antitesting bandwagon, but that's not so. I often do extensive tests, including some rare ones, when people come to me with troublesome chronic complaints that haven't responded to treatment. Some tests should be done much more routinely than they are. They include:

• Ultrafast CAT scan of the heart. This is a way to detect calcium deposits in the coronary arteries, as an indicator of atherosclerosis.

• Magnetic resonance angiography (MRA). Now under development, MRA promises to be a noninvasive test that will assess the health of arteries and the degree of atherosclerosis. We'll be able to use this test to confirm whether an intervention program of diet and exercise has been successful.

• The PET scan for cardiovascular imaging and other early warnings. This is a noninvasive test that goes beyond the "plumbing diagram" that ordinary dye studies of the arteries depict. Rather, it shows patterns of energy use and nutrient uptake in rapidly metabolizing parts of the body like the brain and the heart. Patterns of PET scan abnormalities are beginning to be used to analyze progression towards Alzheimer's disease and other neuro-degenerative conditions as well as subtle changes in heart function. The PET scan was used recently to document improvements in heart function with nutritional and lifestyle changes patterned after the recommendations of Dean Ornish.

• A more complete cardiovascular panel. Although cholesterol levels without HDL are really meaningless, many doctors and hospitals are doing "mini–blood panels" that don't include HDL levels in an effort to contain costs. Everyone should demand an HDL test, especially if there's been any discussion about lowering cholesterol levels. The expanded cardiovascular panel should ideally include lipoprotein A and B (which normally parallel cholesterol levels but provide additional information), fibrinogen (which assesses thickness and clotting tendency of blood), lp(a) and homocysteine (independent measures of susceptibility to vascular disease).

• The ferritin blood test, which reveals stored levels of iron in the blood. High levels suggest iron excess, which is sometimes linked with heart disease and even cancer. Low levels can indicate iron deficiency.

• Additional nutritional parameters. There are already some nutritional parameters, such as iron and potassium, in the normal blood test. Albumin levels are an index of the amount of protein you are absorbing and synthe-sizing. Magnesium is a very useful indicator that's often not included; low magnesium levels are often associated with chronic fatigue or sensitivity to stress. In women vitamin D levels are useful to know, since low levels are a risk factor for osteoporosis. In both sexes it's important to assess vitamin B_{12} levels. Deficiencies can be devastating and can cause symptoms that resemble those of Alzheimer's disease, to say nothing of weakness and fatigue. Folic acid is an important cancer-protective nutrient that's good to check.

• New tests to assess antioxidant levels in the bloodstream and measure the extent of free-radical damage in the body. These can provide a very strong indicator of someone's overall health and long-term prognosis. They can provide a definite basis on which to recommend antioxidants. These are among the more significant tests of the future and are probably more important than some of the standard blood tests as a prognosticator of general health, since the oxidation process has been associated with heart disease, cancer, and the aging process itself. Unfortunately, they are not now covered by insurance and are at this time fairly expensive.

• Impedance plethysmography, a test of the fat-to-lean ratio of overall body composition. It can give an indication of one of the main parameters of aging, which is marked by a loss of lean body mass and susceptibility to weight gain through increased fat mass. The procedure is an electronic measurement of the fat percentage of body, and it can be done in a doctor's office. A very, very weak electric current is sent through the body, and the results are compared with different norms for men and for women. The test can reveal aspects that are not obvious; for example, a chunky person may have a good ratio of muscle to fat, while a thin person may have too high a fat percentage. We can then use the test to measure someone's progress in slowing the natural decline of lean body mass with aging.

• The glucose tolerance test with insulin, an extremely important test that's unfortunately very rarely done. In fact, it's done mostly to indulge what doctors see as a patient's fears of hypoglycemia. The problem is that the criteria for normalcy are so broad that the value of the test is limited. The glucose tolerance test is also rarely performed with insulin, which makes the test much more useful, since the reading of insulin levels can indicate whether someone is on the path to Syndrome X and becoming prediabetic.

• A more comprehensive stool test, which can be very useful to someone who has gastrointestinal problems or even such apparently unrelated symptoms as fatigue, malaise, arthritic aches and pains, or allergies. The basic stool tests are normally performed only in patients with serious GI problems in whom parasites are suspected. If parasites are ruled out, the doctor may well dismiss the GI tract as a problem area, even though a more comprehensive stool test may suggest additional problems there. The comprehensive test can indicate an imbalance of intestinal bacteria, which can cause an immune reaction and allergic symptoms.

• For women, a bone density test at the time of menopause, to determine

whether there's a risk of accelerated osteoporosis. We have the capability
for early warning of osteoporosis, which we can help prevent through
calcium supplements or sometimes hormone replacement therapy. It's
really not responsible to start estrogen replacement therapy without doing
this test to evaluate a woman's real risk of osteoporosis, but it's done. Most
doctors will go along with doing this test if asked. A new urine test looks
for byproducts of bone turnover that help establish the rate of progression
of bone loss.

It can sometimes be difficult to ask for some of these tests, since there's
always the chance that a doctor will take umbrage and think you're telling
him or her how to practice. They may not all be covered by standard health
insurance either. While you may find that your doctor is willing to do these
tests, you should also try to judge whether she is really interested in
interpreting them, and is not just going along to humor you. Without the
interpretation, the results are not going to be that meaningful. If you get a
blank look or a resigned sigh when you ask for these tests, you may be better
off with a physician who is more familiar with them and interested in using
them.

The key criterion that should be applied to all medical tests is not just
whether they can provide information but whether the information is
medically useful for you, the patient.

Surgery: Let the Buyer Beware

Any fool can cut off a leg; it takes a surgeon to save one.

GEORGE G. ROSS (NINETEENTH-
CENTURY BRITISH SURGEON)

*Tis the Chyrurgions's praise and height of Art, not to cut off,
but cure the vicious part.*

ROBERT HERRICK (1591–1674)

Clara, a fifty-two-year-old woman, came into my office looking tired,
haggard, and overweight, but it was clear that she had been beautiful. Five
years previously, she had been told that she needed a hysterectomy because
of bleeding fibroids. Her doctor had convinced her that she didn't need her
ovaries, either, because they would cause trouble later. By their surgical

removal, she would reduce the risk of ovarian cancer. After the surgery, she gained forty-five pounds and her sex drive vanished. I'm always saddened when I see someone who's been affected like this, because her surgery was unnecessary. Clara should have had a myomectomy, a surgery involving only removal of the fibroids themselves with conservation of the uterus and ovaries.

Surgeons as a group probably command the highest respect of any medical specialists, and certainly the highest salaries. They are the miracle workers, and there seems no limit to the ways they can patch people up and put them back together. They certainly do perform miracles of "biological engineering," and many lives have been saved by advances in modern surgical techniques. As a holistic doctor, I often see people who come to me for an alternative to surgery but have to tell them, "No, there is no 'alternative' treatment for a brain tumor, or a thyroid mass. Go and have the surgery, now."

At the same time, it's clear that surgery is a big business, and a good business for hospitals, surgeons, and anesthesiologists. In some areas there is real competition for patients, and too many procedures seem to have taken on a life of their own and are performed as the "standard procedure" whether or not they're in the best interests of the patient. I think it's just fine for people to have a healthy skepticism about surgery and to look for alternatives, especially to the so-called elective procedures. In our current craze for surgery we may well be ignoring a basic principle: the inviolate nature of the body. The body is not just silly putty to be manipulated and reshaped without consequence. Surgery should remain an extreme measure, a treatment of last resort. It is no light thing to invade the human body with saws and scalpels, and there may be long-term repercussions that are subtle and not generally recognized.

It's been suggested, for example, that there are "neural networks" that traverse the body and follow nodes of the autonomic nervous system. When we interrupt these circuits with incisions and surgery scar lines, this can disturb the functioning of the body. It's not uncommon for someone who has acquired a large appendix scar to have pain that is perceived in the right shoulder (this is known as referred pain, because it is felt in a place other than the source). Scars also tend to cause contraction of muscles and to send feedback signals to the autonomic nervous system, which can cause additional disturbances. The European practice of neural therapy provides dramatic evidence of the relationship between surgical scars and seemingly unrelated pain. In this practice, injection of a local anesthetic to a scar can cause immediate relief of referred pain in a distant area of the body. Furthermore, many surgical procedures, especially abdominal surgery, cause adhesions as an aftereffect. These are painful internal tangles of scar tissue and fibrous tissue that develop as the body's attempts to "wall off" the injured area, and they can cause painful internal tugs and pulls.

No surgery is to be undertaken lightly. Even if the complication rate is very low, it's still a factor.

A Caveat: Don't Write Off All Surgery

In spite of my own skepticism about quite a few popular surgical procedures, the last thing I would want to do is reinforce anyone's individual anxiety about surgery to the point where he or she would always refuse it and insist on an alternative. Because of my views I'm sometimes used as the "Say it ain't so" doc when it comes to surgical procedures. But while surgery is often performed excessively, in certain instances you really need to find out what's going on. Someone once came in to my office with an operable brain tumor, looking for a herbal treatment or some other alternative to surgery. I did my best to get him signed up with a good hospital and surgeon as quickly as possible. In a more common instance, someone comes in with thyroid nodules, tells me surgery has been recommended, and wants me to recommend an alternative treatment such as a vitamin protocol. But a thyroid specialist who recommends a biopsy is doing so on the basis of suspicious nodules, and while the vast majority of these turn out to be harmless, the risk of leaving a smoldering cancer in place is great enough to justify the preemptive strike.

A recommendation of surgery by a very conservative physician — one who really considers the alternatives — is particularly weighty. In fact, that's probably the way the need should be determined: not by the surgeons who are going to perform the surgery but by physicians who are schooled in the indications for surgery but critical of surgical excess. A primary care physician might play an important role in this process. A second opinion by another surgeon is more likely to support the first surgeon's opinion, but a second opinion by another primary physician may offer a truly independent point of reference.

How to Select a Surgeon and a Hospital

If you do determine that you really do need surgery, you certainly want to know that you're getting a competent surgeon in a hospital with a good support system. In most cases, someone matches you to a surgeon. Your primary care physician will give you a reference, and most people don't go beyond that. But in this area, too, people are beginning to take a more active role in their own medical care, and this is all to the good, considering the seriousness of the matter. You can certainly interview several surgeons, ask for information about their background and experience, and check up on hospital records of complication rates for a given procedure. You should also be aware of some general trends in the medical profession and the health care industry that have a great deal of influence on quality of care.

One of these trends is rather troubling: surgeons are becoming increasingly competitive, angling for patients and procedures to fill up their schedules. The reason is that we have simply created too many surgeons for the general populace, and they have not been allocated on any rational basis to different parts of the country where they might be needed. Instead, a great many surgeons live and work in desirable parts of the country — the east and west coasts, and big cities like Boston, New York, Los Angeles, San Francisco, and Seattle. At the same time there is a shortage of surgeons in rural areas and parts of the west and the middle west. In these surgical "hot spots," there's a lot of competition, and surgeons try to master the latest techniques very quickly — sometimes too quickly. Conversely, in the less populated areas, the local surgeons may be called upon to perform procedures that they do very infrequently, without a lot of background experience, just because they are the only surgeons available.

Another troubling trend is that new techniques are sometimes mainstreamed too quickly, so that your surgeon may not be that experienced or thoroughly trained in the procedure. For example, there was a real concern about procedural quality as surgeons started to learn laparoscopic surgery, in which they use lasers to resect organs, working through a "keyhole" incision. Some studies were done, and it turned out that there was an extraordinary disparity in skill and knowledge between surgeons. The more competent surgeons had trained in a hospital setting through residency and fellowship programs at university hospitals. Much less competent were the community-based surgeons, often working in more underserved areas, with no university hospitals, who learned this technique either through three-day seminars or in some instances simply from salespeople or support personnel from the equipment manufacturers.

Specialization is another important issue in surgery. The government has actually cracked down on some regional hospitals or smaller hospitals that have been performing very challenging or specialized types of surgery. There's an incentive for smaller hospitals to flaunt their crown jewels: a transplant unit or a sophisticated cardiovascular unit. This has a trickledown effect for the hospital, since these units attract big-ticket patients, with long hospital stays, who use a lot of drugs and often have complications, and require consultations with specialists from other departments. It's financially very desirable for a hospital to have this kind of unit. The problem is that relatively few patients may use it, so that none of the surgeons or other specialists may be that experienced with the procedures.

If you're considering surgery and you live in one of the big urban centers with several teaching hospitals, this should make you feel better, since the city will be teeming with surgeons and state-of-the-art technical support and training. In fact, you may at times need to fend off the whole community of surgical specialists who need a good steady crop of candidates for the operating room to keep them all in business. However, there are pluses and minuses to teaching hospitals. On the positive side, they are centers of excellence, the training is better, and the standards are much more rigorous, not just for the residents but also for the attending physicians. The minus side is that sometimes you will be subject to the ministrations of inexperienced medical students and residents, and this is part of the game. To a certain extent, though, you don't have to play this game. If you're in a bed in a teaching hospital and a rag-tag band of young people in white coats approaches you and wants to interview you or perform a specific exam or even a procedure on you, you don't have to assent. This is part of the Patient's Bill of Rights.

On the positive side for the community hospitals and small regional hospitals, they are distinguished by the quality of their nursing care, which is generally more personal and more caring. The nurses may be people from your community, and they're likely to treat you less like a room number and more like a person. There certainly are some very good surgeons with a lot of training and practice who work in these hospitals, though perhaps not in every area of specialization.

Now that you have a sense of the lay of the land, let's consider what you should specifically look for in a surgeon and a hospital.

• Interview the surgeon who's been recommended to you, and ask the right questions.

It is certainly fair for you to ask whether the surgeon in question is experienced in the type of surgery you need. You can ask this of your personal physician, you can ask it of the surgeon directly, and you can ask it of the hospital. You should get a clear answer. If you don't get an answer, you should complain. More specifically, you want to know what percentage of his practice consists of the type of surgery you're considering, and how many times he's performed this type of surgery. If you are having a rare and esoteric type of surgery, perhaps involving a very new technique, your surgeon may well say, "Look, I want you to give fully informed consent to this. We've only done five of them, but four out of five have been successful, and we think it's going to be successful for you." Then you can consult with another physician, if you like, and make your best judgement.

On the other hand, if you're about to have your gallbladder taken out by a surgeon who has performed laser laparascopic cholecystectomy only three or four times, you might well say, "No thank you; I'd rather have this done by a doctor who's done it fifty times, or a hundred times." You can ask how many times the surgeon has performed the operation. Doctors are at liberty to say, "No, I'm not going to tell you," but at their own peril if it's a competitive marketplace.

• Don't be swayed by charm alone.

While most people prefer a physician who's sensitive and caring and has a good bedside manner, this should not be the most important criteria. Credentials and experience should be. If you're having major surgery, the really important activity will go on while you're knocked out with an anesthetic, and what you want is a highly skilled and competent physician who will be doing careful and cautious work.

• Get the hospital's statistics for the procedure you're going to have.

You can find out about the success rate of the surgical procedure you're considering at the specific hospital you'd be going to. If you're about to undergo a coronary artery bypass graft, for example, you can find out your hospital's success rate is for this specific procedure, as well as the complication rate and the mortality rate. This is public information. Be careful in assessing what this means, however, since you may see statistics that show fairly high complication rates or a somewhat higher death rate in what are supposed to be some of the finest hospitals. This doesn't necessarily mean that those hospitals do it less well. They may be getting referrals of the very tough, borderline cases precisely because they do have a very skilled staff. These tough cases are bound to generate worse statistics.

You may see a very high complication rate at an obscure smaller hospital in the hinterlands, somewhat lower rates at a respected regional hospital, and higher rates again at a respected teaching hospital in a big city. At the small hospital, this may reflect a real lack of experience with the procedure. At the big-city teaching hospital, it may simply mean that they are doing lots of emergency surgery, and taking on riskier, sicker patients that other hospitals don't even want to deal with.

You can get hospital statistics from organizations for medical consumers, which exist in a number of states, and also from your state health department. Several national organizations can provide help (see the Resource section).

How Safe Are Hospitals?

In 1984, the parents of Libby Zion, a college freshman, brought their daughter to the emergency room of one of the finest hospitals in the country because she had had a persistent ear infection and was running a high fever. The resident performed an initial examination and admitted Libby to the hospital for further monitoring. She was in the care of a top medical team with the most advanced high-tech facilities in the world. Eight hours later, Libby's parents were notified that she had died.

The case triggered one of the most publicized malpractice trials of the decade. Libby's father, Sidney Zion, a well-known journalist, still contends that the hospital's system of delivering care was at fault, that the overworked and overburdened residents who were entrusted with Libby's care were unable to properly supervise her medical management, and that a series of medical mishaps ensued in which Libby was given powerful medications without thought of their possible interactions. In a sense, Libby's "person-hood" became lost in a medical maze. She was given sedating drugs that interacted with her other medications, lapsed into a coma, and died of cardiac arrest. (A jury finally decided that both the hospital and Libby herself were partially responsible, because she hadn't told the doctors about her occasional cocaine use, which *could* have caused an interaction with one of the drugs she was given.)

The drama of this malpractice suit was played out in the full view of the American public — it was actually shown on *Court TV.* It was quite compelling, and the case had a lot of resonance, because many Americans do distrust hospitals, sometimes to the extent of refusing essential care. This kind of mistrust can be fatal. The painter Andy Warhol refused for thirteen years to go into a hospital for a gallbladder operation because he feared that he would die there. When he finally had to be admitted because of a crisis, his health had failed to such a point that his prophecy came true. Still, many people do wonder whether a trip to a hospital for a relatively minor problem will entail the risk that they will succumb to a catastrophe like Libby's and become victims of a medical system gone awry.

In spite of the horror stories, there's no question that lives are saved in hospitals, major health problems are solved, and many people are restored to full functioning and quality of life. To some extent, the inherent problems that led to Libby's death have been addressed. The duty hours of medical residents have been reduced, so it's less likely that a resident you encounter during your hospital visit will be working into his 120th hour of weekly responsibilities. By the same token, it's felt that this may result in less continuity of care for the patient. There are now sometimes fewer medical personnel in the hospital at a given time, and medical residents may have more responsibilities because they have to monitor the care of more patients, especially during long overnight or weekend duty.

Some critics also contend that the quality of nursing care has declined as hospitals are forced to cut corners to contain rising costs. And it's the nurses who provide a second line of defense against cursory or inadequate medical monitoring. They're the backup to cover for the inexperience of young residents whose faces change each year in the hospital, while the more stable nursing staff remains in place.

If you do have to spend time in a hospital, how can you optimize your care? Some contend that since hospitals are not perfect, and since there are problems inherent in the system, it's incumbent upon patients or their families to demand higher standards of care. When I was a harried, exhausted resident myself, I used to dread the approach of demanding relatives during visiting hours, because they really were an impediment to my racing through my many chores and responsibilities. On the other hand, they often did push me to provide better care or address specific issues regarding their relatives that the medical staff had generally ignored. From my perspective, I do think it's true that you can overcome some of the systemic flaws in hospital care by being a demanding patient, having your relatives present, and insisting on sufficient communication with your doctor.

Personalize Yourself

If you go into the hospital for a few days or longer, for a serious medical problem, anything you can do to make yourself more of an individual to the medical staff will help you get more careful attention. The hospital staff, from nurses to doctors, will tend to look at you as "a surgery" or "a disease" and not as an individual with hopes and fears and a whole life beyond your health problem. It's especially hard for them to make this leap if you're in intensive care with tubes coming out of you, sedated, mute, and not really "yourself."

To present yourself as a human individual, adorn your hospital room (perhaps with a friend's or relative's help) not just with flowers, but with personal things — pictures of the family, special books or magazines even if you don't feel like reading them, something that evokes your profession or life outside the hospital. This could be a law journal if you're a lawyer, a picture of your class if you're a teacher or of your children if you're a homemaker, or something you've made if you're a hobbyist or craftsperson. Or just bring a few pictures of you that show you working or enjoying life, so that the staff can see what you look like when you're not in a hospital gown. This will humanize you to the medical staff, and you'll probably get better care.

Miracle Drugs or Mystery Medicine?

Probably the greatest seismic shift in medicine for the baby-boomer generation was the advent of miracle drugs. This was the first generation that was really raised on antibiotics, beginning in childhood, and the first to be protected by convenient vaccines from fearful, crippling diseases like polio. From childhood, we've expected the doctor to have a medicine for every ailment, a pill for every pain. The drug companies and medical researchers have been working overtime for thirty years to meet this expectation. Doctors are swamped with ads and samples from drug companies touting their wares, and a vast array of new "miracle medications" is available for the prescribing. The new focus on biomolecular medicine has provided a field day for drug developers. There's scarcely an illness that doesn't have a least one drug therapy available, sometimes several different kinds, working through different biochemical pathways.

It's a world of miracle drugs, but some haunting questions remain. How many of these new drugs have really been proved to improve long-term outcomes, without potentially dangerous side effects? They all *do* something; there's no doubt about that, and they may improve test results or symptoms. But how many really contribute to an improved overall health outlook? What are the potential risks we run in using high-powered chemicals to alter our body's metabolism? How can the average physician keep up with the avalanche of new medications, clearly understand the guidelines for using them, and be prepared for potential side effects or interactions with other drugs? This question becomes more troubling when you consider the source of drug information for most doctors: the drug companies themselves, who stand to make millions from getting a new drug out into the medical marketplace.

This is not a theoretical issue. A recent study published in the *Journal of the American Medical Association* shows that fully one in four elderly patients receives the wrong drugs. The author of the study, Dr. Steffi Woolhandler of Harvard Medical School, says, "A lot of the problem is that doctors frequently ascribe side effects of drugs to old age. If a patient loses memory or loses balance, they says it's old age."

Indeed, the potential for mayhem is great, given all the permutations of modern medical interventions, their firepower, and their unforeseen interactions. This issue is raised in a different form by Michael Crichton, in his book *Jurassic Park* and in the subsequent blockbuster movies. Crichton is an intelligent writer, a physician himself, and although he wraps his message in a fascinating cavalcade of special effects, rampaging dinosaurs, and squashed jeeps and people, *Jurassic Park* is intended to convey an important reflection on the nature of technological advance. That message is articulated by the character of Dr. Malcolm, a mathematician, played by Jeff Goldblum in the movie, who philosophizes at length about chaos theory. As he explains it, chaos theory predicts that when three or more variables are present in a natural system, outcomes can no longer be predicted with certainty. Chaos theory is actually currently in vogue among mathematicians seeking to characterize an unpredictable universe. A classic illustration of chaos theory is the example of the butterfly that unleashes a tornado. It's a parable of the unpredictability of complex natural systems. A butterfly gently beats its wings, sending a puff of pollen from a nearby flower into the air, which causes a rabbit to sneeze. The sneeze surprises a bird, which takes flight, startling a large flock. The flock begins to encircle the sky, setting up a circling current of air, which affects other currents, until local weather patterns are perturbed, eventually giving rise to a tornado. This is Malcolm's message in *Jurassic Park*: that the whole artificially created ecosystem is so complex that it is ultimately unpredictable. He maintains that it is sheer hubris and all-too-human arrogance to believe that we can tamper unscathed with these complicated natural systems.

The current furor over cloning is a reflection of our fear of science and medical technology that is outstripping our ability to control it. While the popular imagination focuses on the scary implications of cloning—such as loss of individuality, eugenic manipulation of personality and physical traits, and the harvesting of spare body parts from clones—cloning is just a logical extension of our shifting pharmaceutical paradigm. Drugs of the future will no longer be synthesized from petroleum residues in mixing vats; rather, they will be harvested from designer tissue cultures derived from specially cloned animals and—yes—humans. Blocker and booster drugs will be supplanted by hormones, growth and repair factors, and "informational" drugs that will correct aberrant genetic coding for disease.

In some ways, our current medical system is like *Jurassic Park*. We have developed an elaborate biomolecular picture of how the body works. This molecular model is harnessed to a technology that attempts to alter the very chemical reactions that give us life. These reactions are of such complexity that a single drug may operate on multiple systems at once, creating unpredictable side effects. While it may seem that we are managing chaos, surprising new manifestations of disease may ultimately arise.

A clear example of this is the medical diagnosis of polypharmacy, which sometimes appears on medical charts when patients are admitted to a hospital for reactions to the numerous drugs they have been taking. It has become an increasing problem, ranking with many common diseases as a cause of hospital admissions and as a contributing factor to spiraling medical costs. I commonly treat polypharmacy in patients who come to me for a second opinion after conventional treatment for their problems hasn't worked or has created problems of its own.

An example of polypharmacy is the following case. I recently treated a seventy-four-year-old woman whom I was initially reluctant to see, because it sounded as if I probably wasn't going to be able to help her very much. I had received a plaintive phone call from her son saying that his mother had suddenly taken a turn for the worse — that she was depressed, had stopped eating, and had lost the will to live. I reminded the son that sometimes people reach the limits of their natural life span in this fashion, and I suggested to him that the prognosis was poor if his mother was uninterested in placing the phone call to me herself and perhaps was not motivated to get better. But the son was insistent that this was a recent development and that six months ago his mother had been healthy, robust, and jovial. Obviously something had happened, so I agreed to see her.

I was struck by the woman's tired-looking face and emotional flatness. She indeed seemed ready to die. Yet, nothing seemed medically wrong with her. The results of prior blood tests, which her son showed me, seemed to be normal. A physical exam could reveal no evidence of underlying serious disease. I inquired about her medical history. The son told me that she had recently been diagnosed as having high blood pressure, which had not responded to the initial drug she was given, so she was given a second. It struck me that this occurred just when she began to lose her appetite and feel depressed and fatigued. Her personal doctor had not noted this, suggesting instead that she see a psychiatrist. Indeed, depression is common among the elderly. The woman was then given an antidepressant medication along with a remedy for anxiety that would help her sleep. When she came to see me, she was taking all four of these medications. One interesting feature was that she experienced dry mouth and change of taste, so that food tasted "ashen" to her, causing a near-complete loss of appetite. Quickly checking the *Physicians' Desk Reference* for each of the four medications she was taking, I noted that every one of them was known to have the potential to cause taste disturbance and loss of appetite. One might well imagine the combined effects of all four medications when used simultaneously.

I ran additional tests to assess her nutritional status and then shared my hunch with mother and son. I told them that in my opinion she was suffering from polypharmacy and suggested that she try a diet to moderate her blood pressure while gradually tapering off her medications. I told her we needed to do this carefully and did not ask her to stop taking all her medications at once. She then went home with supplements and instructions to come in twice a week for intravenous infusions of vitamins and minerals, which were administered by my nursing staff.

Three weeks later we reconvened. The woman looked absolutely transformed. Her expressionless face was animated, and there was rosy color in her cheeks. She was gregarious and smiling, in dramatic contrast to the first visit, during which she had barely uttered a word and her son had spoken on her behalf. I asked her about her progress in tapering off the two of the four medications I had wanted her to target first. To my surprise and somewhat to my dismay, she told me she had stopped all medications after the second week because she had felt so good after getting off one or two of them. My staff had checked her blood pressure prior to this return visit, and I was satisfied that it was now normal. I could see what the son had meant when he said his mother had been a vibrant person until just a few months earlier. I could also see why he was so determined to get her out of her trough of despondency rather than let her sink slowly into decline and ultimately into death.

What this case illustrates is that nutritional intervention should be tried first in the treatment of medical problems like high blood pressure, and doctors should be aware that patients' complaints may be attributable to the very medications they use to treat their conditions. It's easy to add drugs as new symptoms arise, but few physicians have the inclination, or frankly the guts, to taper off medications and see what really is the underlying cause of their patients' problems.

Side Effects

Many doctors are frustrated when they write out a prescription and their patients immediately go out and consult the *Physicians' Desk Reference*, or some family version of it, and come back and report every obscure known side effect to the doctor. I think this is fine. I encourage more public awareness of the side effects of the many drugs that are offered in the medical marketplace, and I'm happy to discuss these issues with patients. It's the physician's job to be aware of this. On the other hand, it's true that busy physicians are swamped with a deluge of information about the great numbers of new drugs on the market place, and it's increasingly difficult to keep up on all the details, especially side effects and potential drug interactions.

One way to avoid drug-induced problems in the future will be computerized systems widely available in the doctor's office or the pharmacy that will spit out areas of potential interaction between drugs. The pharmacist, who may actually be more familiar with side effects and interactions and warnings than some doctors, can play an important role here. Many pharmacies even now can give you a printout of such information when you get a prescription filled.

One contributor to polypharmacy is the deep flaw in the whole system of reporting side effects, which is a government-managed procedure. The system is based on an initial drug trial, usually with a restricted population, such as healthy men between the ages of twenty and forty. The initial trial may have been conducted with just a few thousand individuals. The most exacting reporting stops there. Then, other side effects will naturally tend to occur in the general populace, where millions of people take a drug. Some people may have very individual responses to drugs that are quite different from the norm. Ideally, these responses are supposed to be reported, and added to the mass of data about the drug.

The way the database gets amplified is that research physicians write articles to medical journals and report on new side effects, and individual physicians can fill out forms that are sent to the FDA about new side effects they observe. Most doctors have in their desks a whole sheaf of blank FDA forms, but even the reasonably conscientious doctors, who are attuned to side effects, may not sit down at the end of a busy day and methodically fill out these forms and mail them to the FDA. So a lot of individual reactions and side effects may not get posted to the database on a drug. Even so, you can find hundreds of side effects actually recorded for one generally used antihypertensive drug that is considered fairly innocuous. They can range from mild malaise to full-blown hepatitis.

Don't go overboard, though, and become pharmaphobic. Every drug has its side effects. On the other hand, side effects should make us think twice about whether a particular drug is really needed, especially when it's subject to long-term, casual use. Some of the most commonly used drugs do have potentially serious side effects, such as antibiotics, anti-inflammatory pain-relievers like ibuprofen, and nasal sprays. These shouldn't be treated so lightly, whether they're readily prescribed or available over the counter.

How Safe is Modern Medicine?

We tend to think that modern medical practice is pretty safe in comparison with earlier times. Yet, the statistics show otherwise. One study found a high level of error in medical practice, so high that if all the errors that occurred in a year — many of them fatal — were reported in the news media, it would be comparable to the simultaneous crash of several jumbo jets. These errors don't make the news because they're underreported, they're disparate iso-lated events, they occur sporadically, they occur to individuals rather than groups, and they occur in hundreds of different hospitals well away from the public view. Where jumbo jets are concerned, we have an incredible number of fail-safe systems and cross-checking routines to reduce error to a very small percentage. In medicine, this isn't done. We actually have a two-digit percentage of errors — a figure that would never be permitted in the airlines industry.

Why not create more orderly fail-safe systems in medicine, with orderly chains of command, double-checking, and computerized backup systems? Instead, we treat medical errors in a whole different way: everyone agrees they shouldn't happen, but they do, and not all errors lead to malpractice suits. Patients suffer, and doctors themselves are devastated by errors.

We have this notion that medicine is an inexact science, and we just can't have the standards we expect from our transportation technology. It's true that bodies sometimes simply fail or react unpredictably. Still, there are ways in which we could implement better controls, such as a cross-check by the pharmacist for drug interactions, or a fail-safe system for catching errors. This could start with a different fundamental philosophy of simply using fewer drugs and taking more seriously the choice of whether or not to use them.

Many medical blunders are perpetrated because the orientation of modern medicine is to suppress symptoms with multiple drugs. Perhaps medicine of the future will recognize the need to reestablish homeostasis in the body rather than to introduce numerous new variables into the equations that reflect our incredibly complex biochemistry.

The New Era for Patients and Doctors

While we may have nostalgic memories of the age of paternalistic medicine, that kind of passivity and compliance was never ideal. We need to take on the same kind of personal responsibility for our medical care that we do in every other important aspect of our lives. We need to think through our health care options in a careful, rational way, avoiding both irrational fears of the medical establishment and slavish dependency on every pronouncement by a medical professional. Taking an active, involved role in your own health care is the foundation for intelligent medicine: a goal to be pursued not only by baby-boomer-aged patients and physicians but by future generations as well.

Notes

CHAPTER FOUR

1. Kathy Keaton, *Longevity: The Science of Staying Young.* (New York: Viking, 1992).
2. Ibid.
3. R. K. Chandra, "Immunodeficiency in Undernutrition and Overnutrition," *Nutritional Reviews* 39, no. 6 (1981).
4. R. K. Chandra, "Micronutrients and Immune Functions: An Overview," *Annals of the New York Academy of Sciences* 587 (1990).
5. R. K. Chandra, "Nutrition and Immunity — Practical Applications," *Contemporary Nutrition* 11, no. 12 (1986).
6. J. Wesley Alexander, "Nutrition and Infection: New Perspectives for an Old Problem," *Archives of Surgery* 121 (August 1986).
7. Kenneth A. Bock, "Chronic Fatigue in Lyme Disease," Audiotape: Tape #2. 1992 Fall Conference of American College for Advancement in Medicine, Colorado Springs, CO. Insta-Tape, Inc. P.O. Box 1729, Monrovia, CA 91017-5729.
8. Yukinori Kusaka, Hiroshi Kondou, and Kanehisa Morimoto, "Healthy Lifestyles Are Associated with Higher Natural Killer Cell Activity," *Preventive Medicine* 21 (1992) 602–15.
9. A study of healthy young men showed that lowering the amount of fat in their diet to 30 percent of total calories caused an increase in NK cell activity. The effect was even greater in those who consumed less than 25 percent of their calories as fat. (Total calories were also reduced in this study.) Jeanine Barone, James R. Hevert, and Mohan M. Reddy, "Dietary Fat and Natural-Killer-Cell Activity," *American Journal of Clinical Nutrition* 50 (1989): 861–7.
10. Michael D. Lieberman, Jian Shou, et al., "Effects of Nutrient Substrates on Immune Function," *Nutrition* 6 no. 1 (January/February 1990).
11. J. Wesley Alexander, "Nutrition and Infection: New Perspectives for an Old Problem," *Archives of Surgery* 121 (August 1986).
12. Studies have shown that supplements of beta-carotene, vitamin E, and vitamin B_6 in amounts higher than the recommended daily allowance have increased immune response. "Pumping Immunity," *Nutrition Action Health Letter* (April 1993): 5–7. "Immune Function: Nutritional Supplementation," Review from *CP Currents*, 3, no. 6 (June 1993).
13. One study gave a single multivitamin a day to well-nourished elderly people who were not sick, and found it reduced their days of infection by one-half, in comparison with a control group whose members did not receive the vitamin.

This was a minimal dosage of several nutrients. Simin Kikbin Meydani, "Vitamin/Mineral Supplementation, the Aging Immune Response, and Risk of Infection," *Nutrition Reviews*, 51, no. 4 (1989).

14. Ibid.

15. Hoffman-La Roche Newsletter regarding Vitamin C: Shorter duration of cold symptoms may be related to effect on phagocytic cell activity with secondary bacterial invaders rather than direct antiviral effects. W. R. Beisel, *American Journal of Clinical Nutrition* 35 (supplement) (1982): 417–68.

16. Kathy Keaton, *Longevity: The Science of Staying Young* (New York: Viking, 1992).

17. Ibid.

18. Mouse studies with zinc in older mice caused lymphocytes to produce five to twelve times more antibody.

   Dr. Jean Duchateau at Saint Pierre University Hospital, Brussels, gave 220 milligrams of zinc sulfate twice daily for a month to members of a group aged over seventy whose average age was eighty-one. Then, given tetanus vaccine, they showed much higher antibody levels than those in a control group.

   Nicola Fabris, scientific coordinator of the Gerontological Research Department of the Italian National Centers on Aging, gave daily oral zinc supplements of 15 milligrams to members of a group over sixty and found that the production of thymic hormones was restored.

   John Bogden of the New Jersey Medical School, Newark, found that natural killer cell activity was improved in people taking 100 milligrams per day. Keaton, *Longevity*.

19. A doctor in Austin, Texas, prescribed zinc lozenges to suck on for a three-year-old girl who was having trouble swallowing the zinc capsules she needed to correct a deficiency. Her parents noticed that she stopped having her usual frequent colds and runny nose. In a double-blind followup study in Texas, zinc lozenges or a placebo were given to 146 volunteers. When they had colds, those taking the placebo averaged 10.8 days of infection; those taking the zinc lozenges averaged 3.9 days, with reduced symptoms. Twenty percent of the subjects recovered completely within one day!

20. Ibid.

21. Michael A. Schmidt, "Antibiotics: Is it Time to Reassess Their Role in Medicine?" *Journal of Advancement in Medicine*, 6, no. 1 (Spring 1993).

22. Frederick B. Rudolph, Anil D. Kulkarni, et al., "Role of RNA as a Dietary Source of Pyrimidines and Purines in Immune Function," *Nutrition* 6, no. 1 (January/February 1990).

23. A German study of 49 AIDS patients, half of whom engaged in a six-month program of two supervised physical exercise sessions a week, while the other half did not exercise, found no opportunistic infections or deaths in the group that exercised, and measurable psychological benefits. C. Schlonzig, M. Wehrenberg, et al., "The Role of Physical Exercise in the Treatment of Patients with HIV Disease," 9th International Conference on AIDS, Berlin, June 1993.

24. Yukinori Kusaka et al., "Healthy Lifestyles Are Associated with Higher Natural Killer Cell Activity."

25. "Nutrition, Immunity, And Exercise: A Fundamental Connection," *The Nutritional Supplement* 7, no. 1 (1992).

26. Ton-Fon Chin, Jaung-Geng Lin, and Shu-Yu Want, "Induction of Circulating Interferon in Humans by Acupuncture,"

27. Russell Jaffe, "Immune Defense and Repair Systems: Clinical Approaches to Immune Function Testing and Enhancement,"

28. Ibid.

29. Lawrence Steinman, "Autoimmune Disease," *Scientific American* 269, no. 3 (September 1993).

30. Thierry Boon, "Teaching the Immune System to Fight Cancer," *Scientific American* 266, no. 3 (March 1993).

31. Steven A. Rosenberg, "Adoptive Immunotherapy for Cancer," *Scientific American Special Issue/1993: Medicine.*

CHAPTER FIVE

1. "Combination Therapy with Acetyl-L-Carnitine, Ginkgolide Extract and Thiamine Tetrahydrofurfuryl Disulfide in the Treatment of Alzheimer's Disease and Other Cerebrovascular Pathologies," *Research Perspectives in Neuropharmacology.*

2. Study by Dr. Merrill Elias, psychologist at the University of Maine, reporting to Society for Behavior Medicine in Boston, April, 1994. Also analysis of Framingham Heart Study: Merrill Elias, *The American Journal of Epidemiology* (September 1993).

3. Blass and colleagues at Cornell University Medical College discovered that Alzheimer's patients who received 3 grams a day of thiamine hydrochloride showed significant improvement on standard cognitive tests, compared with a control group that received a placebo. Other types of thiamine compounds are expected to have a similar effect, with much lower doses. J. P. Blass, et al., "Thiamine and Alzheimer's Disease: A Pilot Study," *Archives of Neurology* 45 (1988), 833–5.

4. A. L. Bernstein and Jamie S. Dinesen, "Brief Communication: Effect of Pharmacologic Doses of Vitamin B_6 on Carpal Tunnel Syndrome, Electroencephalographic Results, and Pain," *Journal of the American College of Nutrition*, 12, no. 1 (1993) 73–6.

CHAPTER NINE

1. Ronald L. Hoffman, *Seven Weeks to a Settled Stomach* (New York: Simon & Schuster, 1990), 71.

2. Theodore B. Van Itallie, "Health Implications of Overweight and Obesity in the United States," *Annals of Internal Medicine* 103, no. 6 (1993), Pt. 2, 983.

3. Kay Sheppard, *Food Addiction—The Body Knows* (Deerfield Beach, Fla.: Health Communications, Inc., 1993), 63.

4. Jules Hirsch, NIH Consensus Development Panel, "Health Implications of Obesity," *Annals of Internal Medicine* 103, no. 6 (1985), Pt. 2, 1074.
5. Hoffman, *Seven Weeks to a Settled Stomach*, 131.
6. K. Heaton, P. Emmett, C. Symes, and F. Braddon, "An Explanation for Gallstones in Normal-weight Women: Slow Intestinal Transit," *The Lancet* 341 (January 2, 1993), 8–10.
7. Sandra Boodman, "Colon-cancer Screening: Results Puzzle Researchers," *The Washington Post* (June 1, 1993).
8. Elaine Gottschall, *Breaking the Vicious Cycle* (Kirkton, Ont.: The Kirkton Press, 1994), 7.

CHAPTER TEN

1. Vicki Hufnagel and Susan K. Golant, *No More Hysterectomies*, (New York: Penguin Books/Women's Health, 1989), 26–32.
2. Dena E. Harris and Helene MacLean, *Recovering From a Hysterectomy*, (New York: Harper Paperbacks, 1992), 1–2.
3. Hufnagel and Golant, *No More Hysterectomies*, x.
4. Ibid, 63.
5. "Hysterectomy for Benign Disorders Still High," *Family Practice News*, November 1, 1995; 16.
6. Ibid, 25.
7. A. H. Follingstad, "Estriol, the Forgotten Estrogen?" *Journal of the American Medical Association* 239, no. 1 (1978), 29–30.
8. Gilbert W. Gleim, *Journal of the American College of Nutrition*, 12, no. 4 (1993), 363.
9. Robin Marantz Henig, "Are Women's Hearts Different?" *The New York Times Magazine* (October 8, 1993).
10. Sidney M. Wolfe, *Health Letter* 7, no. 6 (June 1991).
11. *Internal Medicine News*, (November 1–14, 1986), 44.
12. Harris and MacLean, *Recovering From a Hysterectomy*, 133.
13. *American Journal of Clinical Nutrition* 49 (1989), 1179–83.
14. *Journal of the National Cancer Institute* 9 (1993), 722–6.
15. Janice Hopkins Tanne, *New York Magazine*, (October 11, 1993), 57.
16. Natalie Angier, *New York Times* (July 12, 1994), Section C, 12.
17. Dan Hurley, *Medical Tribune* (May 13, 1993).
18. Angier, 12.
19. Maxine Rock, *Medical Tribune* (May 27, 1993), 13.
20. J. H. Tanne, *New York Magazine*, (October 11, 1993), 57.
21. Hufnagel and Golant, *No More Hysterectomies*, 252.
22. J. J. Michnovicz, *How to Reduce Your Risk of Breast Cancer* (New York: Warner Books, 1994), 102–6.
23. Roger L. Wolman, *British Medical Journal* 309 (1994), 401.
24. Herbert Goldfarb, *Hoffman Center News*, vol 2, no. 2 (1993), 5.

CHAPTER ELEVEN

1. Johan Braekman, "The Extract of Serenoa Repens in the Treatment of Benign Prostatic Hyperplasia: A MultiCenter Open Study," *Current Therapeutic Research* 55, no. 7 (1994), 776–85.

CHAPTER TWELVE

1. American Heart Association, "Heart and Stroke Facts: 1996 Statistical Supplement."
2. B. Bower, "Depressing News for Low-Cholesterol Men," *Science News* 143 (January 16, 1993), 37.
3. Uffe Ravnskov, *British Medical Journal* 305, 6844:15; July 4, 1992.
4. Cal Beverly and Cindy Eckhart, "Low Cholesterol Benefits Are Questioned" *Natural Healing Newsletter* 4, no. 45, reporting on Ravnskov, note 3.
5. Thomas B. Newman, "Carcinogenity of Lipid-Lowering Drugs," *Journal of the American Medical Association* 275, no. 1 (1996), 55–60.
6. Beverly Eckhart, "Low Cholesterol Benefits Are Questioned."
7. Don Davis, "Cholesterol, Fat and Heart Disease: A Scientific Boondoggle?" *Health Hunter Newsletter* 7, no. 1 (January 1993). *New England Journal of Medicine* 325 (1991), 373.
8. Richard A. Kronmal, et al., "Total Serum Cholesterol Levels and Mortality Risk As a Function of Age: A Report Based on the Framingham Data," *Archives of Internal Medicine* 153 (May 10, 1993).
9. Ibid.
10. One recent study by Dr. Taylor and his colleagues at Harvard showed that reducing cholesterol levels reduced mortality from heart disease by an average of 6.7 percent. However, Dr. Taylor's statistical analysis showed other interesting figures: For people at low risk of heart disease, the effect of lowering cholesterol would be to add only three days to three months to life expectancy. Even more interesting, the effect for high-risk people would be to add only eighteen days to twelve months to life expectancy. *Annals of Internal Medicine* (April 1987).
11. "More Research Exposes The Great Cholesterol Myth," *Health Facts* 17, no 16 (September 1992).
12. Marjorie Shaffer, "Lipid controversy Builds Up," *Medical World News* (October 1992).
13. Ibid.
14. "More Research Exposes The Great Cholesterol Myth."
15. Jill Stein, "Measure HDL Routinely in Postmenopausal Women," *Internal Medicine World Report* 8, no. 1 (January 1–14, 1993).
16. A group was encouraged to eat two eggs daily and as much butter as they liked for three months, and then as much margarine as they liked. There were no significant changes in blood cholesterol or HDL whether the subjects ate butter or margarine. The subjects who began with low cholesterol counts ended the study with slightly higher levels, while the subjects who began with

higher levels actually saw their cholesterol levels decline. "Butter vs. Oleo Made No Difference in Cholesterol," *Internal Medicine News* 21, no. 14 (July 15–31, 1988).

17. Michael Mogadam et al., "Within-Person Fluctuations of Serum Cholesterol and Lipoproteins," *Archives of Internal Medicine* 150 (August 1990). Lisa Bookstein et al., "Day-to-Day Variability of Serum Cholesterol, Triglyceride, and High-Density Lipoprotein Cholesterol Levels."

18. Andrea Bonanome and Scott M. Grundy, "Monounsaturated Fatty Acids for Plasma Cholesterol-Lowering Diets," *Nutrition & the M.D., A Continuing Education Service for Physicians and Nutritionists* (January 1989).

19. Elaine Blume, "Why Oxidized Fats Are in Your Food and Why You Wish They Weren't," *Nutrition Action Healthletter* (December 1987).

20. Walter C. Willett, et al., "Intake of *trans* fatty acids and risk of coronary heart disease among women," *The Lancet* 341 (March 6, 1993).

21. *Journal of Nutrition Education* 20, no. 33 (1988).

22. *The Lancet* (1978).

23. G. E. Fraser, et al., "A Possible Protective Effect of Nut Consumption on Risk of Coronary Heart Disease — The Adventist Health Study," *Archives of Internal Medicine* 152, no. 7 (1992), 1416–24.

24. In one study, men with a high cholesterol level (over 250) ate 100 grams a day of fiber in the form of hot oatmeal cereal or muffins, or 115 grams of fiber in the form of pinto or navy beans. At the end of the study, they showed an average 19 percent reduction in total cholesterol level and a 20 percent reduction in LDL. "Hypocholesterolemic Effects of Oat Bran," *Nutrition & the M.D., A Continuing Education Service for Physicians and Nutritionists* (January 1989).

25. In one study, when 26 men aged thirty to sixty-five with moderate to high cholesterol levels took 3 teaspoons a day of mucilloid with meals, they experienced a 14.8 percent drop in total cholesterol and a 20.2 percent drop in LDL. There was no effect on blood pressure, body weight, HDL, or triglycerides. (*Archives of Internal Medicine* 148, no. 292 (1988). "Psyllium for Hypercholesterolemia?" *Nutrition & the M.D., A Continuing Education Service for Physicians and Nutritionists* (January 1989).

26. One study of a low-fat diet replaced 50 percent of dietary protein with soy protein, along with additional soy fiber, in baked goods such as fruit bars, muffins, and bread. The combination diet lowered total cholesterol by 12 percent and LDL by 11.5 percent. Susan M. Potter, et al., "Depression of Plasma Cholesterol in Men by Consumption of Baked Products Containing Soy Protein," *American Journal of Clinical Nutrition* 58 (1993), 501–6.

27. *Journal of the American Medical Association* 268, no. 7 (1992), 877.

28. L. D. Greenberg, et al., *American Journal of Clinical Nutrition* 6 (1958), 635.

29. Mildred S. Seelig, *Magnesium Deficiency and the Pathogenesis of Disease: Early Roots of Cardiovascular, Skeletal and Renal Abnormalities.*

30. A study by Dr. Jukka T. Salonen in Finland from 1984 to 1989 on the effect of high levels of stored iron on 1931 white men, aged forty-two to sixty found no signs of heart disease beginning in 1984. In 1981, fifty-one had heart attacks;

they had significantly higher levels of stored iron (ferritin) than those without heart problems or attacks.

Laura N. Beverly, "Building up Your Iron Supply Could Be Tearing Down Your Heart," *Circulation* 86, no. 3 (September 1992), 803. *Natural Healing Newsletter* 4, no. 45 (19XX).

Scientist Jerome L. Sullivan of the Medical University of South Carolina in Charleston suspects that lowering stored iron can reduce the risk of heart attacks. *Science News* 142, no. 12, (1992), 180.

31. The effect is dose-related. In one study, a daily supplement of 75 milligrams of zinc gluconate decreased HDL slightly; 160- and 300-milligram supplements decreased it significantly. Margaret Black, Denis Medeiros, Emery Brunett, and Ruth Welke. "Zinc supplements and serum lipids in young adult white males," *American Journal of Clinical Nutrition* 47 (1988), 970–5.

32. B. S. Raheja, S. M. Sadikot, and R. B. Phatak, "Insulin Resistance in Syndrome X" [Letters to the Editor], *The Lancet* 342 (August 28, 1993).

33. *The Lancet* (December 1993). NPR radio report.

34. Anne Geller with M. J. Territo, *Restore Your Life: A Living Plan for Sober People* (New York: Bantam Books, 1991).

35. "Happy birthday . . . maybe," *Science News* 143, no. 15 (April 10, 1993).

36. Prakash C. Deedwania, "New Clue to Morning Heart Risk," *Science News* 143, no. 15 (April 10, 1993).

37. Ronald P. Mensink, Mary-Christel Janssen, and Martjin B. Katan, "Effect on Blood Pressure of Two Diets Differing in Total Fat but Not in Saturated and Polyunsaturated Fatty Acids in Healthy Volunteers" *Internal Medicine World Report* 8, no. 1 (January 1–14, 1993).

38. "The Relationship of Bone and Blood Lead to Hypertension," *Journal of the American Medical Association* 275 (1966), 1171–6.

39. J. P. Buchet, et al., "Renal Effects of Cadmium Body Burden of the General Population," *The Lancet* 336 (19XX), 669–702.

40. M. N. Morris, et al., "Exercise in Leisure Time: Coronary Attack and Death Rates," *British Heart Journal* 63, no. 6 (1990), 325.

41. *New England Journal of Medicine* (December 1993).

42. "Antianginal Efficacy of Exercise Training: A Comparison with Beta Blockade," *British Heart Journal* 64, no. 1 (1990), 14.

43. M. A. Smutok, et al., "Aerobic Versus Strength Training for Risk Factor Intervention in Middle-Aged Men at High Risk for Coronary Heart Disease," *Metabolism* 42, no. 2 (February 1993), 177–84.

44. "Antianginal Efficacy of Exercise Training."

45. "Too Many Coronary Angiograms?" *Internal Medicine Alert* 15, no. 1 (January 15, 1993); T. B. Greyboys, et al., *Journal of the American Medical Association* 268 (1992), 2537–40.

46. "Long-Term Outcome of Bypass Surgery," *Journal Watch* 10, no. 4 (August 15, 1992). "Eighteen-Year Follow-Up in the Veterans Affairs Cooperative Study of Coronary Artery Bypass Surgery for Stable Angina," *Circulation* 86 (1992), 121–30.

47. Nicolas Danchin, "Is Myocardial Revascularisation for Tight Coronary Stenoses Always Necessary?" *The Lancet* 342 (July 24, 1993).

CHAPTER THIRTEEN

1. Lawrence M. Lichtenstein, "Allergy and the Immune System," *Scientific American* 269, no. 3 (September 1993).
2. Roger Field, "Air Pollutants May Worsen Allergies," *Medical Tribune* (May 27, 1993).
3. *Allergy-Asthma Shopper,* Allergen Control Products, Fate, Texas.
4. Jennifer K. Peat, Rene H. van den Berg, Wesley F. Green, Craig M. Mellis, Stephen R. Leeder, and Ann J. Woolcock, "Changing Prevalence of Asthma in Australian Children," *British Medical Journal* 308 (June 18, 1994), 1595.
5. Kaliner, Michael A. "Asthma Deaths: A Social or Medical Problem?" *Journal of the American Medical Association,* April 21, 1993; 269 (16): 1994–1995.
6. Julian Crane, et al., "Worldwide Worsening Wheeze: Is the Cure the Cause?" *The Lancet,* March 28, 1992; 339: 814.
7. *The Nutritional Supplement* 6, no. 2 (1991).

CHAPTER FOURTEEN

1. A. I. M. Bartelds, et al., "Acute Otitis Media in Adults: A Report from the International Primary Care Network. *Journal of American Board of Family Practice* 6 (July/August 1993), 333–9.
2. American Tinnitus Association, quoted by *The Capitol Times* (May 24, 1994).
3. *Scientific American* (July, 1993).
4. David A. Newsome, et al., "Oral Zinc in Macular Degeneration," *Archives of Ophthalmology* 106 (February 1988).

CHAPTER SIXTEEN

1. *New York Times* (April 13, 1993), C9.
2. *Environmental Nutrition* 15, no. 12 (December 1992).
3. Sherry Rogers, *Health Letter* (Summer 1993).
4. *Environmental Nutrition* 15, no. 12 (December 1992).
5. A study published in the American Heart Association's publication *Circulation* (September 1992) cites iron as the second leading cause of heart disease!

CHAPTER SEVENTEEN

1. Jack K. Leiss and David A. Savitz "Home Pesticide Use and Childhood Cancer: A Case-Control Study," *American Journal of Public Health,* February 1995; 85 (2): 249–252.

Resources

CHAPTER 4. SELF AND NONSELF: THE IMMUNE SYSTEM

Books and Periodicals

Better Bones, Better Bodies by Susan Brown (New Canaan, CT: Keats Publishing, 1997)

Professional and Support Organizations

Immune Deficiency Foundation
P.O. Box 586
Columbia, MD 21045
(410) 461-3127
Provides support and education.

Immunosciences Laboratory
1801 La Ciegna Boulevard
Los Angeles, CA 90035
(310) 287-1884
Provides testing.

Web Site

http://www.best.com/~immune   Immune mailing list

Health Products

Super Immuno-Tone: PhytoPharmica, Green Bay, WI 54311
Zinc Echinacea Lozenges: Quantum, Inc., Eugene, OR 97402 (800) 448-7448
Grifron Maitake: Fiji Tea Co., San Rafael, CA 94912-2056
Ester C: Allergy Research Group, San Leandro, CA 94577
Oscillococcinum (homeopathic flu remedy): Distributed by Boiron/Borneman, Newtown Square, PA 19073
Echinacea Concentration (cold preventive and treatment, immunity booster): McZand Herbal, Inc. Santa Monica, CA 90409

CHAPTER 5. NERVES AND BRAIN: MEMORY AND THE ENERGY PATHWAYS

Books and Periodicals

Brain: The Future in Repair and Regeneration by Dr. David S. Steenblock, M.S., D.O.

The Multiple Sclerosis Diet Book by Roy Swank and Barbara Dugan (Garden City: Doubleday & Company, 1987)

Brain Longevity by Dharma Singh Khalsa, M.D. (New York: Warner Books, 1997)

Professional and Support Organizations

Alzheimer's Prevention Foundation
11901 E. Coronado Road
Tucson, AZ 85749
(520) 749-8374

American Association of Retired Persons
(206) 517-2322

Web Sites

http://www-hbp.scripps.edu/home.html	Human Brain Project
http://maui.net/~jms/brainuse.html	Mysteries of the Brain
http://www.neuroguide.com	Neurosciences links

Health Products

Brainstorm: Allergy Research Group, San Leandro, CA 94577

Phoschol: Phillips Nutritionals, Laguna Hills, CA 92653

PhosSerine: Allergy Research Group, San Leandro, CA 94577

Marinol (dronabinol) (useful in treating anorexia, reducing disturbed behavior, improving mood in Alzheimer's disease): Unimed Pharmaceuticals, (847) 541-2525

Aricept (donepezil): A newly released drug that seems to improve thought and memory in some patients without the side effects of Cognex. Recently approval by FDA. Manufactured by Pfizer. For information, call (800) 438-1985.

Brain Synch Tapes: Brain Synch Corp., (800) 984-7962

CHAPTER 6. ENDOCRINE SYSTEM

Books and Periodicals

Enter The Zone, A Dietary Road Map by Barry Sears, Ph.D., with Bill Lawren (New York: Regan Books, HarperCollins, 1995)

Grow Young with HGH by Ronald Klatz (New York: HarperCollins, 1997)

Professional and Support Organizations

The Broda Barnes Foundation
(203) 261-2101

Diagnos-Tech Clinical and Research Laboratory
6620 South 192nd Place
Kent, WA 98032
(800) 878-3787

Web Site

http://www.endocrine.org   All-over resources

Health Products

DHEA-25: PhytoPharmica, Green Bay, WI 54311
Hopewell Pharmacy: Innovative formulator of natural hormone preparations,
    (800) 792-6670

CHAPTER 7. THE INFRASTRUCTURE: MUSCLES, BONES, AND JOINTS

Books and Periodicals

Preventing Computer Injury: The Hand Book by Stephanie Brown (New York:
    Ergonome, [212] 222-9600) (also available in software)
Pain Free by Luke Bucci, Ph.D. (Summit Group, [800] 875-3346)
The Arthritis Cure by Jason Theodasakis (New York: St. Martin's Press, 1996)
Hold It! You're Exercising Wrong by Edward J. Jackowski (New York: Fireside,
    1995)
Athlete's Guide to Mental Training by Dr. Robert M. Nideffer (Human Kinetics,
    P.O. Box 5076, Champaign, IL 61825-5076. [800] 747-4457)

Professional and Support Organizations

Arthritis Foundation
P.O. Box 19000
Atlanta, GA 30326
(800) 283-7800

National Acupuncture Foundation
1718 M Street, Suite 195
Washington, DC 20036
(202) 332-5794

Web Sites

http://www.visitorinfo.com/health/arthritis.htm   Links to arthritis sites
http://www.pathway.net/hws/muscles.html   Muscle charts of the
                                             human body

Health Products

Glucosamine Sulfate (for arthritis): Allergy Research Group, San Leandro, CA 94577-0489
Super EPA: Phillips Nutritionals, Laguna Hills, CA 92653
Super Malic (for fibromyalgia): Biomicotek, P.O. Box 3378, Torrance, CA 90510
Sprain Care (tincture of arnica): Weleda, Congers, NY 10920

CHAPTER 8. KEEPING BONES VITAL: OSTEOPOROSIS

Book

Better Bones, Better Bodies by Susan Brown (New Canaan, CT: Keats Publishing, 1997)

Professional and Support Organization

National Osteoporosis Foundation
1150 17th St. N.W., Suite 500
Washington, DC 20036-4603
(202) 223-2226

Web Sites

http://www.dundee.ac.uk/orthopedics/link/welcome.htm   Links to other sites
http://www.nof.org   National Osteoporosis Foundation

Health Products

Osteo Prime: PhytoPharmica, Green Bay, WI 54311
Osteomark (a simple urine test to measure bone loss): Provided by OSTEX, 800-99-OSTEX
Fosamax (oral alendronate): Manufactured by Merck
Miacalcin (nasal spray): College Pharmacy, Colorado Springs, CO, (800) 888-9358
Natural estrogen: Women's International Pharmacy, (800) 279-5708

CHAPTER 9. BASIC PLUMBING: THE GASTROINTESTINAL TRACT

Books and Periodicals

Breaking the Vicious Cycle by Elaine Gottschall (Kirton Press, 1995, [505] 466-3656)
Stop The Heartburn, by Dr. David Utley (Lagado Publishing, PO Box 620891, Woodside, CA 94062, [415] 562-3800)
The Yeast Connection, by Dr. William Crook (Jackson, TN: Professional Books, Inc., 1997)

Seven Weeks to a Settled Stomach by Ronald L. Hoffman (New York: Pocket Books 1991)

Professional and Support Organizations

Crohn's and Colitis Foundation (CCFA)
444 Park Avenue South, 11th Floor
New York, NY 10016
(800) 932-2433
A national organization with 90 chapters

Web Sites

http://www.niddk.nih.gov/Digestivedocs.html   National Institutes of Health
                                                pamphlets
http://members.aol.com/jokersaf/noni.   Self-help for sufferers of IBS
                                                and related diseases

Health Products

Rhizinate (source of DGL): PhytoPharmica, Green Bay, WI 54311
Aloe Vera Liquid: Allergy Research Group, San Leandro, CA 94577-0489
Artemesia: Allergy Research Group, San Leandro, CA 94577-0489
Enteric-coated Peppermint: Enzymatic Therapies, Green Bay, WI 54311

CHAPTER 10. MOSTLY FOR WOMEN

Books and Periodicals

No More Hysterectomies by Dr. Vicki Hufnagel (New York: Penguin Books, 1989)
Better Bones, Better Bodies by Susan Brown (New Canaan, CT: Keats Publishing, 1997)
Estrogen Replacement Therapy, Yes or No by Dr. Elizabeth Kaimen ([800] 889-5767)
Strength Training for Women by James Peterson & Cedric Bryant (Champaign, IL, Human Kinetics, [800] 747-4457)
Women's Bodies, Women's Wisdom by Christiane Northrup, M.D. (New York: Bantam Books, 1994)
Breast Health by Charles B. Simone, M.D. (Garden City Park, NY: Avery, 1995)
Women's Sports & Fitness Magazine
A Consumer Guide to Midwifery, (Public Citizen, 1600 20th St., N.W., Washington, DC 20009)

Professional and Support Organizations

Women—Midlife & Menopause (WMM)
7337 Morrison Drive
Greenbelt, MD 20770

Vulvar Pain Foundation
(910) 226-0704
National support group for sufferers of vulvodynia

Resolve
Boston, MA
(617) 623-1156
Infertility information

Gynecare, Inc.
235 Constitution Drive
Menlo Park, CA 94025
(415) 614-2500
Information on nonsurgical alternatives to hysterectomies

Web Sites

http://www.echonyc.com/~wham	WHAM — Women's Health Action and Mobilization: All around health information and resources
http://www.ppfa.org/ppfa/menopub.html	Planned Parenthood on menopause
http://nysernet.org/bcic/	Breast cancer information

Health Products

Pro-Gest Body Cream for PMS and menopausal symptoms: Transitions for Health, Portland, OR 97205
Key E Suppositories (for vaginal dryness): Carlson, Arlington Hts., IL 60004-1985
Osteo Prime: PhytoPharmica, Green Bay, WI 54311

CHAPTER 11. MOSTLY FOR MEN

Books and Periodicals

The Natural Way to a Healthy Prostate by Michael Schachter, M.D. (New Canaan, CT: Keats Publishing, 1996)
Reclaiming Male Sexuality by George Ryan (New York: M. Evans & Co., 1997)
Dave Barry's Complete Guide to Guys, by Dave Barry (New York: Random House, 1995)
Men's Health Magazine
Men's Fitness Magazine

Professional and Support Organizations

National Men's Health Foundation
14 E. Minor Street
Emmaus, PA 18098-0099
(610) 967-8620

National Men's Resource Center
PO Box 800-SH
San Anselmo, CA 94979-0800
(415) 453-2839

Web Sites

http://www.vix.com/pub/men/health/health.html General men's health
http://www.manslife.com General men's health
http://www.comed.com/prostate Prostate information
http://www.cinenet.net/~prostate/awareness Cooking and prostate
 cancer
http://www.erols.com/gtodorov/impotenc.html Impotence

Health Products

Palmetto Complex II (for prostate): Allergy Research Group, San Leandro, CA
 94577
Stinging Nettle (for prostate diseases): Available at health-food stores

CHAPTER 12. THE HEART OF THE MATTER

Books and Periodicals

Heartbreak and Heart Disease by Stephen Sinatra (New Canaan, CT: Keats
 Publishing, 1996)
Bypassing Bypass: The New Technique of Chelation Therapy by Elmer Cranton,
 M.D. (Trout Dale, VA: Medex Publishing, Inc., 1995)
Steering Clear of Highway Madness: A Driver's Guide to Curbing Stress and Strain
 by John A. Larson, M.D. (Wilsonville, OR: BookPartners, Inc., 1996) (Book on
 heart attacks) ([503] 682-9821)
Heart Frauds by Charles T. McGee, M.D. (Coeur d'Alene, ID: MediPress, 1993)

Professional and Support Organizations

American College for Advancement in Medicine (ACAM)
23121 Verdugo Drive, Suite 204
Laguna Hills, CA 92653
(714) 583-7666
Referrals to doctors certified in chelation techniques

American Heart Association
(800) 242-8721 (800-AHA-USA1)

Institute for HeartMath
14700 W. Park Avenue
Boulder Creek, CA 95006
(408) 338-8700

Web Sites

http://www.hearthome.com	Heart info from private med center
http://www.heartdisease.org/	Heart info from nonprofit service, covering disease, cholesterol
http://www.heartinfo.com	Heart disease prevention, other info, with links to other sites
www.heartmath.org	Alternative approaches to heart health
www.acam.org/	Detailed information on chelation therapy, referrals.

Health Products

Niacin Time (time-released niacin for cholesterol reduction): Carlson, Arlington Heights, IL 60004
Co-Q10 — Amni (800) 437-8888

Chapter 13. The Breath of Life: The Respiratory System

Professional and Support Organizations

Health & Fitness Outdoors, Inc.
P.O. Box 515
Montvale, NJ 07645
(201) 930-0557
Provides courses in "breathing awareness"

Clean Air Conservatory (formerly INHALE)
Cleveland, OH
(800) 228-9247

Web Sites

http://www.njc.org/mfhtml/mflist-subj.html	Information from National Jewish Center for Immunology and Respiratory Medicine
http://www.maricopa.gov/medcenter/links	Links to organizations and publications concerned with respiratory health

Health Products

Ginseng (for chronic respiratory diseases): Yeh Grace, Inc., Cliffside Park, NJ 07010

N.A.C. (N-acetylcysteine, a natural mucus-reducer): Allergy Research Group, San Leandro, CA 94577

Breathe Right Nasal Strips
Provide relief for those suffering from deviated septum; gently pull nostrils open, decreasing airflow resistance 31 percent; available from CNS, Inc., and in many stores.

AirWatch
A pocket-sized airway monitor, records how hard and how much air a patient can blow, hooked to a telephone jack, transmits data to a central computer, report immediately faxed to a physician's office.

SO_2 Certificate
Lets you "retire," in the name of a loved one, the right of companies to pollute the air with SO_2. With your purchase of a certificate, the Clean Air Conservatory buys pollution allowances, thus taking them out of circulation and preventing companies from polluting.

CHAPTER 14. SIGHT AND HEARING

Book

Nutrition And The Eyes by William Sardi (Health Spectrum Publishers, [800] 809-2219)

Professional and Support Organizations

Vision Foundation
818 Mt. Auburn Street
Watertown, MA 02172
(617) 926-4232

National Association for the Visually Handicapped
22 W. 21st Street
New York, NY 10010
(212) 889-3141

Association for Macular Diseases, Inc.
210 E. 64th Street
New York, NY 10021
(212) 605-3719

Health Education for Rockers (HEAR)
(415) 441-9081
Organization set up by Ted Nugent and Peter Townshend for prevention and treatment of noise-induced hearing disorders

Web Sites

http://www.eyeinfo.com	General information
http://vanbc.wimsey.com/~jlyon/index.html	Resources; links for the vision impaired
http://www.com/~houtx	Hearing loss resources

Health Product

Ocudyne (for eyes): Allergy Research Group, San Leandro, CA 94577-0489

CHAPTER 15. NOT ONLY SKIN DEEP: SKIN, HAIR, NAILS

Books and Periodicals

Healing Psoriasis: The Natural Alternative by Dr. John O. A. Pagano (The Pagano Org., Inc., [800] 919-4001)
Skin Cancer Foundation Journal, 245 5th Avenue, Suite 1403, New York, NY 10016 (212) 725-5176; (800) 754-6490 (800) SKIN-490

Professional and Support Organization

The Pagano Organization
(201) 947-4001
Information about psoriasis

Web Sites

http://www.derm-infonet.com	General information clearinghouse on skin
http://mindlink.bc.ca/sjacobs	Hair loss
http://biomed.nus.sg/nsc/hair.html	Hair loss information from National Skin Center

Health Products

Glycort (topical preparation for eczema, derived from licorice, acts like a natural steroid application without the side effects of synthetic steroidal creams): Allergy Research Group, (800) 545-9960
Exorex (for psoriasis, uses combination of coal tar and fatty acids from bananas, for long-term remission): IMX Corporation, (800) 617-3545
Skin Cap Shampoo (for dandruff and seborrhea): Progressive Laboratories, Irving, TX 75038-7962
SoftLight Laser System (Introduced by the Laser and Skin Surgery Center of New York as a safe way to remove unwanted facial and body hair): 317 E. 34 Street, New York, NY 10016, (212) 686-7306

Chapter 16. Eating for Health and Pleasure

Books and Periodicals

Native Nutrition: Eating According to Ancestral Wisdom by Dr. Ronald Schmid (Rochester, VT: Healing Arts Press, 1993)

Enter The Zone, A Dietary Road Map, by Barry Sears, Ph.D., with Bill Lawren (New York: Regan Books, HarperCollins, 1995) (Includes glycemic index)

Professional and Support Organization

Overeaters Anonymous
(213) 542-8363
An organization based on the twelve-step principles of Alcoholics Anonymous (the cheapest weight loss program you'll ever try—it's free!)

Web Sites

http://www.blonz.com/blonz/index.html   Nutrition information
                                                                        gateway

http://www.veg.org/veg   Vegetarianism

Health Products

Beefalo or bison organic and wild game meats:
Coleman Beef Company
U.S. Bison Company
The Organic Foods Warehouse (703) 631-0881

Jamar Foods (800 597-8325)

Chapter 17. External Medicine: Coping with a Hostile Environment

Books and Periodicals

Pesticide Alert, by Lawrie Mott and Karen Snyder (San Francisco: Sierra Club Books, 1988) (An informative guide to pesticide residues in common fruits and vegetables) ([800] 935-1056)

Raising Children Toxic Free, by Dr. Philip J. Landrigan and Dr. Herbert Needleman (New York: Avon Books, 1995) (How you can keep your children safe from environmental toxins)

Staying Well in a Toxic World, by Lynn Lawson (Evanston, IL: Lynnwood Press, 1994) (How you can protect your family and yourself from toxins)

The Enemy Within: The High Cost of Living Near Nuclear Reactors by Dr. Jay M. Gould (New York: Four Walls Eight Windows, 1996) (How you can protect yourself from radiation exposure)

Professional and Support Organizations

The American Academy of Environmental Medicine
P.O. Box 1606
Denver, CO 80206
(303) 622-9755
For information about MCS

HEAL (Human Ecology Action League)
P.O. Box 49126
Atlanta, GA 30359-1126
(404) 248-18980
National support group for people suffering from chemical sensitivities

Environmental Protection Agency
(800) 426-4791
Water safety hotline

American College for Advancement in Medicine
23121 Verdugo Drive, Suite 204
Laguna Hills, CA 92653
(714) 583-7666
To find a doctor certified in chelation techniques

Great Smokies Diagnostic Lab
63 Zillicoa Street
Asheville, NC 28801-1074
(800) 231-9197

Food & Water
(800) EAT-SAFE
For information about pesticides

The Rachel Carson Council, Inc.
(301) 652-1877
For information about pesticides

Web Sites

http://www.niehs.nih.gov	Environmental health information from the National Institute of Health
http://www.EnvPrevHealthCtrAtl.com/	Environmental and Health Center of Atlanta — great all-around diagnostic information about environmental medicine
http://ace.orst.edu/info/extoxnet/	Pesticide and environmental information

http://atsdrl.atsdr.cdc.gov:8080/toxfaq.html   Frequently asked questions about
                                                 toxic substances
http://www.uky.edu/waterResource/   Water resource information from
                                                 the University of Kentucky
http://www.gov/travel/foodwatr.htm   Drinking water travelers' advisory
                                                 from the Centers for Disease
                                                 Control and Prevention

Health Products

Home lead-testing kits: Frandon Lead Alert Kit, (800) 359-9000; Lead-check
    Swabs, (800) 262-LEAD
Kit for home testing of water, air, and soil for a wide variety of common pesticides,
    at a fraction of laboratory costs: RCI Environmental 2701 West 15th Street, Suite
    250, Plano, TX 75075, (214) 250-6706
Shower and water filters, customized for your home if necessary: National Ecologi-
    cal and Delivery System (N.E.E.D.S.), (800) 634-1380
Water-purification units for your pool, or for country wells, that don't use toxic
    chlorine: Withers Mill Company, P.O. Box 347, Hannibal, MO 63401, (800)
    223-0858.
Ultra Clear (Detoxifying drink recommended by Dr. Jeffrey Bland): HealthComm
    International, Inc., 5800 Soundview Drive, Gig Harbor, WA 98335, (206)
    851-3943
On-site evaluations of environmental hazards in the home or workplace: Micro
    Ecologies, Inc., 141 East 61st Street, 2nd Floor, New York, NY 10021, (212)
    755-3265

CHAPTER 18. DOCTORS AND MEDICINE: HOW TO COPE

Books and Periodicals

Examining Your Doctor by Dr. Timothy B. McCall (New York: Carol Publishing
    Group, 1995) (How you can learn more about your doctor)
Dr. Tom Linden's Guide To Online Medicine by Dr. Thomas Linden (New York:
    McGraw Hill, 1995); *Health Online* by Thomas Ferguson, M.D. (New York:
    Addison-Wesley, 1996) (Two great books providing numerous Internet sources
    for consumer health information)
Hospital Smarts by Theodore Tyberg, M.D., and Ken Rothaus, M.D. (New York:
    Hearst Books, 1995) and *Health Care Rights* by Nancy Levitin, Esq. (New York:
    Avon Books, 1996) (To find out what rights you have as a patient)
Simple Diagnostic Tests You Can Do At Home by Martha M. Christy (Scottsdale,
    AZ: Self Healing Press, 1994)
The People's Guide To Deadly Drug Interactions by Joseph Graedon, Ph.D, and
    Teresa Graedon, Ph.D (New York: St. Martin's Press, 1995) (How to take
    medicines safely)
The Center For Medical Consumers Ultimate Medical Answerbook by Maryann
    Napoli, and Carl Sherman (New York: Philip Lief Group, 1995)

Good Operations, Bad Operations: The People's Medical Society's Guide to Surgery
   by Charles B. Inlander (New York: Viking, 1993) (If you're considering surgery
   for anything)

Professional and Support Organizations

To find a holistic doctor, contact one or more of the following organizations and
ask for a list of members in your area:

American College for the Advancement of Medicine
Laguna, CA
(800) 532-3688

American Holistic Medical Association
4101 Lake Boone Trail, Suite 201
Raleigh, NC 27607
(919) 787-5181

The American Academy of Environmental Medicine
Box CN 1001-8001
New Hope, PA 18938
(215) 862-4544; FAX: (215) 862-4583

The American Academy for the Advancement of Anti-Aging Medicine
1510 W. Montana
Chicago, IL 60614
(773) 528-1000

To obtain hospital statistics and complication rates for surgical procedures, ask the
organizations for medical consumers that exist in several states, or ask your state
health department. See also the following:

Public Citizen's Health Research Group
Sidney M. Wolfe, M.D., Director
1600 20th Street, N.W.
Washington, D.C. 20009
(202) 588-1000
Conducts research and analyses of data obtained from the government and other
sources to produce reports that educate the public about important health care
issues

People's Medical Society
462 Walnut Street
Allentown, PA 18102
(610) 770-1670
A nonprofit consumers' medical rights group

American Preventive Medical Association
(800) 230-2762
Advocacy organization for medical freedom, especially regarding use of complementary and alternative therapies

Center for Medical Consumers
237 Thompson Street
New York, NY 10012
(212) 674-7105
A free library for general medical and health information, open to the public
(Monday–Friday, 9–5)

Web Sites

http://www.hotwired.com/drweil	Dr. Andrew Weil (author of *Spontaneous Healing*) answers questions from alternative perspective
http://www.healthanswers.com/	General medical information
http://www.medscape.com/	Articles on a variety of health topics
http://www.hooked.net/users/wcd/cmsotw.html	Interesting medical sites selected by Dr. Bil.
http://www.drhoffman.com	Dr. Hoffman's own web site, with articles, newsletters, nutritional advice, information about the Hoffman Center.
AOL's AHH Forum	America Online's Alternative Health & Healing site. Articles, resources, on-line discussions.

Index

Breaking the Vicious Cycle (Gottschall), 194,
195
breast cancer, 11, 37, 42, 215–21
alcohol and, 214, 218, 291
causes of, 37, 167, 214, 215–16, 217–19,
291
childbirth and, 218–19
diet and, 37, 167, 214, 218, 220, 221
ERT and, 160, 161, 207, 210, 211
genetic predisposition to, 11, 215–16, 218
prevention of, 219–20, 395, 412
screening for, 212, 216, 219
treatment of, 221
breast-feeding, 218
immunity conferred by, 6, 165, 166
breast implants, 64, 216
breasts:
cystic, 212, 213, 215, 216–17
male, 214, 240–41
self-examination of, 219
surgical removal of, 216, 221
tenderness and swelling of, 202, 210, 213,
215, 216–17
breathing, 87–88, 131
difficulties with, 74, 78–79, 310, 347
normal rates of, 79
see also respiratory system
breathing exercises, 79, 91, 340
Breneman, James, 190
brewer's yeast, 413
bronchial tubes, 63, 329, 330
bronchitis, 61, 82, 329, 330, 333
bronchodilators, 334, 338, 340
bulimia, 169
Burkitt, Colin, 394
Burkitt, Dennis, 176
Burns, George, 394
bursitis, 135, 143
B vitamins, 39–40, 62–63, 90, 406

cadmium, 34, 302, 423
caffeine, 75, 77–78, 169–70, 216, 303, 346
calcium, 121, 166, 298
absorption and storage of, 155–56, 157,
160, 162, 169
deficiencies of, 89, 129, 156, 157
dietary, 156–57, 161, 176
magnesium and, 283–84, 299, 319, 323
supplements of, 89, 155, 156–57, 160, 161,
162, 176, 197, 209, 319, 323, 408
calcium channel blockers, 84, 318–19
calories, 37–38, 111, 112, 204, 277, 278, 385–86
from fats, 277, 278, 279

Canadian Air Force Program for Physical
Fitness, 307
cancer, 7, 14, 20, 27, 28, 141, 417
aging and, 28, 66–67
chemotherapy for, 18, 149, 220–21, 351,
378
dietary factors in, 9, 35, 37–38, 39, 67, 167,
214, 218, 220, 221, 222–23
exercise and, 43–45
immune system and, 28, 29, 48, 66–67
metastasis of, 33, 45, 66
midlife, 66–67
prevention of, 177, 196–97
screening and testing for, 196
smoking and, 343
terminal, 48, 67
see also specific cancers
Candida albicans, 51, 53, 54, 74, 75, 168,
174–75, 184, 185–86, 197, 225, 226–
228, 331, 373, 376, 377
CA125 blood test, 223–24
capsaicin, 152–53
carbohydrates, 106–11, 130, 175
complex, 36–37, 38, 102, 104, 106, 108,
109–10, 115, 322
craving of, 21, 100, 104, 105–6, 110, 114–
118, 185, 203, 346
exclusion of, 111
and rate of conversion to sugar, 104, 108–
111, 112, 113, 116
refined, 88, 102–5, 108, 390
supplements of, 183
therapeutic diet based on, 183, 194
see also grains; sugar; vegetables
carbon dioxide, 78–79, 329, 423
carbon monoxide, 289–90, 344, 423
cardiology, 310–16
cardiovascular disease, 84, 86, 256–57
see also heart disease; high blood pressure
cardiovascular system, xiii, 22, 35, 38, 256–
327
see also heart; *specific conditions*
carotenoids, 38–39, 49, 139, 176, 220, 223,
323, 329, 356, 405, 408, 411
carotid arteries, 84, 316
carpal tunnel syndrome, 88–89, 129–31
cartilage, 122, 127, 128, 146, 152, 312
cataracts, 357–60
prevention of, 357–59, 360
surgical removal of, 357–58, 359–60
CAT scans, 70, 83, 84, 316
cells, 12, 13, 31–32
cancer, 33, 37, 39, 41, 43, 45, 66